Methods in Molecular Biology

Series Editor
John M. Walker
School of Life and Medical Sciences
University of Hertfordshire
Hatfield, Hertfordshire, AL10 9AB, UK

For further volumes:
http://www.springer.com/series/7651

Reporter Gene Imaging

Methods and Protocols

Edited by

Purnima Dubey

Department of Microbial Infection and Immunity, The Ohio State University, Columbus, OH, USA

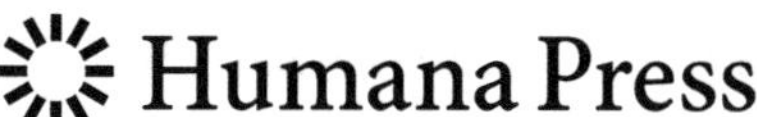

Editor
Purnima Dubey
Department of Microbial Infection and Immunity
The Ohio State University
Columbus, OH, USA

ISSN 1064-3745 ISSN 1940-6029 (electronic)
Methods in Molecular Biology
ISBN 978-1-4939-9306-2 ISBN 978-1-4939-7860-1 (eBook)
https://doi.org/10.1007/978-1-4939-7860-1

Printed on acid-free paper

This Humana Press imprint is published by the registered company Springer Science+Business Media, LLC part of Springer Nature.
The registered company address is: 233 Spring Street, New York, NY 10013, U.S.A.

Preface

Advances in the field of molecular imaging have provided biologists with tools to noninvasively follow fundamental biology processes with unprecedented ease and sensitivity. Noninvasive imaging techniques include radioactive, magnetic, and light-based methods to visualize cell movement, cell-cell communication, and gene expression.

The strength of reporter gene-based molecular imaging lies in the ability to track both the movement and function of cell populations in living subjects. Furthermore, the use of more than one imaging modality provides complementary information. This volume begins with a discussion of the advantages and limitations of combining fluorescent, bioluminescent, and radioisotopic reporter genes into one construct. This comprehensive review is followed by a method for creating a dual modality imaging reporter gene construct. Bioluminescent imaging using various luciferase genes is now a workhorse technique widely used in preclinical models of cancer and infectious disease. A detailed protocol for conducting a bioluminescent or fluorescent imaging experiment is followed by chapters that use light-based imaging to track immune system reconstitution, hypoxia, bacterial colonization, and macrophage localization and function. Widespread use of positron emission tomography (PET) imaging began with the advent of ^{18}F-FDG and is now a standard clinical diagnostic tool. Development of thymidine kinase (TK) as a PET reporter expanded the utility of this imaging modality to track specific cell populations and cellular functions in vivo. Protocols for detecting cancers using TK and responding immune cells using ^{18}F and ^{124}I-based tracers for TK and other nuclear reporters are described. Apoptosis is an important measure of cancer therapeutic efficacy. A comprehensive protocol for synthesis and use of an ^{18}F tracer for detection of caspase 3 as a readout for apoptosis is provided. Also included are protocols for emerging techniques such as the preclinical evaluation of PET radiotracers by Cerenkov imaging and the use of silver nanoparticles as cancer therapies.

Each chapter begins with an introduction to the topic, followed by a list of materials and detailed methods to conduct the procedure. Vendors are listed only where the equipment or reagent from a specific source is required.

This volume provides an introduction for the scientist who is new to the field of molecular imaging, as well as detailed methods for experts in other areas of molecular imaging.

Finally, I thank the colleagues who contributed their knowledge and expertise and John Walker for his advice and patience during the compilation of this volume.

Columbus, OH, USA *Purnima Dubey*

Contents

Contributors

MARIETTE BARBIER • *Department of Microbiology, Immunology and Cell Biology, West Virginia University School of Medicine, Morgantown, WV, USA*

JUSTIN BEVERE • *Department of Microbiology, Immunology and Cell Biology, West Virginia University School of Medicine, Morgantown, WV, USA*

SANTOSH K. BHARTI • *JHU ICMIC Program, Division of Cancer Imaging Research, The Russell H. Morgan Department of Radiology and Radiological Science, The Johns Hopkins University School of Medicine, Baltimore, MD, USA*

NIKUNJ B. BHATT • *Department of Cancer Biology, Wake Forest University Health Sciences, Winston-Salem, NC, USA*

ZAVER M. BHUJWALLA • *JHU ICMIC Program, Division of Cancer Imaging Research, The Russell H. Morgan Department of Radiology and Radiological Science, The Johns Hopkins University School of Medicine, Baltimore, MD, USA; Sidney Kimmel Comprehensive Cancer Center, The Johns Hopkins University School of Medicine, Baltimore, MD, USA*

ZIXIN CHEN • *Molecular Imaging Program at Stanford, Departments of Radiology and Chemistry, Stanford University, Stanford, CA, USA*

JEFFREY D. CIRILLO • *Department of Microbial Pathogenesis and Immunology, Texas A & M University Health Science Center, Bryan, TX, USA*

F. HEATH DAMRON • *Department of Microbiology, Immunology and Cell Biology, West Virginia University School of Medicine, Morgantown, WV, USA*

PIERRE DANHIER • *JHU ICMIC Program, Division of Cancer Imaging Research, The Russell H. Morgan Department of Radiology and Radiological Science, The Johns Hopkins University School of Medicine, Baltimore, MD, USA*

JOHN DAVID • *Pfizer, La Jolla, CA, USA*

ABHIJIT DE • *KS325, Molecular Functional Imaging Lab, Tata Memorial Centre (TMC), Advanced Centre for Treatment Research and Education in Cancer (ACTREC), Navi Mumbai, Maharashtra, India*

WILLIAM A. DEZARN • *Department of Radiation Oncology, Wake Forest University Health Sciences, Winston-Salem, NC, USA*

AJIT DHADVE • *Imaging Cell Signaling & Therapeutics Lab, Tata Memorial Centre (TMC), Advanced Centre for Treatment, Research and Education in Cancer (ACTREC), Navi Mumbai, Maharashtra, India; Homi Bhabha National Institute, Mumbai, Maharashtra, India*

PURNIMA DUBEY • *Department of Microbial Infection and Immunity, The Ohio State University, Columbus, OH, USA*

ANNE E. GIBBONS • *Department of Radiology, Center for Molecular Imaging, University of Michigan, Ann Arbor, MI, USA*

WILLIAM H. GMEINER • *Department of Cancer Biology, Wake Forest University Health Sciences, Winston-Salem, NC, USA*

STUART B. GOODMAN • *Orthopaedic Research Laboratories, Department of Orthopaedic Surgery, Stanford University School of Medicine, Stanford, CA, USA*

SAMATA KAKKAD • *JHU ICMIC Program, Division of Cancer Imaging Research, The Russell H. Morgan Department of Radiology and Radiological Science, The Johns Hopkins University School of Medicine, Baltimore, MD, USA*

YING KONG • *Department of Microbiology, Immunology, and Biochemistry, University of Tennessee Health Science Center, Memphis, TN, USA*
BALAJI KRISHNAMACHARY • *JHU ICMIC Program, Division of Cancer Imaging Research, The Russell H. Morgan Department of Radiology and Radiological Science, The Johns Hopkins University School of Medicine, Baltimore, MD, USA*
JASON T. LEE • *Memorial Sloan Kettering Cancer Center, New York, NY, USA*
TZU-HUA LIN • *Orthopaedic Research Laboratories, Department of Orthopaedic Surgery, Stanford University School of Medicine, Stanford, CA, USA*
GARY D. LUKER • *Department of Radiology, Center for Molecular Imaging, University of Michigan, Ann Arbor, MI, USA; Department of Biomedical Engineering, University of Michigan, Ann Arbor, MI, USA; Department of Microbiology and Immunology, University of Michigan, Ann Arbor, MI, USA*
KATHRYN E. LUKER • *Department of Radiology, Center for Molecular Imaging, University of Michigan, Ann Arbor, MI, USA*
ARIJIT MAL • *KS325, Molecular Functional Imaging Lab, Tata Memorial Centre (TMC), Advanced Centre for Treatment Research and Education in Cancer (ACTREC), Navi Mumbai, Maharashtra, India*
FRANK C. MARINI • *Department of Cancer Biology, Wake Forest University Health Sciences, Winston-Salem, NC, USA*
MELISSA N. MCCRACKEN • *Institute for Stem Cell Biology and Regenerative Medicine, Stanford University School of Medicine, Stanford, CA, USA; Ludwig Center for Cancer Stem Cell Research and Medicine, Stanford University School of Medicine, Stanford, CA, USA; Stanford Cancer Institute, Stanford University School of Medicine, Stanford, CA, USA*
MAXIM A. MOROZ • *Memorial Sloan Kettering Cancer Center, New York, NY, USA*
JUKKA PAJARINEN • *Orthopaedic Research Laboratories, Department of Orthopaedic Surgery, Stanford University School of Medicine, Stanford, CA, USA*
DARPAN N. PANDYA • *Department of Cancer Biology, Wake Forest University Health Sciences, Winston-Salem, NC, USA*
VLADIMIR PONOMAREV • *Memorial Sloan Kettering Cancer Center, New York, NY, USA*
JIANGHONG RAO • *Molecular Imaging Program at Stanford, Departments of Radiology and Chemistry, Stanford University, Stanford, CA, USA*
MAITREYI RATHOD • *KS325, Molecular Functional Imaging Lab, Tata Memorial Centre (TMC), Advanced Centre for Treatment Research and Education in Cancer (ACTREC), Navi Mumbai, Maharashtra, India*
PRITHA RAY • *Imaging Cell Signaling & Therapeutics Lab, Tata Memorial Centre (TMC), Advanced Centre for Treatment, Research and Education in Cancer (ACTREC), Navi Mumbai, Maharashtra, India; Homi Bhabha National Institute, Mumbai, India*
RAVI SINGH • *Department of Cancer Biology, Wake Forest School of Medicine, Winston Salem, NC, USA; Comprehensive Cancer Center of Wake Forest Baptist Medical Center, Winston Salem, NC, USA*
DAVID STOUT • *D&D Design, Culver City, CA, USA*
JESSICA SWANNER • *Department of Cancer Biology, Wake Forest School of Medicine, Winston Salem, NC, USA*
BHUSHAN THAKUR • *Imaging Cell Signaling & Therapeutics Lab, Tata Memorial Centre (TMC), Advanced Centre for Treatment, Research and Education in Cancer (ACTREC), Navi Mumbai, Maharashtra, India; Homi Bhabha National Institute, Mumbai, India*

PIERRE L. TRIOZZI • *Department of Hematology and Oncology, Wake Forest University Health Sciences, Winston-Salem, NC, USA*
THADDEUS J. WADAS • *Department of Cancer Biology, Wake Forest University Health Sciences, Winston-Salem, NC, USA*
PAT ZANZONICO • *Memorial Sloan Kettering Cancer Center, New York, NY, USA*
DAWEN ZHAO • *Department of Biomedical Engineering, Wake Forest University Health Sciences, Winston-Salem, NC, USA*

Chapter 1

Dual Modality Imaging of Promoter Activity as a Surrogate for Gene Expression and Function

Ajit Dhadve, Bhushan Thakur, and Pritha Ray

Abstract

Molecular functional imaging with optical reporter genes (both bioluminescence and fluorescence) is a rapidly evolving method that allows noninvasive, sensitive, real-time monitoring of many cellular events in live cells and whole organisms. These reporter genes with optical signatures when expressed from gene-specific promoters or Cis/Trans elements mimic the endogenous expression pattern without perturbing cellular physiology. With advanced recombinant molecular biology techniques, several strategies for optimal expression from constitutive or inducible, tissue-specific and weak promoters have been developed and used for dynamic and functional imaging. In this chapter, we provide an overview of the applications of this powerful technology for imaging gene expression in living cells and rodent models.

Key words Noninvasive imaging, Dual modality, Luciferase, Fluorescence, Gene expression

1 Introduction

Over the last few decades, identification of molecular interactors of various signaling cascades and their regulation has significantly advanced our knowledge of multiple cellular and biological processes. However, the complexity of molecular determinants increases with the number and kinetics of interactions in living subjects and requires real-time and/or in vivo monitoring of biological processes and novel strategies. Molecular imaging is one such emerging approach, which comprises visualization, characterization, and measurement of biological processes at the molecular and the cellular level in preclinical animal models and humans. Both anatomical (computed tomography and magnetic resonance imaging) and functional (radionuclide and optical imaging) imaging approaches are routinely used to trace molecular signatures in living subjects [1, 2].

Functional molecular imaging could be achieved either via direct imaging (interaction of endogenous target and target-specific probe) or through indirect imaging (expressing exogenous

Purnima Dubey (ed.), *Reporter Gene Imaging: Methods and Protocols*, Methods in Molecular Biology, vol. 1790, https://doi.org/10.1007/978-1-4939-7860-1_1, © Springer Science+Business Media, LLC, part of Springer Nature 2018

reporter gene and respective probe) strategies. Although the direct imaging approach is most desirable, it is impossible to develop specific probes against all endogenous targets. Thus, reporter genes play a crucial role by modeling endogenous gene expression. The only caveat of reporter-based indirect imaging approach is that cells must be labeled exogenously or transduced with reporter genes, either by viral transduction/transfection, or creation of transgenic mice. Reporter genes that emit light when excited (variants of fluorescent protein) or through substrate catalysis (luciferase enzymes) offer unique sensitivity and temporal resolution since as low as 10^{-15} to 10^{-17} mol/L of reporter protein can be detected over a period of nano-seconds to few hours. However, deep tissue attenuation and lack of anatomical information limit certain applications.

Optical reporter genes include light emitting luciferase enzymes and fluorescent proteins. Luciferases are a class of oxidative enzymes derived from diverse natural sources such as beetles, marine organisms (e.g., sea pansy), and luminous bacteria that oxidize respective substrates and emit light at different wavelengths. Most commonly used luciferase reporters are Firefly [3], Renilla [4], Gaussia [5], and Oplophorus luciferase [6]. Following the discovery of green fluorescent protein by Osamu Shimomura in 1960, GFP cDNA was cloned and extensively utilized as a reporter for cell imaging [7]. Various mutants of GFP and DsRED fluorescent proteins such as YFP, CFP, eGFP, mCherry, Dronpa, TagRFPs, KFP, IrisFP are available that emit light at different wavelengths of visible spectra [8]. Fluorescence proteins are well suited for single cell imaging and cell lineage tracking; however [9, 10], they suffer from high background due to tissue autofluorescence [11, 12]. On the other hand, luciferases that emit light after reacting with specific substrates have minimal or no background signal. Therefore, the combination of both fluorescence and luciferase imaging offers synergistic advantages for both in vivo and cellular level detection.

Cellular homeostasis is maintained by intrinsic or extrinsic factor-driven changes in the transcript and/or protein levels of critical genes. Promoter and cis-trans acting elements are the key "sensors" of these genes, which modulate their expression in response to stimuli. Promoters and cis acting elements harbor distinct and multiple response elements, which bind an array of transcription factors and co-factors. A gene at a given time but under various stimuli behaves differently based on its promoter and transcription factor interaction. While all these events can be well studied in vitro, it is straightforward to monitor DNA and protein interactions in vivo [13]. Imaging of RNA molecules is possible with special probes but is not widely used due to the complexity of design and inherent instability of the RNA complexes

[14, 15]. Noninvasive imaging of promoter and cis acting element activity also provides indirect information on gene-specific transcriptional modulation through a reporter gene. A wide range of promoters such as constitutive [16], tissue-specific [17], and development stage-specific [18, 19] promoters have been validated and utilized to understand the biology in the preclinical setting through functional molecular imaging. In general, tissue-specific promoters are weak in nature; however, with the help of two step transcriptional activators (TSTA) and a reporter gene, the signal can be enhanced [20].

2 Applications

Early efforts to visualize and track organ development, tumor growth, and metastasis in animal models laid the groundwork necessary to develop different ways of labeling cells. Use of *E. coli* beta galactosidase as a reporter gene was first used to visualize biological processes in mouse models [21–25]; however, this approach was limited by the inability to monitor biological evens in real time and laborious histological preparations. The field of reporter gene imaging achieved a milestone with the identification of fluorescent proteins, light emitting luciferase enzymes and SPECT/PET reporters along with their specialized substrates. The concurrent development of high end detectors enabled noninvasive, real-time, and repeated measure of biological processes [26–29]. Among various molecular imaging modalities, optical imaging systems are cost effective and time efficient, easily manipulated and require minimal resources compared to PET or MRI.

Promoters and cis-trans acting elements act at the core of differential gene regulation. Promoters driving reporter gene expression provide information on promoter modulation under various physiological conditions. Cis-acting elements are enhancers or repressors that affect distant promoter activity while trans-acting elements are transcription factors that bind to cis elements on promoters of various genes. Reporter genes used to monitor both promoter and cis-trans elements aid in unraveling the complexity of gene regulation. These reporter genes are ideal candidates to portray individual gene expression in a temporal and spatial manner when driven by gene-specific promoter/response elements. In the next section, certain examples pertinent to in vivo imaging of biological and molecular events using different gene regulatory elements and multi modal optical reporter genes are discussed.

3 Kinetic Monitoring of Tumor Growth, Development and Metastasis

Cancer cells stably expressing luciferase and fluorescence proteins are important tools for noninvasive monitoring of tumor development in small animals. Constitutively active CMV promoter, the simian virus 40 (SV40) early promoter, ubiquitin C promoter (UBC) have been used to develop optical reporters to monitor in vivo tumor growth [16, 30–34]. The first report of a florescence-bioluminescence fusion protein to visualize gene expression in cells and animals noninvasively came from Wang et al. in 2002. A fusion of rluc and GFP was used to noninvasively image single cells in culture and live animals [35]. Ray et al. for the first time described construction and validation of a novel bifusion reporter system consisting of an optical bioluminescence (*rluc*) and positron emission tomography (mutant herpes simplex virus type 1 thymidine kinase (HSV1-sr39tk)) reporter to noninvasively monitor tumor xenograft in live mice [30]. Early detection of metastasis has been difficult in mice; however bioluminescence with high sensitivity enables detection of as few as 10,000 cells [32, 36, 37]. Using luciferase tagged cells, many groups have used bioluminescence imaging to detect micro metastases in nodes and distal organs. For example, Feng et al. used *fluc* and GFP multimodality reporter to develop a xenograft peritoneal orthotopic model of malignant mesothelioma. GFP was used to select cells expressing the multimodal reporter whereas luciferase was used to monitor tumor growth in vivo. They also tested an immunotoxin therapy in this xenograft mouse model and used luciferase imaging to detect drug response in vivo [38]. Another group used a similar strategy to develop a retinoblastoma tumor and metastasis model. They detected micro metastases in lymph node, brain, and bones using BLI which were further confirmed by histopathological staining [39]. Kim et al. used a subcutaneous tumor model of rat prostate cancer cells stably expressing *fluc* and GFP and monitored tumor growth by both BLI and fluorescence [40]. Peiris et al. used 4T1 cells stably expressing luciferase and GFP to monitor breast cancer micro metastases and evaluated the efficacy of $\alpha_v\beta_3$ integrin targeted doxorubicin loaded nanoparticles to impair metastatic progression [41].

4 Reporter Genes as Indirect Measure of Endogenous Gene Expression

Although it is difficult to image functional aspects of each gene, it is possible to indirectly measure gene expression by using gene-specific regulatory sequences. Often this indirect strategy generates important information required for disease management and drug treatment. Lymphangiogenesis is a dynamic process and factors including vascular endothelial growth factor receptor 3 (VGFR3) play an important role in this process. This receptor is expressed on the surface of lymphatic endothelial cells and is an important marker for lymphangiogenesis. A pioneering study by Martinez-Corral et al. reported construction of an optical reporter, GFP-Luciferase (*fluc*) under control of the VGFR3 promoter to monitor lymphangiogenesis in vivo under various physiological conditions. This construct allowed tracking of vasculature, lymphatic vessel development during embryogenesis, wound healing, around tumor periphery, and at the lymph node metastasis [42]. Such reporter systems are valuable tools to rapidly screen efficacy of both inducers and inhibitors of lymphangiogenesis. Aberrant PIK3CA/Akt signaling plays an important role in ovarian cancer progression and chemoresistance. Our group for the first time monitored the effect of cisplatin and paclitaxel, the standard first-line drugs for ovarian cancer, on this signaling cascade using a PIK3CA promoter-driven *fLuc2* and *tdt* dual reporter. Attenuation of PIK3CA promoter activity (detected as a reduced luciferase signal) in response to the drugs was found in two ovarian cancer cells (PA1 and A2780) both in vitro and in vivo using a subcutaneous tumor model. We further showed that the promoter attenuation was mediated through binding of p53 to the PIK3CA promoter and mutation of the p53 binding sites in the promoter prevented attenuation of luciferase activity [43]. This study demonstrates the ability of optical reporter genes to noninvasively monitor the effect of chemotherapeutic drugs on gene expression.

Malaria is a worldwide epidemic killing millions of people every year [44]. A major challenge in the treatment of this disease is the presence of dormant parasites in the liver during the life cycle of the parasite, which is not yet drug targetable and leads to re-emergence of the disease. Ploemen et al. identified a liver stage-specific gene regulatory element in *P. berghei* parasite and used it to dissect the liver-specific stages of the parasite life cycle. Transgenic parasites with this regulator element driving GFP-luc fusion protein served as a model for in vivo parasite imaging and drug screening [45].

5 Reporter Gene to Monitor Transcriptional Activity of Proteins

Transcription factors (TF) are sequence-specific DNA binding proteins which modulate gene expression when bound to the promoter or enhancer of a gene. TATA binding proteins are general TFs that form a preinitiation complex important for RNA polymerase to bind to promoter controlling basal transcriptional activity, whereas other TFs are important in controlling the cell cycle during development and pathogenesis. Reporter genes driven by a promoter consisting of minimal TF binding sites (response element) are an important tool to evaluate activity of TFs during various physiological conditions. NF-κB is an important TF with roles in the innate and adaptive immune system. In addition, it drives an important signaling cascade that protects cancer cells from apoptosis and aids proliferation [46]. A recent study by Kim et al. showed that higher disease recurrence was associated with Myd88 positive tumors; however, a population of MyD88 negative patients relapsed and 65% of these were NF-κB positive [47]. In order to understand the role of NF-κB in acquisition of cisplatin, paclitaxel, or combination treatment resistance in the absence of MyD88, our group used a bi-fusion reporter construct consisting of NF-κB response elements driving Renilla luciferase-eGFP to monitor transcriptional activity of NF-κB in Myd88 negative acquired drug resistant cell lines. A2780 (MyD88 negative) acquired cisplatin resistant cells when treated with cisplatin showed increased NF-κB nuclear localization and increased NF-κB reporter activity. However, in A2780 acquired paclitaxel or combination drug resistant cells, both nuclear localization and NF-κB reporter activity decreased after treatment with paclitaxel and combination treatment respectively. Interestingly, following cross treatment of cisplatin and paclitaxel resistant cells, cisplatin-treated paclitaxel resistant cells showed increased NF-κB reporter activity. Subcutaneous tumors of cisplatin resistant A2780 cells stably expressing NF-κB-RL-eGFP, when treated with cisplatin showed 14-fold increased NF reporter activity. To confirm that the acquisition of cisplatin resistance depends on NF-κB activation independent of TLR-4/Myd88 signaling, we assessed NF-κB activity in an intrinsically cisplatin resistant ovarian cancer cell line SKOV3 (MyD88 positive), after shRNA-mediated Myd88 knockdown. MyD88 knockdown SKOV3 cells showed increased NF-κB activity after cisplatin treatment arguing for MyD88 independent activation of NF-κB. Using an NF-κB reporter construct we showed that NF-κB signaling is important to maintain cisplatin resistance in the absence of active TLR-4/MyD88 signaling [48]. Recently, Buckley et al. reported construction of a TF-reporter lentiviral library. The library consists of different TF responsive elements driving expression of an Fluc-eGFP fusion protein. Each construct is a reporter system to assess transcriptional activity of a TF under various physiological conditions. They validated 16 different TF-reporter constructs, which included TFs such as p53, STAT3, HIF, FOXO, and NF kB. They also validated specificity and showed that there was no cross activation of NF kB and SMAD2/3 biosensors with in vivo imaging [49]. Construction of TF-responsive reporter library with different combinations of reporter genes is achievable with current cloning methods. Cell lines established with such TF-reporters are valuable tools to effectively and rapidly screen drugs against these TFs.

6 Inducible Reporter Systems

Inducible reporter systems are valuable tools when expression of trans-genes needs to be tightly controlled. Tetracycline ON/OFF system is the most widely used method to control expression of trans-genes [50, 51]. Tet system consists of two major elements, tetracycline controlled trans-activator (tTA) element and specific tTA responsive promoter element (Ptet). Tetracycline trans-activator (tTA) protein is a fusion of TetR (tetracycline repressor) and the activation domain of protein VP16. Ptet promoter consists of the tetracycline operator placed upstream of a minimal promoter such as CMV. The transgene is cloned downstream to Ptet. In the Tet OFF system tTA binds to the promoter (Ptet) and positively regulates transgene expression in the absence of tetracycline. When doxycycline, a derivative of tetracycline, is added to the system, it prevents binding of Tta to promoter and thus inhibits trans-gene expression. Schonig et al. used a TET OFF transgenic rat with a forebrain-specific Ca2+/calmodulin-dependent protein kinase IIa (CaMKIIα) promoter driving expression of tTA. The CaMKIIα mice were used to generate double transgenic mice with a bidirectional and inducible Ptet promoter driving expression of *fluc* and GFP. Using this double transgenic rat, the authors detected brain-specific trans-gene expression, which was turned off using doxycycline treatment [14]. Such an on/off tissue-specific transgene expression provides an opportunity to monitor development-specific gene expression in a spatial and temporal manner using an inducer (doxycycline).

7 Stem Cells and Gene Therapy

Stem cell therapy is a promising strategy for regenerative medicine, cardiac and neurological diseases, and cancer treatment. However, behavior, differentiation, fate, and homing of stem cells to the target tissue after injection into the living subject remain unclear due to the inability to monitor these events in vivo in real time. Recent advances in reporter genes enable tagging of stem cells to monitor their movement and localization in vivo. We describe a few current examples related to cancer research in this section. Sasportas et al. evaluated the fate and efficacy of engineered mesenchymal stem cells (MSCs) designed to deliver TNF-related apoptosis-inducing ligand (TRAIL) for cancer therapy. First, they confirmed survival of MSCs in the host in the presence and absence of glioma. MSCs labeled with fLuc-GFP were injected into the brain with or without glioma cells Gli36-EGFRvIIIl (Gli36 expressing a constitutively active variant of EGFR) and showed that at day 14, 60% of the MSCs were viable when co-injected with glioma cells, whereas no BLI signal was observed from MSCs alone. Then a secreted TRAIL-GLuc fusion was expressed in fLuc-GFP labeled MSCs. The homing of MSCs to the tumor site was monitored using fLuc imaging and the amount of secreted TRAIL was measured through secreted Gluc activity. MSCs engineered to deliver TRAIL for glioma cancer therapy improved median survival of mice from 54.5 to 72 days [52]. Alieva et al. used an orthotopic model of glioblastoma U87 cells expressing double fusion reporter of fLuc-eGFP and adipose-derived MSCs labeled with triple fusion reporter rLuc-RFP-TK (TK stands for thymidine kinase, a PET reporter gene) as therapeutic cells to target glioblastoma. The substrate specificity of Fluc and Rluc allowed monitoring of cell survival and proliferation of both tumor and MSCs in the same animal before and after initiation of stem cell therapy. MSCs expressing the triple fusion reporter (rLuc-RFP-TK) were tagged with another bi-fusion reporter fLuc-eGFP driven by an endothelial-specific promoter (PECAM/CD31 promoter). Using BLI imaging of epithelial promoter-driven luciferase expression, the authors observed that at day 7 after MSCs implantation most of the MSCs died. The ratio of PECAM/CD31 promoter-regulated fluc activity to constitutively expressed rluc increased by 92-fold, indicating that a subpopulation of the implanted MSCs had differentiated to the endothelial lineage. In addition, fluorescence microscopy of tumor sections showed close association of the differentiated MSCs with the tumor microvasculature. Upon ganciclovir treatment TK labeled MSCs inhibited tumor growth [53].

8 Transgenic Mice

Gene knockout and knockin mice are used extensively to identify gene functions and their role in development and other physiological conditions. Transgenic mice with reporter genes have further improved our understanding of gene function with the ability to noninvasively image gene function in real time. Here, we discuss a few promoter-reporter-based transgenic animal models to study gene or promoter activity. Ju et al. reported generation of a transgenic mouse model for two oncogenes $p53^{R172H}$ and $KRAS^{G12D}$ with Fluc and eGFP as reporter genes under control of the Cre-Lox system. This multimodality reporter consists of two oncogenes and fluc-eGFP linked by self-cleaving peptide 2a sequences and driven by a constitutive promoter that is flanked by LoxP sites with a stop codon. Using tissue-specific Cre-mediated expression of the oncogenes the authors monitored induced tissue-specific activation of oncogenes. Fluc-eGFP reporter was used to monitor tumor incidence and tumor growth upon oncogene activation [54]. Growth-associated protein-43 (GAP-43) is associated with neuronal development and early synapse formation; however, its role in injured adult nervous stem remains unclear. Gravel et al. developed a transgenic luc-gfp mouse model driven by the GAP-43 promoter. This mouse model was validated with endogenous expression of GAP-43 and served as a means to study the ability of adult nervous stem cells to regenerate after injuries [55]. Wang et al. used transgenic mice constitutively expressing fLuc-eGFP reporter gene to obtain labeled MSCs, which were further used to monitor tumor homing and fate of MSCs at tumor site [15]. Transgenic mice with ubiquitous or tissue-specific reporter gene expression have expanded the ability to monitor biological events in real time and significantly reduced the number of animals required for study. They are also a valuable source of uniformly labeled cells for in vitro drug screening and stem cell isolation.

9 Summary and Future Aspects

At the center of developmentally or environmentally triggered genetic circuits are the promoters and associated cis and trans acting elements, which together control the spatial and temporal expression of genes. Fluorescent and bioluminescent optical reporter genes provide an excellent means to noninvasively and repeatedly monitor these events in single cells and living subjects. Promoter-optical reporter genes have been used to map core promoter regions of various endogenous genes and to map distal cis acting elements that influence gene expression [56, 57]. With advances in molecular biology it is now possible to generate promoter-based optical reporters which have accelerated in vivo studies. Multiplexing of these promoter strategies and promoter reporter-based transgenic animals provides excellent preclinical models to study disease pathology and drug responses. Epigenetic modifications control chromatin structure and in turn control access to transcriptional machinery conferring another complex layer of gene regulation. Maternal or paternal imprinting of genes is an important phenomenon during development. Strategies to image these modifications using optical reporter genes are under development, and imaging the combination of promoter modulation along with epigenetic modifications is a future area of research to extend the applications of reporter gene-based imaging.

Continued efforts to improve the signal and reduce the background of fluorescent and optical reporters are underway. Luciferase enzymes are codon optimized to make luciferases with longer wavelength light output to improve deep tissue imaging [58]. Fluorescent proteins with emission in the near infrared region have been developed for better in vivo imaging [59]. Substrates for luciferase enzymes are undergoing modification to yield better sensitivity and light output in the far red region [60]. Development of computational advances will allow optical imaging to provide anatomical information and 3D images. Until then PET reporter genes, which provide deep tissue imaging with spatial and anatomical information, can be multiplexed with optical reporter genes to overcome the limitations of optical imaging [61]. New and improved versions of reporter genes and multiplexed modalities, along with improved gene delivery methods, will continue to play an important role in biomedical and basic research.

References

1. Massoud TF, Gambhir SS (2003) Molecular imaging in living subjects: seeing fundamental biological processes in a new light. Genes Dev 17(5):545–580
2. Thakur B et al (2015) Molecular imaging of therapeutic potential of reporter probes. Curr Drug Targets 16(6):645–657
3. Thorne N, Inglese J, Auld DS (2010) Illuminating insights into firefly luciferase and other bioluminescent reporters used in chemical biology. Chem Biol 17(6):646–657
4. Shimomura O (1985) Bioluminescence in the sea: photoprotein systems. Symp Soc Exp Biol 39:351–372
5. Tannous BA (2009) Gaussia luciferase reporter assay for monitoring biological processes in culture and in vivo. Nat Protoc 4(4):582–591
6. Inouye S et al (2000) Secretional luciferase of the luminous shrimp Oplophorus gracilirostris: cDNA cloning of a novel imidazopyrazinone luciferase(1). FEBS Lett 481(1):19–25
7. Shimomura O, Johnson FH, Saiga Y (1962) Extraction, purification and properties of aequorin, a bioluminescent protein from the luminous hydromedusan, Aequorea. J Cell Comp Physiol 59:223–239
8. Chudakov DM, Lukyanov S, Lukyanov KA (2005) Fluorescent proteins as a toolkit for in vivo imaging. Trends Biotechnol 23 (12):605–613
9. Sato S et al (2016) Single-cell lineage tracking analysis reveals that an established cell line comprises putative cancer stem cells and their heterogeneous progeny. Sci Rep 6:23328
10. Carlson AL et al (2013) Tracking single cells in live animals using a photoconvertible near-infrared cell membrane label. PLoS One 8(8): e69257
11. Choy G et al (2003) Comparison of noninvasive fluorescent and bioluminescent small animal optical imaging. Biotechniques 35 (5):1022–1030
12. Swenson ES et al (2007) Limitations of green fluorescent protein as a cell lineage marker. Stem Cells 25(10):2593–2600
13. Brogan J et al (2012) Imaging molecular pathways: reporter genes. Radiat Res 177 (4):508–513
14. Schonig K et al (2012) Conditional gene expression systems in the transgenic rat brain. BMC Biol 10:77
15. Wang H et al (2009) Trafficking mesenchymal stem cell engraftment and differentiation in tumor-bearing mice by bioluminescence imaging. Stem Cells 27(7):1548–1558
16. Qin JY et al (2010) Systematic comparison of constitutive promoters and the doxycycline-inducible promoter. PLoS One 5(5):e10611
17. Yang G et al (2015) Development of endothelial-specific single inducible lentiviral vectors for genetic engineering of endothelial progenitor cells. Sci Rep 5:17166
18. Huang BL, Brugger SM, Lyons KM (2010) Stage-specific control of connective tissue growth factor (CTGF/CCN2) expression in chondrocytes by Sox9 and beta-catenin. J Biol Chem 285(36):27702–27712
19. Dussmann P et al (2011) Live in vivo imaging of Egr-1 promoter activity during neonatal development, liver regeneration and wound healing. BMC Dev Biol 11:28
20. Iyer M et al (2001) Two-step transcriptional amplification as a method for imaging reporter gene expression using weak promoters. Proc Natl Acad Sci U S A 98(25):14595–14600
21. Friedrich G, Soriano P (1991) Promoter traps in embryonic stem cells: a genetic screen to identify and mutate developmental genes in mice. Genes Dev 5(9):1513–1523
22. Bonnerot C, Nicolas JF (1993) Application of LacZ gene fusions to postimplantation development. Methods Enzymol 225:451–469
23. Maretto S et al (2003) Mapping Wnt/beta-catenin signaling during mouse development and in colorectal tumors. Proc Natl Acad Sci U S A 100(6):3299–3304
24. Watson CM et al (2008) Application of lacZ transgenic mice to cell lineage studies. Methods Mol Biol 461:149–164

25. Bengtsson NE et al (2010) lacZ as a genetic reporter for real-time MRI. Magn Reson Med 63(3):745–753
26. Akin O et al (2012) Advances in oncologic imaging: update on 5 common cancers. CA Cancer J Clin 62(6):364–393
27. Barsanti C, Lenzarini F, Kusmic C (2015) Diagnostic and prognostic utility of non-invasive imaging in diabetes management. World J Diabetes 6(6):792–806
28. Dweck MR et al (2016) Imaging of coronary atherosclerosis – evolution towards new treatment strategies. Nat Rev Cardiol 13 (9):533–548
29. Garland M, Yim JJ, Bogyo M (2016) A bright future for precision medicine: advances in fluorescent chemical probe design and their clinical application. Cell Chemical Biology 23 (1):122–136
30. Ray P, Wu AM, Gambhir SS (2003) Optical bioluminescence and positron emission tomography imaging of a novel fusion reporter gene in tumor xenografts of living mice. Cancer Res 63(6):1160–1165
31. Lehmann S et al (2009) Longitudinal and multimodal in vivo imaging of tumor hypoxia and its downstream molecular events. Proc Natl Acad Sci U S A 106(33):14004–14009
32. Kim JB et al (2010) Non-invasive detection of a small number of bioluminescent cancer cells in vivo. PLoS One 5(2):e9364
33. Liu H et al (2010) Cancer stem cells from human breast tumors are involved in spontaneous metastases in orthotopic mouse models. Proc Natl Acad Sci U S A 107 (42):18115–18120
34. Puaux AL et al (2011) A comparison of imaging techniques to monitor tumor growth and cancer progression in living animals. Int J Mol Imaging 2011:321538
35. Wang Y et al (2002) Renilla luciferase-Aequorea GFP (Ruc-GFP) fusion protein, a novel dual reporter for real-time imaging of gene expression in cell cultures and in live animals. Mol Gen Genomics 268(2):160–168
36. Klerk CP et al (2007) Validity of bioluminescence measurements for noninvasive in vivo imaging of tumor load in small animals. Biotechniques 43(1 Suppl):7–13, 30
37. Stabenow D et al (2010) Bioluminescence imaging allows measuring CD8 T cell function in the liver. Hepatology 51(4):1430–1437
38. Feng M et al (2011) In vivo imaging of human malignant mesothelioma grown orthotopically in the peritoneal cavity of nude mice. J Cancer 2:123–131
39. Ji X et al (2009) Noninvasive visualization of retinoblastoma growth and metastasis via bioluminescence imaging. Invest Ophthalmol Vis Sci 50(12):5544–5551
40. Kim Y et al (2011) Sensitive optical detection of an early metastatic tumor using a new cell line with enhanced luminescent and fluorescent signals. J Anal Sci Technol 2(2):83–90
41. Peiris PM et al (2014) Treatment of cancer micrometastasis using a multicomponent chain-like nanoparticle. J Control Release 173:51–58
42. Martinez-Corral I et al (2012) In vivo imaging of lymphatic vessels in development, wound healing, inflammation, and tumor metastasis. Proc Natl Acad Sci U S A 109(16):6223–6228
43. Gaikwad SM et al (2013) Non-invasive imaging of phosphoinositide-3-kinase-catalytic-subunit-alpha (PIK3CA) promoter modulation in small animal models. PLoS One 8(2): e55971
44. Cibulskis RE et al (2016) Malaria: global progress 2000-2015 and future challenges. Infect Dis Poverty 5(1):61
45. Ploemen IH et al (2009) Visualisation and quantitative analysis of the rodent malaria liver stage by real time imaging. PLoS One 4(11): e7881
46. Hoesel B, Schmid JA (2013) The complexity of NF-kappaB signaling in inflammation and cancer. Mol Cancer 12:86
47. Kim KH et al (2012) Expression and significance of the TLR4/MyD88 signaling pathway in ovarian epithelial cancers. World J Surg Oncol 10:193
48. Gaikwad SM et al (2015) Differential activation of NF-kappaB signaling is associated with platinum and taxane resistance in MyD88 deficient epithelial ovarian cancer cells. Int J Biochem Cell Biol 61:90–102
49. Buckley SM et al (2015) In vivo bioimaging with tissue-specific transcription factor activated luciferase reporters. Sci Rep 5:11842
50. Gossen M et al (1995) Transcriptional activation by tetracyclines in mammalian cells. Science 268(5218):1766–1769
51. Lewandoski M (2001) Conditional control of gene expression in the mouse. Nat Rev Genet 2 (10):743–755
52. Sasportas LS et al (2009) Assessment of therapeutic efficacy and fate of engineered human mesenchymal stem cells for cancer therapy. Proc Natl Acad Sci U S A 106(12):4822–4827
53. Alieva M et al (2012) Glioblastoma therapy with cytotoxic mesenchymal stromal cells optimized by bioluminescence imaging of tumor

and therapeutic cell response. PLoS One 7(4): e35148

54. Ju HL et al (2015) Transgenic mouse model expressing P53(R172H), luciferase, EGFP, and KRAS(G12D) in a single open reading frame for live imaging of tumor. Sci Rep 5:8053
55. Gravel M, Weng YC, Kriz J (2011) Model system for live imaging of neuronal responses to injury and repair. Mol Imaging 10 (6):434–445
56. Del Vecchio I et al (2009) Functional mapping of the promoter region of the GNB2L1 human gene coding for RACK1 scaffold protein. Gene 430(1-2):17–29
57. Zou MX et al (2004) Characterization of functional elements in the neurofibromatosis (NF1) proximal promoter region. Oncogene 23 (2):330–339
58. Wu C et al (2009) In vivo far-red luminescence imaging of a biomarker based on BRET from Cypridina bioluminescence to an organic dye. Proc Natl Acad Sci U S A 106 (37):15599–15603
59. Levin RA et al (2014) An optimized triple modality reporter for quantitative in vivo tumor imaging and therapy evaluation. PLoS One 9(5):e97415
60. Jathoul AP et al (2014) A dual-color far-red to near-infrared firefly luciferin analogue designed for multiparametric bioluminescence imaging. Angew Chem Int Ed Engl 53 (48):13059–13063
61. Ray P et al (2004) Imaging tri-fusion multimodality reporter gene expression in living subjects. Cancer Res 64(4):1323–1330

Chapter 2

Construction of Dual Modality Optical Reporter Gene Constructs for Bioluminescent and Fluorescent Imaging

Ajit Dhadve, Bhushan Thakur, and Pritha Ray

Abstract

Dual modality reporter genes are powerful means of tracking cellular processes in cell culture systems and whole animals. In this chapter, we describe the methods for construction of a plasmid reporter gene vector expressing a fluorescent and a bioluminescent gene and its validation by in vitro assays in mammalian cells as well as by noninvasive imaging methods in small animal models.

Key words Dual modality, Optical imaging, Bioluminescent, Fluorescent, Reporter gene, Two-step transcriptional activator

1 Introduction

The preceding chapter provided an overview of the strengths and limitations of light-based imaging methods that utilize fluorescent and bioluminescent reporter genes. Here, we will provide a new user with the tools required to (a) create a reporter gene construct that contains a green or red fluorescent reporter gene along with a cell expressed or secreted luciferase gene, (b) efficiently transduce cells of interest, (c) validate gene expression, and (d) detect in vivo expression of both reporters in living subjects.

Strategies for the creation of a multimodality optical reporter for monitoring promoter/response element activity:

1. *Two-promoter bearing vector system*: Two reporter genes expressed under the control of two different promoters present in a single vector resulting in the production of two transcripts and two translational products. The promoters could both be constitutive or one constitutive and the other tissue-specific. Competition and availability between transcriptional regulators for the promoters may lead to differential expression of the two reporters (Fig. 1a).

Purnima Dubey (ed.), *Reporter Gene Imaging: Methods and Protocols*, Methods in Molecular Biology, vol. 1790,
https://doi.org/10.1007/978-1-4939-7860-1_2,

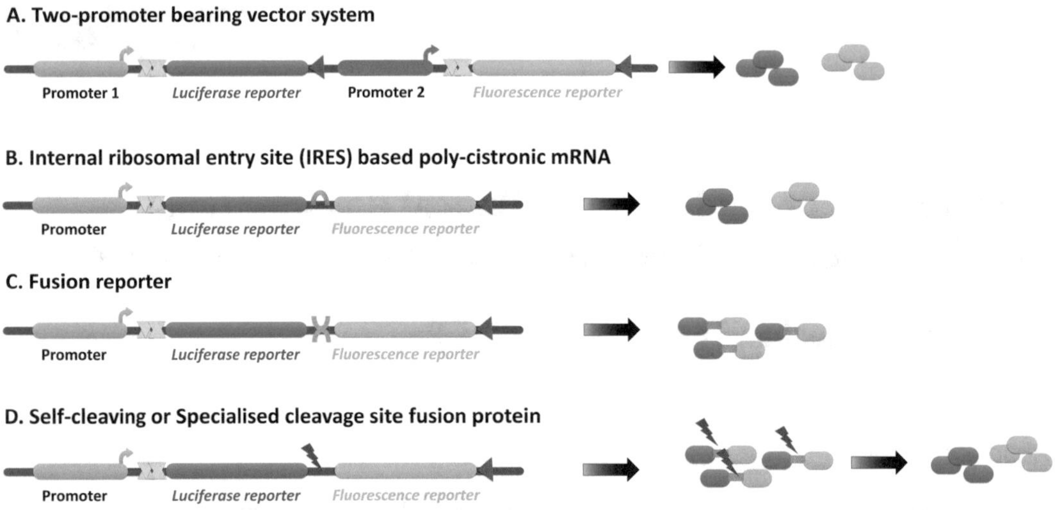

Fig. 1 Schematic representation of various strategies of multimodality optical reporter vector construction. (**a**) A two promoter-based vector system where two reporter genes are driven by two individual promoters which can be same or different types from single vector. (**b**) A single promoter-based vector system driving expression of two reporter genes linked by an IRES, which leads to synthesis of single mRNA but two proteins. (**c**) A single promoter-based vector system driving expression of two reporter genes linked by a linker leading to synthesis of single RNA and a fusion protein. (**d**) A single promoter-based vector system driving expression of two reporter genes linked by a self-cleaving sequence such as peptide 2a producing fusion protein which undergoes self-cleaving after synthesis or linked by a special cleavage sequence such as DVED, which is recognized by active caspase, hence such a system serves as a sensitive tool for detecting caspase activation and apoptosis

2. *Internal ribosomal entry site (IRES)-based poly-cistronic mRNA*: In this strategy, a single promoter drives expression of two or more reporter genes linked using an IRES sequence. This construct expresses a poly-cistronic transcript, which translates into two or more peptides. IRES-based vectors often display down-regulation of the second cistron due to lower efficiency of ribosome binding and initiation of translation from the IRES sequence (Fig. 1b).

3. *Self-cleaving fusion protein*: The self-cleaving fusion protein construct comprises two or more reporter protein sequences fused by an 18 amino acid long 2A self-cleaving peptide sequence derived from foot-and-mouth disease virus (FMDV). During translation, this peptide causes skipping of its "C"-terminal peptide bond and hence results in the production of two separate peptides from the same poly-cistronic mRNA (Fig. 1d).

4. *Fusion reporter*: In this strategy, two or more reporter coding sequences are fused directly or through a small linker and are expressed under a single promoter. This construct produces a single transcript and a hybrid protein. One must take care to

delete the stop codon/s of the first/second reporter and maintain the triplet codon sequence in frame. This fusion reporter may possess attenuated activity due to steric hindrance between the two polypeptides. Following are the few strategies for fusing two or more reporter genes:

(a) *Linker-based fusion protein*: Two reporters linked through a short peptide sequence express a single cistron. Choice of amino acids (such as glycine, serine but not cysteine or proline) (*see* **Note 1**) and the peptide length determine flexibility of two reporters in a fused form. However, longer linker peptide is more vulnerable for protease cleavage (Fig. 1c).

(b) *Specialized cleavage site fusion reporter*: The linker sequence described above can have specialized cleavage sites for proteases such as the DEVD sequence of caspase 3 or the MMP target sequences. Activated proteases cleave the fusion reporter at corresponding cleavage sequence into individual reporter proteins and thereby cause dramatic increase in each reporter activity compared to the fused form. This strategy helps indirectly to measure the protease activation constitutively or in a tissue-specific manner depending upon the nature of the inducer or experiment (Fig. 1d).

Choice of promoter for construction of promoter reporter:

The choice of promoter depends on the requirement of the assay system. For example, to identify specific transcription factor binding cis-acting element/s, clone a gene-specific promoter of interest upstream of the reporter gene. Reporter activity measured from various mutant or/and deletion promoter constructs identifies the binding cis-acting element sequence. For other studies such as cell trafficking or monitoring tumor growth kinetics, use a constitutively active promoter such as cytomegalovirus (CMV) promoter, the simian virus 40 (SV40) early promoter, and ubiquitin C promoter (UBC) (Fig. 2a). Use a tissue-specific promoter to investigate expression of a reporter gene specific to a tissue type under variable conditions (Fig. 2b). In general, tissue-specific promoters are weak in nature; however, using a two-step transcriptional approach (TSTA), the reporter gene expression is improved for weak promoters [1]. The TSTA reporter system consists of a weak promoter, which drives expression of a transcription factor and a second promoter consisting of multiple transcription factor responsive elements driving expression of a reporter gene. Weak promoter-driven TF binds to a second promoter carrying those TF responsive elements and thus gives enhanced reporter gene expression as an indirect measure of endogenous weak promoter activity (Fig. 2c) [1]. An inducible promoter system such as TET ON or TET OFF is helpful to measure context-dependent reporter gene

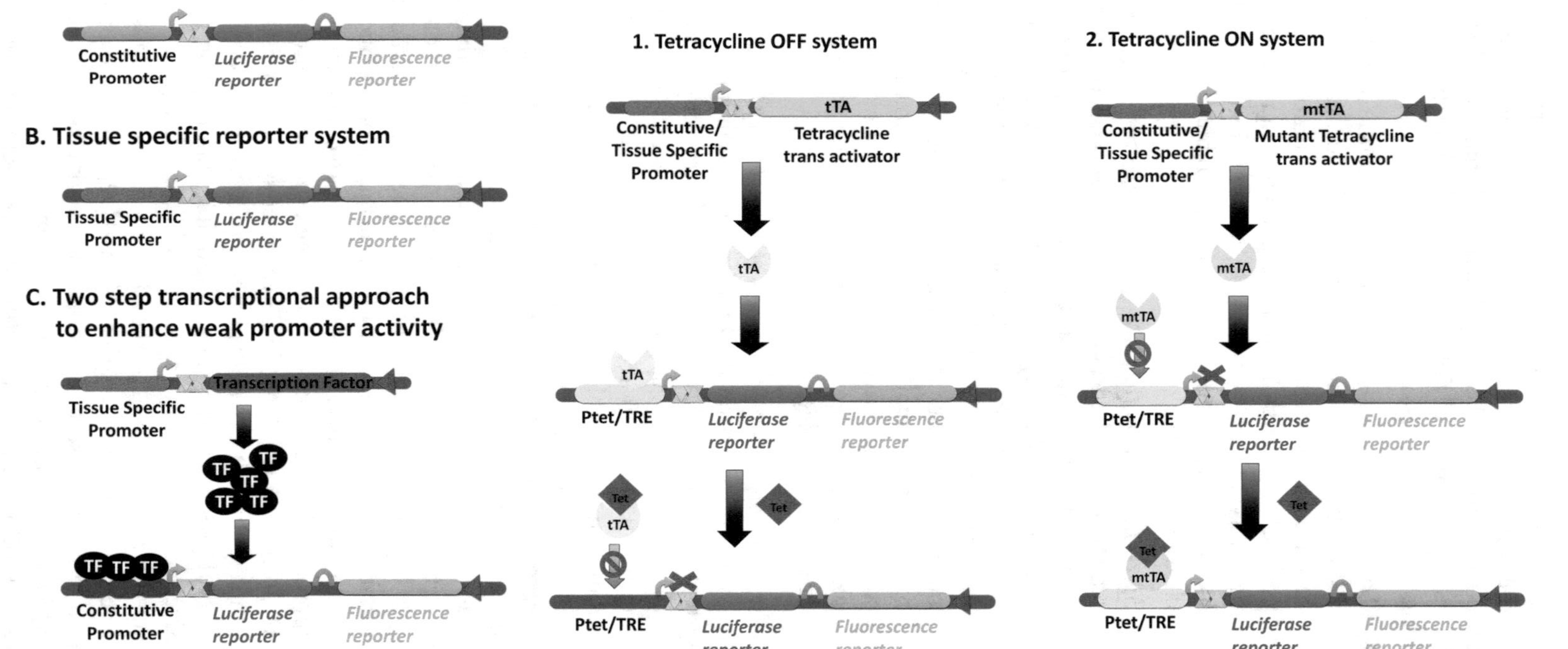

Fig. 2 Schematic representation of various categories of promoters to drive multimodality reporter. (**a**) A constitutive promoter such as CMV, SV40 early promoter, mouse U6 promoter and ubiquitin promoter can be used to obtain constitutive expression of reporter genes in cell or tissue (**b**) A tissue-specific promoter is utilized when expression of the reporter gene is to be restricted to a particular tissue. (**c**) A two-step transcriptional (TSTA) system consists of two vectors, one with a weak promoter driving expression of a transcription factor and the other vector contains a second promoter consisting of multiple responsive elements of the transcription factor which drives expression of the multimodality reporter gene. Low levels of transcription factor expressed from the weal promoter will bind to response elements present in the second promoter and thereby produce enhanced reporter gene expression. (**d**) A tetracycline inducible reporter system consists of two major elements, tetracycline controlled trans-activator (tTA) element and specific tTA responsive promoter element (Ptet). The transgene is cloned downstream to Ptet. In Tet OFF system tTA binds to promoter (Ptet) and positively regulates transgene expression in the absence of tetracycline. When tetracycline is added to the system, it prevents binding of Tta to promoter and thus inhibiting trans-gene expression. In contrast, in the TET ON system due to four amino acid change in tTA sequence, tTA can bind to PTet only when doxycycline is added to the system. Thus, in the TET ON system transgene expression is induced only after the addition of tetracycline to the system

expression. Tet system consists of two major elements, tetracycline controlled trans-activator (tTA) element and specific tTA responsive promoter element (Ptet). Tetracycline trans-activator (tTA) protein is a fusion of TetR (tetracycline repressor) and the activation domain of protein, VP16. Ptet promoter consists of tetracycline operator placed upstream of minimal promoter such as minimal CMV promoter. The transgene is cloned downstream to Ptet (Fig. 2d). In Tet-OFF system, tTA binds to the promoter (Ptet) and positively regulates transgene expression in the absence of tetracycline. By adding doxycycline, a derivative of tetracycline, binding of tTA to the promoter is prevented which inhibits transgene expression (Fig. 2d-1) [2]. The TET-ON system is exactly opposite to TET OFF system due to change in four amino acids present on TetR, which prevents binding of tTA to PTet in the absence of doxycycline, and transgene expression is induced only after the addition of doxycycline to the system (Fig. 2d-2) [3]. Clone an enhancer and/or repressor elements of a gene upstream to the reporter gene similar to promoter reporter to study the activity of cis-regulatory elements.

In this chapter, we will describe construction of a gene-specific and response element-specific promoter-reporter (multimodality). Other examples can be found elsewhere [4–8].

2 Materials

2.1 Cloning

1. Plasmid vectors: pcDNA3.1 (+) vector with neomycin resistance or pcDNA3.1(−) with puromycin resistance.
2. Firefly, Renilla, or Gaussia luciferase containing plasmids to isolate bioluminescent reporter.
3. GFP, mCherry, TdTomato containing plasmids to isolate fluorescent reporter.
4. Gene-specific PCR primers.
5. Taq, Pfu or other similar high fidelity DNA polymerase.
6. Restriction enzymes.
7. T4 DNA ligase.
8. LB media and agar: Make agar pates with 100 μg/mL ampicillin final conastartion.
9. Ampicillin stock (100 mg/mL in water).
10. Horizontal gel electrophoresis unit.

2.2 Cell Culture

1. Fetal bovine serum (FBS-Gibco).
2. Penicillin/Streptomycin (100X-Gibco).
3. 1× PBS.

4. Dulbecco's Minimal Eagles Media (DMEM) (supplemented with 10% fetal bovine serum (FBS), 1% penicillin (100 μg/mL) and 1% streptomycin (292 μg/mL) are used for culturing ovarian cancer cell lines A2780 and A2780-CIS^{LR}.
5. Neomycin (G418) stock, 100 mg/mL in 1× PBS, filter sterilized through 0.2 μm filter.
6. Puromycin stock, 1 μg/mL in 1× PBS, filter sterilized through 0.2 μm filter.
7. Superfect® transfection reagent (Qiagen) or equivalent.

2.3 Western Blot

1. 1× Laemmli sample buffer (32.9 mM Tris–HCl pH 6.8, 13.8% glycerol, 1% SDS) with protease inhibitor cocktail.
2. 100× protease inhibitor cocktail (Sigma).
3. Bradford assay reagent (Sigma).
4. Gel electrophoresis apparatus for polyacrylamide gels.
5. Transfer blot apparatus for western blot.
6. Primary antibodies against reporter genes.
7. HRP-labeled secondary antibodies.
8. Chemiluminescent substrate.
9. Gel documentation system or X-ray film developer machine.

2.4 Bioluminescence and Fluorescence Imaging

1. 5× Passive Lysis buffer (Promega).
2. LAR II (Luciferase Assay Reagent II, Promega): Make LARII substrate and store in −20 °C.
3. Coelenterazine (Biosynth): For measuring renilla activity from cell lysate, prepare 1 mg/mL Coelenterazine stock in Methanol. Dilute this stock 1:100 in 1× PBS just before use. Make a 5 mg/mL stock in methanol for mice imaging. Make a working solution of Coelenterazine by diluting stock at a 1:10 ratio (0.5 mg/mL) in 1× PBS, as direct addition/injection of methanol is toxic to cells and animals.
4. D-luciferin (Biosynth): Dissolve D-luciferin in 1× sterile PBS just before use. Make a 15–30 mg/mL stock and filter through a 0.22 μm filter. Use 100 μL per animal for mice imaging.
5. Female/male nude mice, 8–12 weeks old.
6. Isoflurane inhaled aesthetic.
7. Oxygen cylinder for anesthesia.
8. Anesthesia induction chamber.
9. IVIS® Lumina, IVIS® Spectrum, or equivalent machine to image fluorescent and bioluminescent signals.
10. Live Image software (4.4).

3 Methods

3.1 Vector Construction of Multimodal Optical Reporter (PI3KCA and NF-κB: Sensors)

In addition to using a single reporter gene (either luciferases or fluorescent proteins), a dual- or multi-modality reporter may be used to extend the power of imaging from live cell to live animals. The PI3K/AKT/NF-κB pathway is crucial for the development and maintenance of cisplatin resistance in ovarian carcinoma. For the past few years, we have created sensitive imaging methods to monitor in parallel two diverse molecular events, PIK3CA promoter activity, and NF-κB translational activity [9]. For this, we utilized two different bi-fusion reporter constructs, PIK3CA promoter driving *fl2-tdt* bifusion reporter (Fig. 3a) and NF-κB response element driving *hrl-egfp* bifusion reporter (Fig. 3b).

3.2 Brief Cloning Strategy

1. Use pcDNA™3.1(+) and/or pcDNA™3.1(−) from Invitrogen for high-level stable and transient expression of reporter genes in mammalian hosts. It is a 5.4 kb long vector with a CMV promoter and multiple cloning sites for gene expression.
2. Replace the CMV promoter in pcDNA™3.1(+) background (Neomycin) with a gene-specific promoter of interest to generate the gene-specific promoter-reporter.
3. Digest 3 μg of the pcDNA™3.1(+) vector with BglII and NheI to remove the CMV promoter and get linearized promoter-free vector backbone.
4. Isolate and purify the linearized plasmid vector by DNA gel electrophoresis and gel purification.
5. PCR amplify the gene-specific promoter of interest from genomic DNA. In this case, a 900 bp long PIK3CA promoter sequence is amplified from genomic DNA of ovarian surface epithelial cells using appropriate primers.
6. Design the forward primer with BglII restriction site and reverse primer with NheI restriction site to amplify the gene-specific promoter of interest. Both forward and reverse primers contain 3–4 additional nucleotides at 5′ end, restriction enzyme recognition sites for directional cloning of the insert and exact complement of ~15–20 consecutive bases of a selected target gene.
7. PCR amplify the promoter of interest using primers designed by the above strategy.
8. Check the specific PCR amplification of promoter of interest by DNA gel electrophoresis.
9. Digest 2 μg of PCR amplified product with BglII and NheI.
10. Purify the BglII and NheI digested PCR product by column purification. This will serve as the insert.

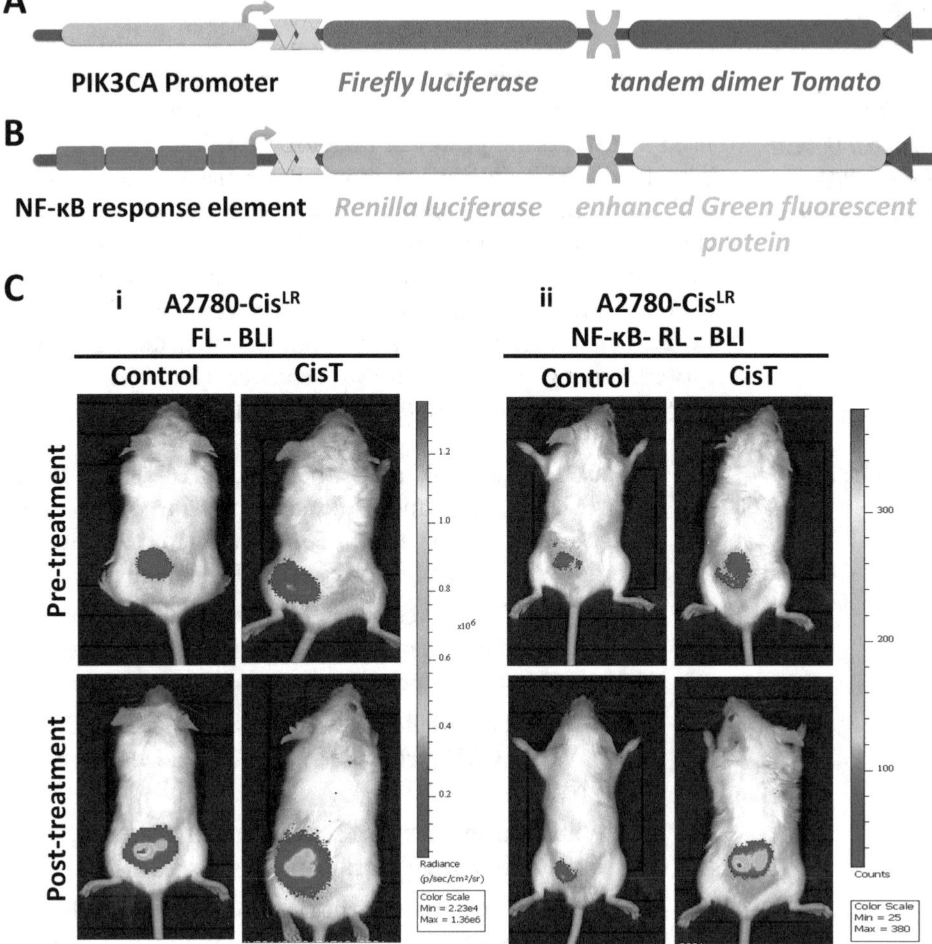

Fig. 3 In vivo imaging of modulation in two diverse molecular events. (**a**) Schematic representation of a PIK3CA promoter sensor driving expression of a firefly luciferase-tandem dimer tomato fluorescent reporter. (**b**) An NF-κB transcriptional activity reporter sensor (four NF-κB response elements) driving expression of a renilla luciferase-enhanced green fluorescent reporter). (**c**) Representative bioluminescence imaging of the PIK3CA promoter activity and NF-κB transcriptional activity in the same mouse bearing A2780-CisLR tumor xenografts. This dual reporter expressing cellular model was used to illustrate the differential modulation of two distinct molecular events, as PIK3CA promoter activity (firefly luciferase activity) and transcriptional activity of NF-κB (renilla luciferase activity) in response to cisplatin treatment. As depicted in the left panel (**c**-i), PIK3CA promoter activity remained stable whereas transcriptional activity of NF-κB escalates post cisplatin treatment (**c**-ii) (Adapted from Gaikwad et al. [9])

11. Ligate the linearized vector and insert DNA using T4 DNA ligase according to the manufacturer's instructions, and transform into bacterial cells and plate on ampicillin containing LB agar plates for selection.
12. Inoculate the bacterial colonies from agar plates into LB media containing ampicillin and grow for overnight incubation.
13. Isolate plasmid DNA from overnight grown culture using the commercially available plasmid DNA isolation kit.

14. Confirm positive clones by restriction digestion and sequencing.
15. Follow the similar strategy to make other reporter constructs. We used a second reporter, the NF-κB sensor (NF-κB-transcription factor response sensor) along with the PIK3CA promoter-reporter.
16. To make NF-κB sensor we used CMV-rl-egfp-pcDNA 3.1(−) with puromycin as a mammalian selection marker.
17. Synthesize the transcription-factor response element sequence available from the literature along with a minimal TA promoter sequence by oligo synthesis. NF-κB response element cassette (four repeats NF-κB response element) of a 50 base pair oligonucleotide was synthesized.
18. Flank the response element sequence with BglII at 5′ and NheI at 3′ end of oligo for cloning.
19. Clone the transcription factor response element oligo with minimal TA promoter into CMV-*rl-egfp*-pcDNA 3.1(−)-*puromycin* DNA by replacing the CMV promoter, as described above for the PIK3CA promoter.
20. Isolation and cloning of cDNA sequences of reporter genes into vector is done similar to that of promoter cloning. Briefly, amplify the cDNA using primes with specific restriction sites and clone the PCR amplified products downstream to the promoter of interest (*see* **Notes 2** and **3**).

PCR amplification of appropriate genes with appropriate restriction digestion, ligation, transformation and screening of the colonies is a common strategy to make these constructs. Finally, transient transfection in mammalian cells confirms luciferase gene expression followed by a luciferase assay and Western blot analysis. Similarly, confirm fluorescent gene expression by fluorescence microscopy and Western blot analysis.

3.3 Validation of Sensors by In Vitro Transient Transfection; and Measuring of Reporter Expression and Activity

3.3.1 In vitro Transient Transfection

1. For luciferase and fluorescence measurement, seed a defined number of cells (2–8 × 10^4 cells/well) into 24-well tissue culture plates a day before transfection and incubate at 37 °C. This cell number results in 50% confluence, which provides optimal transfection efficiency.
2. Next day, transiently transfect the reporter constructs using the Superfect transfection reagent (Qiagen) following the protocol recommended by the manufacturer (*see* **Note 4**).
3. For Western blot, seed cells into 60 mm culture dishes and scale up the cell number accordingly. Transfect the cells as described above with DNA and transfection reagent scaled up appropriately.
4. Incubate the cells at 37 °C for 24–48 h post transient transfection to obtain optimal expression.

3.3.2 Western Blot Analysis

1. Harvest the cells by trypsinization and give a one 1× PBS wash.
2. Lyse the harvested cells Cell lysates in 1× Laemmli buffer.
3. Estimate protein concentration of cell lysates using Bradford protein assay reagent (Sigma) and read absorbance using a spectrophotometer at wavelength 595 nm.
4. Perform a standard vertical polyacrylamide gel electrophoresis and transfer gel resolved proteins to Nitrocellulose or PVDF membrane using trans-blot system.
5. Add respective antibodies against each reporter genes for the detection of reporter gene expression or fusion protein detection.
6. For fusion reporter genes, absence or minimal cleavage of fusion proteins is important.

3.3.3 Bioluminescence and Fluorescence Measurement (from Cells)

1. Wash the reporter-expressing cells (transiently transfected or stable cells) with 1× PBS.
2. Dilute the 5× passive lysis buffer with 1× PBS appropriately and add protease inhibitor cocktail to it.
3. Add 100 μL of 1× passive lysis to each well and rotate on a shaker platform for 10 min at room temperature.
4. Transfer lysates to 1.5-mL micro centrifuge tubes. Centrifuge in a microfuge at 17,000 × *g*, 10 min, 4 °C. Collect supernatants in fresh tubes and discard the pellet.
5. Use LAR II (for fluc assay) or Coelenterazine (for rluc assay) as a substrate for luminescence activity measurement.
6. Use a Birthhold luminometer to measure luciferase and fluorescence activity.
7. *Bioluminescence activity measurement*: In a white 96-well plate, add 100 μL of LAR II (for firefly luciferase activity) or 100 μL of coelenterazine solution (1 mg/mL diluted 1:100 in 1× PBS) to the 10 μL of cell lysate supernatant. As *gluc* is a secretory luciferase, its activity is measurement directly from cell culture media supernatant. For this, add 20 μL cell culture media supernatant into 100 μL of Coelenterazine solution. Luciferase activity of each well is measured using Berthhold luminometer for 1–10 s and expressed as relative light unit (RLU)/s.
8. *Fluorescence activity measurement*: To monitor the fluorescent activity of cells expressing a single or multimodal reporter, lysates are prepared as described for bioluminescence activity. Shine a black 96-well plate containing 1:10 diluted solution of each lysate with light of appropriate excitation spectrum using a Berthhold luminometer. Capture signals at required emission spectrum for 1–10 s and present data as relative fluorescence unit (RFU)/s.
9. Protein concentration for each cell lysate is calculated using Bradford reagent. Reporter activity of each sample is recorded and represented as RLU/μg of protein or RFU/μg of protein.

3.4 Stable Cell Line Generation and In Vivo Imaging

Once the construct/s is characterized by transient transfection by both measuring the reporter activity and western blotting, it is ready for stable cell line establishment and further studies. Stable cell lines expressing reporter genes allow the noninvasive and repetitive imaging of biological functions in live animals.

3.4.1 Stable Cell Line Generation

1. The optimal selection concentration for each cell line needs to be experimentally identified by kill curve of each selection marker.
2. To generate a stable cell line, seed cells into 100 mm culture dishes and scale up the cell number accordingly. Transfect the cells as described above with DNA and transfection reagent scaled up appropriately.
3. After 36 h incubation, split transfected cells into additional culture dishes at 1:3/1:4 ratio (according to the cell size and doubling time) and incubate in the respective selection medium (for neomycin selection marker-G418 and for puromycin selection marker- Puromycin) for 2–3 weeks. A large number of cells die during this period and only cells carrying the reporter vector continue to grow as colony.
4. Allow the individual colony to appear in the plates and pick up individual colony (10–30) and culture them in 96-well plates in a selection medium.
5. Propagate the clones in larger wells and split into duplicate wells.
6. Measure luciferase activity from one of the duplicate wells for each clone as described above. Maintain the duplicate well of the clones with highest activity to use for experiments.
7. For dual stable clone generation, transfect stable cell lines expressing one reporter with a second reporter vector. It is essential that the second reporter vector possesses a different antibiotic selection marker.
8. Maintain the clones in media containing both the antibiotics.
9. Alternatively, if both the fusion reporters contain fluorescent protein component, isolate cells expressing both reporters by flow sorting and then maintain the sorted cells in selection media containing both antibiotics.

3.4.2 Live Cell Imaging (Bioluminescence and Fluorescence)

Bioluminescence imaging in live cells:

1. For live cell imaging, seed desired number of cells expressing the reporter in 96 black well plate.
2. After 24 h, wash cells with 1× PBS and then incubate with the appropriate substrate (Coelentrazine (100 μL of 0.1 mg/mL) for rluc, D-luciferine (1 mg/mL) for fluc) and imaging is done with IVIS spectrum instrument.

3. For gluc measurement, add 10 μL of Coelenterazine directly into culture media.
4. Measure photons emitted from each well for 15 s to 5 min, depending on the intensity of the signal.
5. For dual luciferase imaging, first acquire bioluminescence of whole plate using Coelenterazine (as Coelenterazine signal lasts for shorter time as compared to D-luciferin which can last for hours and may interfere with Coelenterazine signal), then wash with 1× PBS twice followed by imaging with D-luciferin.
6. For analysis, use the Live Image software (4.4), draw region of interest (ROIs) over each well which will give results in the form of relative light units and are measured and quantified as total intensity (photons/s/cm^2/sr).

3.4.3 Fluorescence Imaging in Live Cells

1. Perform fluorescence imaging with respective excitation wavelength and signal is recorded at emission wavelength.
2. The plate can be scanned with epi-fluorescence or trans-fluorescence mode. For the trans-fluorescence method, glass bottom black plates are required, as light will be shinned from the bottom of the plate.
3. For analysis, use the Live Image software (4.4), draw region of interest (ROIs) over each well; this will give results in the form of relative light units and is measured and quantified as total intensity (photons/s/cm2/sr).

In case of an inducible promoter, such as TET ON or OFF, tetracycline derivative doxycycline is either supplemented or removed from the media. Concentration of doxycycline has to be optimized for optimal expression of reporter gene. As per the experimental requirement, a gradient of doxycycline concentration is used to control the amount of reporter expression in a cell.

For tracing a molecular event in response to stimuli or chemotherapeutic drugs, seed cells in duplicates and use one set as control and other as treated with drug or other stimuli. For example, to understand the effect of cisplatin on PIK3CA promoter activity and NF-κB transcriptional activity, dual stable cells expressing both the reporters are treated with cisplatin (with optimized concentration) for specific time periods and then imaged. TNF-α can also be used as an inducer of NF-κB transcriptional activity.

3.5 In Vivo Imaging of Promoter Reporter in Tumor Xenograft

3.5.1 Fluorescence Imaging in Mice

1. First, perform fluorescence imaging as bioluminescence can last long and it can interfere with fluorescence imaging giving false readings.
2. Keep mice on warm stage of IVIS spectrum instrument with constant flow of isoflurane via nose cone.

3. Expose the mice to the respective excitation wavelength for each fluorescent protein and only photons at appropriate emission wavelength are recorded using a specific filter.
4. Either epi-fluorescence or trans-fluorescence mode can be used depending on requirement. Generally, epi-fluorescence scanning is used for imaging signal from surface tissue, while trans-fluorescence scanning mode is advantageous since it provides rapid whole body scan of a mouse. However, photon intensity is reduced in trans-fluorescence scanning due to tissue-specific attenuation.

3.5.2 Bioluminescence Imaging in Mice

1. Use BALB/C nude mice for in vivo fluorescence imaging as mouse fur interferes with fluorescence imaging; while nude or scid both can be used for bioluminescence imaging. Seek approval from your Institutional Animal Care and Use Committee for all the procedures prior to starting experiments.
2. Implant 3–6 $\times$ 10^6 cells (tumor cells) stably expressing luciferase-fluorophore reporter subcutaneously. We implanted 4 $\times$ 10^6 dual stable (PIK3CA-FL2-tdt and NF-kB-RL-eGFP) A2780 and A2780-CisLR cells on either flanks of nude mice subcutaneously (Fig. 3c).
3. Allow tumors to grow up to 5–8 mm.
4. Anesthetize with 2% isoflurane by keeping the animals in an incubation chamber.
5. Acquire whole body imaging of mice in IVIS Spectrum (Perkin Elmer) preclinical in vivo imaging system after injecting respective substrate.
6. For renilla luciferase imaging, anesthetize mice and intravenously inject coelenterazine at a concentration of 50 μg/100 μL in PBS per mouse. Place the mice immediately on the IVIS imaging instrument stage and acquire image. Renilla luciferase shows flash kinetics, which reaches peak signal within 1 min post substrate injection and declines rapidly with time.
7. After 1 h of renilla luciferase imaging, inject 100 μL of D-Luciferin (30 mg/mL) intraperitoneally in mice. Anesthetize mice with isoflurane. Place the mice immediately on the IVIS imaging instrument stage and acquire image. The signal for firefly luciferase peaks from 5 min and remains stable for 30 min. It is always advisable to acquire a background image before D-Luciferin injection.
8. For imaging tumor xenograft bearing mice expressing two luciferases, *rluc* signal is first recorded followed by *fluc* imaging. Post *rluc* imaging a time gap must be given to avoid overlap of renilla activity with firefly luciferase activity.

9. *Gluc activity measurement from mice*: Gluc is a secretory luciferase protein; hence its activity is measured from blood collected from mice. Withdraw blood from either orbital puncture or from tail vain and collected in EDTA vacationer to obtain plasma. Measure Gluc activity by adding 20 μL of plasma into 100 μL of coelenterazine solution 96-well plate. Relative luciferase unit (RLU) of each well was measured using Berthhold luminometer for 10 s.
10. Draw region of interests (ROIs) over each tumor and quantify with the help of Live Image software (4.4). Bioluminescence/Fluorescence signals from each tumor xenografts are recorded as maximum intensity or total intensity (photons/s/cm^2/sr).

4 Notes

1. Serine and Glycine are more commonly used in flexible linkers as they provide good flexibility due to their small sizes, and also help to maintain stability of the linker structure in the aqueous solvent through the formation of hydrogen bonds with water. The length of the flexible linkers can be adjusted to allow for proper folding or to achieve optimal biological activity of the fusion proteins. In contrast, Proline is more rigid and can lead to decrease in optimal biological activity of the fusion proteins. Cysteine can form disulfide bonds with other cysteine residues leading to decreased or no reporter actvity.
2. Bioluminescence reporter genes, CMV-driven firefly luciferase (fluc), or humanized renilla luciferase (rluc) are amplified from plasmid vectors available from Promega (Madison, WI). Gaussia luciferase (gluc) and other fluorescent reporter genes such as enhanced green fluorescent protein (eGFP), mutated red fluorescent protein (mrfp), and tandem dimer tomato (tdt) are amplified from respective plasmid sources.
3. Firefly luciferase and renilla luciferase belong to two diverse classes of luciferases that utilize specific substrates D-luciferine and coelenterazine respectively that do not cross-react. Due to this property, both fluc and rluc are appropriate to monitor two diverse events in living cell/tumor simultaneously fluc and rluc or fluc and gluc are used as a pair for multiplexed imaging. Rluc and gLuc luciferase reporter cannot be used for multiplexing as both catalyze coelentrazine as a substrate.
4. Dilute 1 μg of plasmid DNA in 60 μL serum-free media, and incubate with 5 μL of Superfect reagent for 10 min. Add this complex to 350 μL serum containing media and overlay onto the cells. Incubate the cells under normal growth conditions for 2–3 h. After this change give PBS wash and change media.

References

1. Iyer M et al (2001) Two-step transcriptional amplification as a method for imaging reporter gene expression using weak promoters. Proc Natl Acad Sci U S A 98(25):14595–14600
2. Gossen M, Bujard H (1992) Tight control of gene expression in mammalian cells by tetracycline-responsive promoters. Proc Natl Acad Sci U S A 89(12):5547–5551
3. Gossen M et al (1995) Transcriptional activation by tetracyclines in mammalian cells. Science 268 (5218):1766–1769
4. Neveu MA et al (2016) Multi-modality imaging to assess metabolic response to dichloroacetate treatment in tumor models. Oncotarget 7 (49):81741–81749
5. Dai Y et al (2013) In vivo multimodality imaging and cancer therapy by near-infrared light-triggered trans-platinum pro-drug-conjugated upconverison nanoparticles. J Am Chem Soc 135(50):18920–18929
6. Rumyantsev KA, Turoverov KK, Verkhusha VV (2016) Near-infrared bioluminescent proteins for two-color multimodal imaging. Sci Rep 6:36588
7. Wu T et al (2016) Multimodal imaging of a humanized orthotopic model of hepatocellular carcinoma in immunodeficient mice. Sci Rep 6:35230
8. Dobrucki LW et al (2010) Approaches to multimodality imaging of angiogenesis. J Nucl Med 1 (51 Suppl):669–79S
9. Gaikwad SM et al (2015) Differential activation of NF-kappaB signaling is associated with platinum and taxane resistance in MyD88 deficient epithelial ovarian cancer cells. Int J Biochem Cell Biol 61:90–102

Chapter 3

Optical Bioluminescence Protocol for Imaging Mice

David Stout and John David

Abstract

The presence, growth, or decline of transfected cell populations expressing the enzyme Luciferase can be followed in live mice using bioluminescence optical imaging techniques. This protocol describes how to verify the imaging equipment, options for injecting the substrate Luciferin into mice, image acquisition considerations, and commonly used data analysis techniques.

Key words Bioluminescence, Luciferin, Luciferase, Optical imaging, Mouse, Oncology, Tumor imaging

1 Introduction

Bioluminescent imaging makes use of the enzymatic reaction commonly found in fireflies or deep-sea animals, where light is created from a chemical reaction [1]. A substrate, typically Luciferin, is injected and perfuses to all tissues in the animal. Wherever gene expression of the enzyme Luciferase is present, light is created through a catalytic reaction that also requires oxygen, magnesium, and living cells with energy, in the form of ATP. The most common use of this technique is for oncology research [2], where human tumor cells are transfected with the gene to express Firefly Luciferase (Fig. 1). Tumor cells grow and can be imaged at multiple time points to look at proliferation or declining signal due to various treatments. The imaging technique is noninvasive, requiring injection of the substrate and anesthesia to immobilize the animals for imaging times lasting seconds to minutes. Animals can be imaged many times over weeks or months. Since the entire animal is visible in most optical systems any new or expanded signal locations can be readily identified. Ex vivo imaging is also possible to verify specific organ or tissue uptake, assuming that animals are injected prior to sacrifice, with dissection and imaging completed within a few minutes before the oxygen and ATP levels are depleted.

Purnima Dubey (ed.), *Reporter Gene Imaging: Methods and Protocols*, Methods in Molecular Biology, vol. 1790,
https://doi.org/10.1007/978-1-4939-7860-1_3, © Springer Science+Business Media, LLC, part of Springer Nature 2018

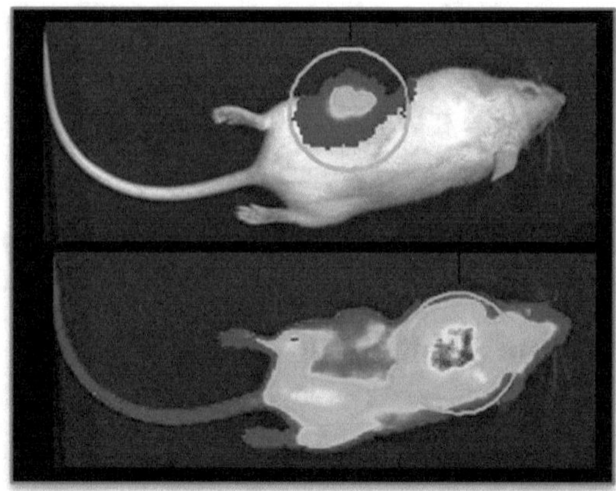

Fig. 1 Bioluminescent mouse image (top) and same mouse with fluorescence imaging (bottom). Note the very specific bioluminescent tumor signal with little background elsewhere in the animal. The fluorescent image shows considerable endogenous background signal coming from fur (green), blood (red), and collagen in the skin (blue). The shaved area around the tumor to improve signal detection is readily visible in the fluorescent image

Because light does not propagate through tissue very well, bioluminescent imaging is ideally suited to small animals such as mice or superficial tissues in larger rodents, for example the rat leg or brain [3]. All the light created is scattered and most of it is absorbed before leaving the body. Only a small fraction of the light closest to the skin surface makes its way out of the animal and can be measured using a digital camera located inside a dark light-tight box. The amount of light leaving the body depends on many factors, including the depth in tissue [4], presence of fur (Fig. 1), background signals, wavelength and efficiency of both the particular substrate and enzyme versions used for the research. Due to the light absorption and diffusion limitations, bioluminescence imaging is a semi-quantitative measurement methodology, able to provide information about the presence or lack of signal, general location and relative trends of increase or decrease in signal intensity over time. An absolute amount of light produced is not possible to measure for many reasons. This discussion is beyond the scope of this document.

2 Materials

1. Optical imaging camera system and knowledge of software operation: Multiple vendors sell optical imaging equipment, thus it is not possible to describe specific instrument operations in this SOP. Typical imaging times are seconds to minutes and the necessary settings, such as binning, exposure, and display settings are instrument specific.

2. Animals expressing bioluminescent gene: Cells expressing Luciferase are injected or implanted to create in vivo optical signaling capability.
3. Imaging chamber or animal holder: Animals are immobilized for imaging and placed in an appropriate reproducible position. The strongest signal producing location is pointed directly toward the camera, which may require taping the animal in place. Low adhesion paper tape is recommended to avoid injuring the skin. Depending on the holder design, it is recommended to place disposable black paper under the animals to minimize any contamination between groups of mice (Fig. 1). This paper must not contain any fluorescent dyes that would give off a background signal.
4. Animal workspace: In the United States, biosafety level 2 or higher conditions are required for animal use space when working with human tumor cell lines or infectious agents in accordance with the Blood Borne Pathogen Act, Biosafety in Microbiological and Biomedical Laboratories (BMBL), federal and local regulations, and institutional policies. Reference institutional policies and local regulations for specifications, as requirements vary. The laboratory space must have all the mechanical and engineering controls required and necessary for rodent work [5]. In particular, the space needs to accommodate heating of animals and cages, anesthesia, injections and recovery. For immune compromised animals, a class II biosafety cabinet is recommended for all handling of animals. Sealed imaging chambers are preferred, where animals are loaded within the biosafety cabinet, transferred and imaged while a barrier is maintained at all times. Sealed chambers serve the dual function protecting research personnel from research pathogen and animals from environmental pathogens.
5. Anesthesia: A gas isoflurane (1–3%) vaporizer with either medical air or oxygen as the carrier gas is preferred. Injected anesthetics such as ketamine/xylazine can be used, however if the optical signal strength is low or perfusion is poor, requiring long imaging times, the mice may start moving and blurred images will compromise the data.
6. Luciferin substrate: Luciferin can be purchased in solution ready to inject, or prepared from powder and frozen until use. Since Luciferin activity is degraded by exposure to light and oxygen, keep the powder and solution frozen at −18 °C in the dark and minimize handling time. For powder, completely dissolve in saline to a concentration of 30 mg/mL, pass through a 0.22 μm sterilizing filter, and store in a −18 °C freezer. After making a stock solution, it is useful to dispense aliquots for individual animal injections into microfuge tubes

and store in a light tight enclosure such as a cardboard box with dividers to hold the tubes. Each mouse will require 100 μL, typically injected into either the intraperitoneal cavity (IP) or via tail vein (IV). For injections, thaw the vial and warm it to at least room temperature before immediate use.

For imaging work utilizing an alternative substrate Coelenterazine, create a stock solution of 2 mg/mL in propylene glycol and store at −18 °C. For injections, dilute 50 μL of stock solution with 450 μL of phosphate-buffered saline (PBS) and inject 100 μL per mouse. Do not filter, as it will remove the substrate. Inject immediately via tail vein and begin acquisition immediately.

3 Methods

1. Animal prep prior to imaging day: Shave the animals over the area of the signal site. Hair blocks light and will reduce the signal measurement, especially black fur. A depilatory cream is useful to remove the fur under the skin. Due to the time and effort required to remove the fur and possible inflammation, this work is best done a day or two prior to imaging. Alternatively, athymic nude mice can be used. Nude mice are widely used for optical imaging studies due to the lack of fur and partial loss of the adaptive immune system that enables transplantation and growth of human tumor cell lines. Recently, additional nude strains with and without immune systems on various common background strains have become commercially available. These strains are especially useful for bioluminescence imaging for a number of study designs. Be wary of pigmented mice. Pigment blunts the light signal and the pigmented patches shift size and location over long studies. Albino mice are preferred for these types of imaging studies.
2. Animal prep immediately prior to imaging: Warm cages of animals for 20–30 min on a 35 °C heating plate or pad prior to anesthetizing and injections (*see* **Note 1**). Animals should be kept warm throughout each step of the imaging process, including recovery.
3. Camera hardware and software test: Acquire a short duration dark field optical image (no objects in field of view) without animals to ensure the instrument is working properly. Look for any signs of light contamination in the image, which may come from materials that may not have been cleaned properly after the previous use. Some instruments require initialization time to cool the charge-coupled device (CCD) camera and stabilize the background signals prior to imaging animals. Typical image correction options include flat field correction for circular lens

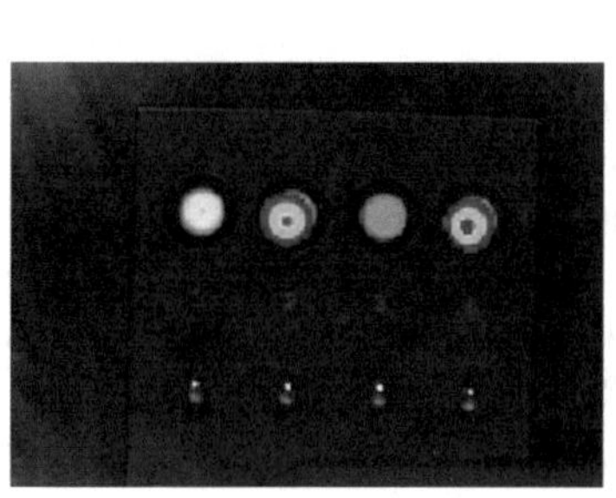

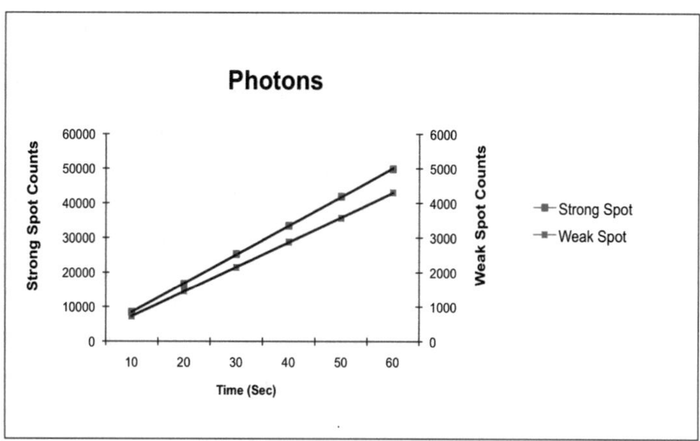

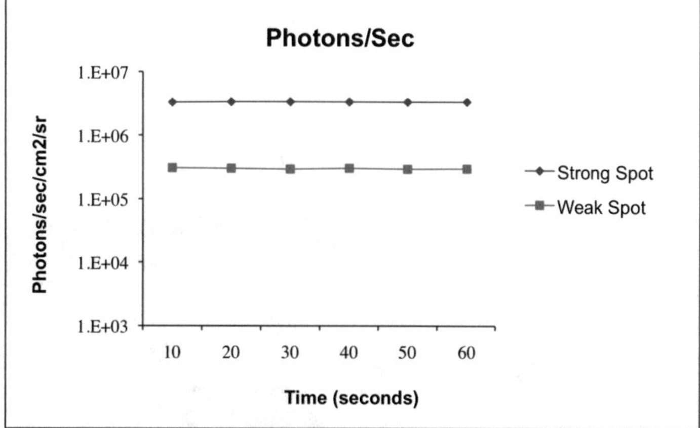

Fig. 2 Quality control light source (photo) and graphs of total light output (top, photons) and light output rate (bottom, photons/s). Total counts measured are dependent on the amount of imaging time, whereas the rate is independent of acquisition time. Using the rate allows for comparison of different duration images, which may be necessary as light signals grow or decrease over the experiment

distortions, cosmic rays, and background subtraction. On a routine basis, either weekly or monthly, acquire images of a calibrated light source to verify accurate and precise measurements [16]. Maintain a log of these values and check that performance is consistent over time (Fig. 2).

4. Image Acquisition: Acquire images where the measurement values are in terms of photons per second, rather than simply a total amount of light measured. By using a rate (photons/sec) rather than a total (# photons), the duration of the imaging session will not be a confounding factor if longer or shorter acquisition times are necessary over the course of the experiment as the optical signal grows weaker or stronger (Fig. 2).
5. Injection syringe prep: Recommend ½ mL 28 g ½ inch ("TB") syringes that have a fixed needle and minimal dead volume. Draw up 100 uL in each syringe and remove any air bubbles.

Try to minimize the time the substrate is exposed to air and light. Note that many institutions have strict policies regarding recapping needles, so it is advisable to inject immediately after drawing each syringe.

6. Anesthesia: Animals can be injected either anesthetized or awake (*see* **Note 2**). For anesthetized animal work, place animals in an induction box and wait at least 2–3 min after movement stops before working with the animals. Ideally there are two induction boxes available, one for induction of anesthesia and one for holding animals after injection (*see* **Note 3**).
7. Injections: Injections can be made either into the intraperitoneal cavity (IP) or tail vein (Fig. 3) (*see* **Note 4**).
   (a) For IP injections, remove mouse from induction box, hold by the scruff and tail in one hand, inject in the IP cavity just lateral of midline to avoid the bladder and cecum. Return mouse to anesthesia box and repeat for each animal being imaged together as a group. If there is no visible light from an animal where signal is expected,

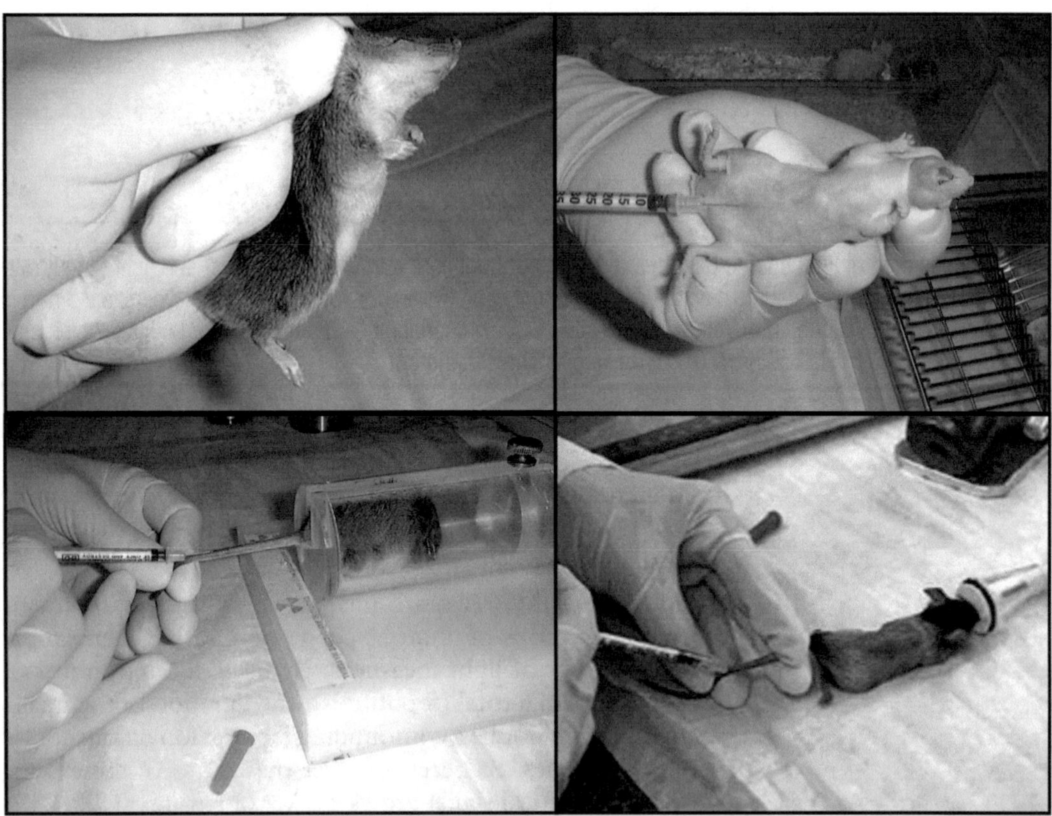

Fig. 3 Injection methods commonly used; Top left: Proper grip for holding mice, Top right: intraperitoneal injection, Bottom left: conscious tail vein, Bottom right: unconscious tail vein. Reproduced with permission from ref. [17]

most likely resulted from an injection into the bowel. This is somewhat common with IP injections, ~5%, and animals can be injected again to look for signal.

(b) For IV injections, it is best to have a warm surface to work on and an anesthesia nose cone to keep the animal anesthetized during the injection process. Place the animal in the nose cone and clean the tail by wiping with an alcohol swab. In some cases, placing a gauze pad soaked in 35–37 °C water is advisable to help increase vasodilation, which facilitates injection. Many users preferred to bend the syringe needle about 20 degrees with the bevel facing up, so the needle can easily slide into the tail vein. Insert the needle into the tail vein at about halfway down the tail and slide into the vein about 3–4 mm. Push the plunger and observe the vein blanching as the blood is displaced by the injection solution. If there is backpressure or swelling forms on the tail, then the syringe is not in the vein and must be repositioned.

(c) For coelenterazine substrate, since light is emitted immediately after injection, animals must be positioned for imaging, injected IV while under anesthesia, and moved to the camera. Imaging should be started as quickly as possible and continued for ~5 min. Only a single acquisition is necessary since the light output decays exponentially over a few minutes.

8. Positioning: After luciferin injection and immobilization, mice must be placed in a holder or positioned and taped onto paper so that the signal location faces the camera.

9. Image Acquisition: Move the animals into the camera and begin image acquisition. The ideal acquisition timing and duration depends on the signal strength, which in turn depends on the injection method, perfusion of the signal site, and amount of Luciferase present. Strong signals may require only a fraction of a second, whereas weak signals may require several minutes. Once the ideal timing is determined, it should be somewhat reproducible for future imaging experiments. However as tumors grow, the perfusion may decrease and change the light output and timing (Fig. 4). It is necessary to acquire multiple images and look quickly at the light output measurement to determine if the peak light output has been reached. It is not necessary to image for the first few minutes, however if one waits too long to start imaging, the peak may be missed. If multiple animals are imaged together, each animal may have a different maximum peak light output time, so check each animal's signal profile.

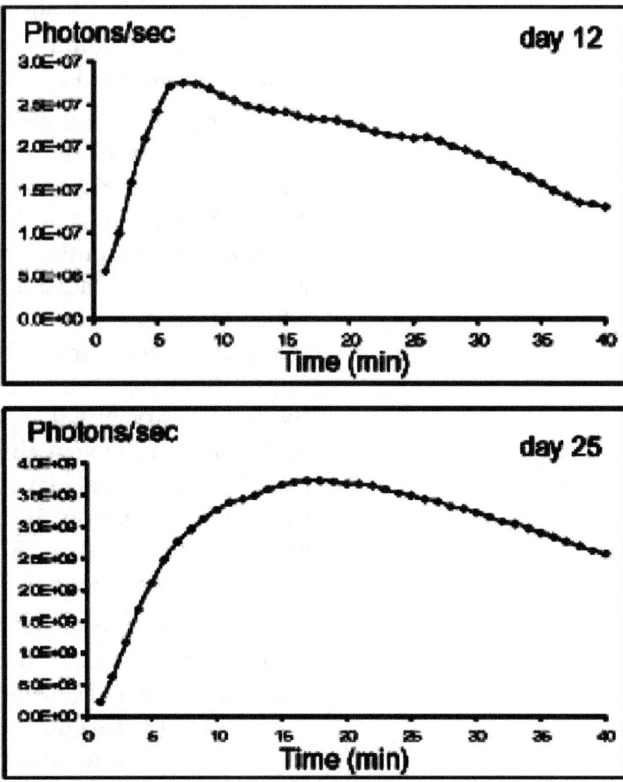

Fig. 4 Peak light output time and intensity from a tumor changes as the tumor grows. Graph shows light output measurements over 40 min at 12 and 25 days post tumor insertion. The peak signal times and shape of the curves are different, demonstrating the need for multiple measurements to determine the ideal measurement value. Reproduced with permission from ref. [6]

10. Image Measurements: Multiple measurements are essential, since the peak light output timing can vary based in the injection, tumor size, and other factors [6] (Fig. 4). In general, the time of the peak light output is shortest with small, well-perfused tumors, and gets longer with larger and more poorly perfused tumors or with poor injections. Acquire at least 3 measurements and measure the light output to see that they are all about the same intensity. If the signal is going up with time, continue acquiring data until a stable plateau is reached. It is likely the ideal imaging timing and duration may lengthen over the duration of an experiment lasting several weeks, both due to poorer perfusion of large tumors and possible loss of signal over time.
11. Animal Recovery: Once measurements are complete, remove the animals from the imaging system and place in a warmed cage for recovery. Animals should be monitored until ambulatory before returning to the vivarium. Consult institutional policies on animal handling and recovery requirements.

12. Cleanup: Clean and disinfect areas where animals touched any surfaces. Discard paper and tape used for securing animals. Specific cleaning requirements are specified by your institution and may include a spray solution of Virkane or Trifectant. Make sure the transparent chamber cover between the animal and camera is clean and clear to get the best picture quality.
13. Data Analysis: Bioluminescent image data is commonly a 2D photograph of light intensity. Regions can be drawn around any observable signals and the amount of light detected can be measured. Some 3D imaging systems require volumetric regions for analysis. Region boundaries are difficult to determine, since all light is scattered and signal strength is depth dependent. Deeper signals mean less light escaping the body and greater scatter, making localization more difficult. Because of the scattering, usually elliptical regions are used to surround any signals. The size will determine the signal measurement, so a consistent method of placing and sizing regions is required. Larger regions may include areas outside of the animal and will have a greater total signal and lower average signal. Smaller regions will have higher average signals and lower total signals, so there is a tradeoff to determine the most appropriate size. The best solution is to avoid this by reporting the maximum signal intensity, which is usually a measure of the signal area closest to the skin surface, reproducible for each measurement time and independent of the region size. This maximum pixel or voxel measurement method is only suitable if multiple detector signals are added together for the measurement (a binning factor of at least 4), otherwise the pixel value may just be the detector element with the greatest baseline noise.
14. Image Interpretation: Optical imaging is a semi-quantitative imaging method because of light scattering and depth-dependent absorption. This method can provide information about the presence or absence of a signal, **relative** changes in intensity, size and location over time. While the amount of light detected by the camera can be accurately and precisely measured, the amount of light emitted within the animal is not completely known. For this reason, care must be taken in interpreting and reporting the results. *In vivo* optical imaging is not a fully quantitative measurement method, unlike *in vitro* optical methods such as flow cytometry-based cell counting. As such, we recommend reporting findings in descriptive terms, such as signal pattern changes and loss or gain of signal rather than absolute light measurement values (*see* **Note 5**).
15. Reporting Results: Because optical signals are so dependent on the exact imaging protocol details used to obtain the data, it is imperative to adequately report the methods used to generate the data [8]. Even if not published, the conditions are essential

to record to replicate work or build upon existing knowledge for future experiments. This includes housing and caging conditions, imaging protocols, equipment and software settings used to acquire and process the data.

4 Notes

1. Optical imaging is dependent on enzymatic reactions that are sensitive to many factors [9], most notably temperature. Warming the animals consistently to a thermoneutral temperature (31–34 °C) enables a stable and reproducible biological signal by bringing animals to a consistent physiological state [10]. Stable physiology has the dual benefit of improving reproducibility between experiments and anesthetic survival in animals that commonly have compromised health status. Animals are often cold stressed in individually ventilated cages [11] which alters the size of tumors and metabolic processes. The blood flow, heart rate, and metabolism of mice can change within a few minutes of changes in temperature; thus moving the cage to a warm area in the imaging location and holding animals for a variable amount of time prior to imaging can result in variable measurements. Other relevant factors that can alter luciferase expression include time of day [12], housing conditions [13], tumor size [7], and plasma protein levels [14]. In addition, handling conditions such as anesthetic agent, position of animal [15], and injection method can alter optical signals [16, 17].
2. Most people find it easier to work with anesthetized animals for injections. Conscious injection is necessary for some study protocols to avoid the physiological changes associated with anesthesia. Conscious injection requires practice and skill to accomplish quickly to minimize stress. With gas anesthesia, animals will begin moving within 20–30 s once removed from the gas, so IP injections need to be done quickly. For IV injections, a nose cone and prep area are ideal so that each animal is handled individually for injections.
3. The use of two anesthesia induction boxes simplifies the injection process. Animals move around and get mixed up when initially exposed to gas anesthesia. Once anesthetized, animals can be taken from the first box, injected and then placed in a separate second box. Because they are no longer moving, animals will stay in place once put in the second box and can be laid out in the order to be imaged or by group type. A second box also helps to prevent confusion between injected and uninjected animals.
4. Intraperitoneal injections will result in slow and more variable perfusion of luciferin into the bloodstream and require a longer time to reach peak light output compared to IV bolus

injections. Tail vein injections are challenging and require skill and practice to do quickly and accurately. The advantage to IV is rapid delivery of the substrate to the blood and less time to reach the peak signal intensity. IV dosing can be especially challenging in animals with compromised health status, which have been repeatedly injected IV, and in strains with low blood pressure (e.g., SCID mice). Both routes of administration will yield results, but will differ in peak time and signal intensity. Thus, one dosing route should be chosen and maintained throughout the entire experiment.

5. Strengths and weaknesses of bioluminescence optical imaging.
   (a) Strengths: low background signal (mice do not normally produce any light); no ionizing radiation required, minimizing costs and regulatory burden; sensitive for measuring small signals, even single cells in some cases; easy to use technology and analysis; relatively low technical skills required; relatively small capital investments; viral labeling vectors for cells and numerous transgenic animal models are commercially available; and ability to image fairly large groups of animals (20+ per hour).
   (b) Weaknesses: only semi-quantitative results, in contrast to other imaging modalities; requirement to remove fur to visualize signal; light scattered and is absorbed based on depth in tissue; little translational value to human clinical settings; works well only in shallow depths of ~1 cm or less; inability to precisely know emission location; and reliance of signal on many factors including perfusion, temperature, and circadian rhythm.
   (c) When to use: When looking for the presence or absence of a signal; to assess changes over time in signal location and amount, for screening animals; large numbers of animals, when working with nude mice. The technique is ideal for implanting transfected cells and looking at growth pattern alterations due to drug, surgical, or other interventions.
   (d) When to avoid: If precise size measurements exact spatial location of signal, quantified light output, or measurement of cell number is required, or when signals originate >1 cm below the skin.

Acknowledgments

This work was made possible by numerous faculty, student, and staff members at the UCLA Crump Institute for Molecular Imaging Preclinical Technology Imaging Center. Waldemar Ladno, DVM and Darin Williams were invaluable with veterinary and logistical help with operations, education, and research work.

References

1. Rice BW, Cable MD, Nelson MB (2001) *In vivo* imaging of light-emitting probes. J Biomed Opt 6(4):432–440
2. Burton JB, Johnson M, Sato M, Koh SBS, Mulholland DJ, Stout DB, Chatziioannou AF, Phelps ME, Wi H, Wu L (2008) Adenovirus-mediated gene expression imaging to directly detect sentinel lymph node metastasis of prostate cancer. Nat Med 14(8):882–888
3. Aswendt M, Adamczak J, Couillard-Despres S, Hoehn M (2013) Boosting bioluminescence neuroimaging: an optimized protocol for brain studies. PLoS One 8(2):e55662
4. Zhao H, Doyle TC, Coquoz O, Kalish F, Rice BW, Contag CH (2005) Emission spectra of bioluminescent reporters and interaction with mammalian tissue determine the sensitivity of detection *in vivo.* J Biomed Opt 10 (4):041210–041219
5. Stout DB, Chatziioannou A, Lawson T, Silverman R, Phelps ME (2005) Small animal imaging center design: the Crump Institute at UCLA. Mol Imaging Biol 7(6):1–10
6. Stout DB (2014) Animal handling and preparation for imaging. Springer
7. Baba S, Cho SY, Ye Z, Cheng L, Engles JM, Wahl RL (2007) How reproducible is bioluminescent imaging of tumor cell growth? Single time point versus the dynamic measurement approach. Mol Imaging Biol 6(5):315–322
8. Stout DB, Berr S, LeBlanc A, Kalen J, Osborne D, Price J, Schiffer W, Kuntner C, Wall J (2013) Guidance for methods descriptions used in preclinical imaging papers. Mol Imaging Biol 12(7):1–15
9. Tremoleda JL, Sosabowski J (2015) Imaging technologies and basic considerations for welfare of laboratory rodents. Lab Anim 44 (3):97–105
10. Gordon CJ (2012) Thermal physiology of laboratory mice: defining thermoneutrality. J Thermal Biol 37:654–685
11. David JM, Knowles S, Lamkin DM, Stout DB (2013) Individually ventilated cage impose cold stress on laboratory mice: a source of systemic experimental variability. J Am Assoc Lab Anim Sci 52(6):738–744
12. Collaco AM, Rahman S, Dougherty EJ, Williams BB, Geusz ME (2005) Circadian regulation of a viral gene promoter in live transgenic mice expressing firefly luciferase. Mol Imaging Biol 7(5):342–350
13. David JM, Chatziioannou AF, Taschereau R, Wang H, Stout DB (2013) The hidden cost of housing practices: using noninvasive imaging to quantify the metabolic demands of chronic cold stress of laboratory mice. Am Assoc Lab Anim Med 63(5):386–391
14. Keyaerts M, Heneweer C, Tchouate-Gainkam LO, Caveliers V, Beattie BJ, Martens GA, Vanhove C, Bossuyt A, Blasberg RG, Lahoutte T (2011) Plasma protein binding of luciferase substrates influences sensitivity and accuracy of bioluminescence imaging. Mol Imaging Biol 13:59–66
15. Virostko J, Chen Z, Fowler M, Poffenberger G, Powers A, Janesen ED (2004) Factors influencing quantification of in vivo bioluminescence imaging: application to assessment of pancreatic islet transplants. Mol Imaging 3(4):333–342
16. Fueger BJ, Czernin J, Hildebrandt I, Tran C, Halpern B, Stout DB, Phelps ME, Weber WA (2006) Impact of animal handling on the results of 18F-FDG PET studies in mice. J Nucl Med 47(6):999–1006
17. Osborne DR, Kunter C, Berr S, Stout DB (2017) Guidance for efficient small animal imaging quality control. Mol Imaging Biol 19:485–498. https://doi.org/10.1007/s11307-016-1012-3

Chapter 4

Dual Reporter Bioluminescence Imaging with NanoLuc and Firefly Luciferase

Anne E. Gibbons, Kathryn E. Luker, and Gary D. Luker

Abstract

Bioluminescence imaging is a powerful, broadly utilized method for noninvasive imaging studies in cell-based assays and small animal models of normal physiology and multiple diseases. In combination with molecular engineering of cells and entire organisms using luciferase enzymes, bioluminescence imaging has enabled novel applications including studies of protein-protein interactions, ligand-receptor interactions, cell trafficking, and drug targeting in mouse models. We describe use of a novel luciferase enzyme derived from *Oplophorus gracilirostris*, NanoLuc, in cell-based assays bioluminescence imaging of tumor-bearing mice. We also combine NanoLuc with another luciferase enzyme, firefly luciferase, to image multiple signal transduction events in one imaging session.

Key words NanoLuc, Bioluminescence imaging, Firefly luciferase, *Oplophorus gracilirostris*

1 Introduction

Over the past decade, bioluminescence imaging has emerged as a powerful, widely utilized method for noninvasive imaging studies in cell-based assays and small animal models of normal physiology and multiple diseases. As compared with other whole-animal imaging modalities, bioluminescence imaging provides unparalleled sensitivity for detecting molecular and cellular events in vivo [1]. Relatively low cost and straightforward operation of commercial bioluminescence imaging instruments make this technology readily accessible to investigators without specific expertise in imaging. In combination with molecular engineering of cells and entire organisms, bioluminescence imaging has enabled novel applications including studies of protein-protein interactions, ligand-receptor interactions, cell trafficking, and drug targeting in mouse models [2–6].

Firefly luciferase (FL) remains the most commonly used reporter enzyme for bioluminescence imaging. Bioluminescence from FL remains relatively constant over an approximately 10–20 min time period, enhancing reproducibility of data from

Purnima Dubey (ed.), *Reporter Gene Imaging: Methods and Protocols*, Methods in Molecular Biology, vol. 1790,
https://doi.org/10.1007/978-1-4939-7860-1_4,

independent cohorts of mice imaged at different times [7]. Luciferin, the substrate for FL, can be delivered readily into mice via intraperitoneal injection, a simple method that facilitates imaging multiple animals at one time. Despite the strengths and widespread use of FL, relying solely on this enzyme for bioluminescence imaging poses a few important limitations. FL provides a single imaging signal, restricting imaging studies to a single molecular event or population of cells. This luciferase requires ATP as a co-factor, making the imaging signal susceptible to changes in intracellular metabolism. Due to reduced concentrations of ATP in the extracellular space, FL functions most efficiently and produces the highest signal when expressed within intact cells. Finally, the relatively large size (about 60 kDa) of FL imposes steric constraints that frequently limit use of this enzyme as a fusion tag for other proteins.

As an alternative or complement to FL and other beetle luciferases, we and other investigators have used different luciferases, such as *Renilla* or *Gaussia* (GL) [6, 8, 9]. In particular, GL has advantages of ATP independence and smaller size (about 20 kDa), making this luciferase a better choice for imaging events in the extracellular space or fusing to another protein as an imaging reporter [6, 10]. Since the substrate for GL (coelenterazine) is distinct from luciferin and FL, GL provides a second, independent imaging signal for molecular and cellular imaging. However, imaging with GL is limited by substantial oxidation of coelenterazine in serum, decreasing overall sensitivity relative to FL and preventing imaging in some organs, such as the liver. In addition, the combination of GL and coelenterazine exhibits flash kinetics, requiring animals to be imaged immediately after injecting substrate. GL also emits blue light with peak admission at 480 nm, which restricts penetration through animal tissues for in vivo imaging.

To provide another bioluminescence imaging signal to complement FL in cell-based assays and living animals, we investigated a recently reported luciferase enzyme, referred to as NanoLuc, developed from the deep sea shrimp *Oplophorus gracilirostris* [11, 12]. NL shares some limitations of GL, including emission of blue light with peak emission of 478 nm and shorter period of bioluminescence emission in animals. NL also is a small (<20 kDa), ATP-independent enzyme with advantages for generating bioluminescent fusion proteins and imaging extracellular events. A key benefit of NL over GL is that the former enzyme utilizes a novel substrate, furimazine, which has markedly lower background signal than coelenterazine. Here, we report our method for expressing NanoLuc in mammalian breast cancer cells for cell-based assays in addition to bioluminescence imaging studies in living mice. We also show our technique for imaging NL and FL sequentially in animal models, focusing on our method for imaging TGF-β signaling through its receptor TGF-βR1 and activation of the TGF-β promoter as an example. More broadly, these same imaging principles can be applied to a wide range of signaling events or cell tracking studies, expanding capabilities for molecular and cellular bioluminescence imaging studies in cell-based assays and mouse models of disease pathogenesis and therapy.

2 Materials

2.1 Molecular Biology

1. Secreted NanoLuc plasmid pNL.1.3 (Promega) (*see* **Note 1**).
2. Firefly luciferase pGL4 plasmid (*see* **Note 2**).
3. Expression vectors with constitutive promoters for expression in mammalian cells.
4. Expression vector and packaging constructs for producing lentiviral vectors.
5. Enzymes, buffers, and equipment for PCR.
6. Restriction digests for DNA and ligations.
7. TGF-β promoter-NL reporter plasmid (Promega) (*see* **Note 3**).
8. FL complementation reporter for kinase activity of TGF-β RI [13].

2.2 Cell Culture

1. HEK 293T cells or other cells that can be transfected easily for the preparation of lentiviruses.
2. Desired cell lines for experiments in cell-based assays and mouse models (*see* **Note 4**).
3. Cell culture supplies: media appropriate for selected cell types, plasticware, and incubators.

2.3 Cell-Based Imaging

1. 96-well plates with black sides, clear bottom, and lid (Corning, Product #3904 or similar).
2. Multichannel pipettes for volumes from 1 to 200 μl.
3. Sterile pipette tips with low adherence coating adherence.
4. Sterile 1× phosphate-buffered saline (PBS) solution.
5. Stock solution furimazine substrate for NL (currently sold as Nano-Glo® Luciferase Assay System, Promega).
6. D-Luciferin powder (Promega or other vendors) (*see* **Note 5**).
7. Recombinant TGF-β.
8. TGF-β inhibitors SB461542 or SD208 (Tocris or other vendors).
9. Bioluminescence imaging system with high sensitivity and software for data quantification and analysis (IVIS, Perkin-Elmer, or similar system).

2.4 Animal Imaging

1. Appropriate mouse strain for experimental system (*see* **Note 6**).
2. Small animal shaver (i.e., Wahl compact cordless trimmer or similar instrument).
3. Depilatory solution (i.e., Nair).
4. 28–30 G insulin syringe for intravenous tail vein injections and intraperitoneal injections in mice.
5. Restraint device for tail vein injection (optional) (Braintree Scientific or other vendors) (*see* **Note 7**).
6. Bioluminescence imaging instrument with isoflurane anesthesia (IVIS or similar instrument).

3 Methods

3.1 Construct Cells Stably Expressing NL and FL Imaging Reporters (See Note 8)

1. For constitutively expressed or inducible NL and FL reporters, stable cells can be generated through methods including transfection or lentiviral transduction with selection for cells stably expressing reporters (*see* **Note 7**). We refer readers to standard texts of cell and molecular biology procedures for techniques used to transfer reporters to lentiviral vectors if desired and isolate stable cell lines.
2. Verify expression of reporter construct(s) in stable cell lines. This can be accomplished by qRT-PCR, Western blotting, and/or bioluminescence imaging assays. We refer readers to standard texts for methods used in qRT-PCR and Western blotting. For functional assays using bioluminescence imaging, see description below for cell-based assays.

3.2 Cell-Based Assays

1. If using separate stock solutions of furimazine and luciferin for cell imaging studies, prepare a stock solution of 15 mg/ml luciferin in PBS and sterile filter. Stocks of luciferin should be stored at −20 °C.
2. Plate cells at 1.5×10^4 cells per well in 96-well, black wall plates 1 day before experiments (*see* **Note 9**).
3. For assays with secreted NL, collect 5 μl of culture medium from stably expressing cells and transfer to a round-bottom, black wall 96-well plate to measure NL bioluminescence. Collect the same volume of culture medium from cells not expressing NL to use as a control (*see* **Note 10**).
4. To measure bioluminescence from secreted NL, add 45 μl PBS with a 1:1000 dilution of furimazine and image plate on an IVIS with open filter, smallest field-of-view (FOV) to capture the entire plate, large binning, and acquisition time of 30 s (*see* **Note 11**).

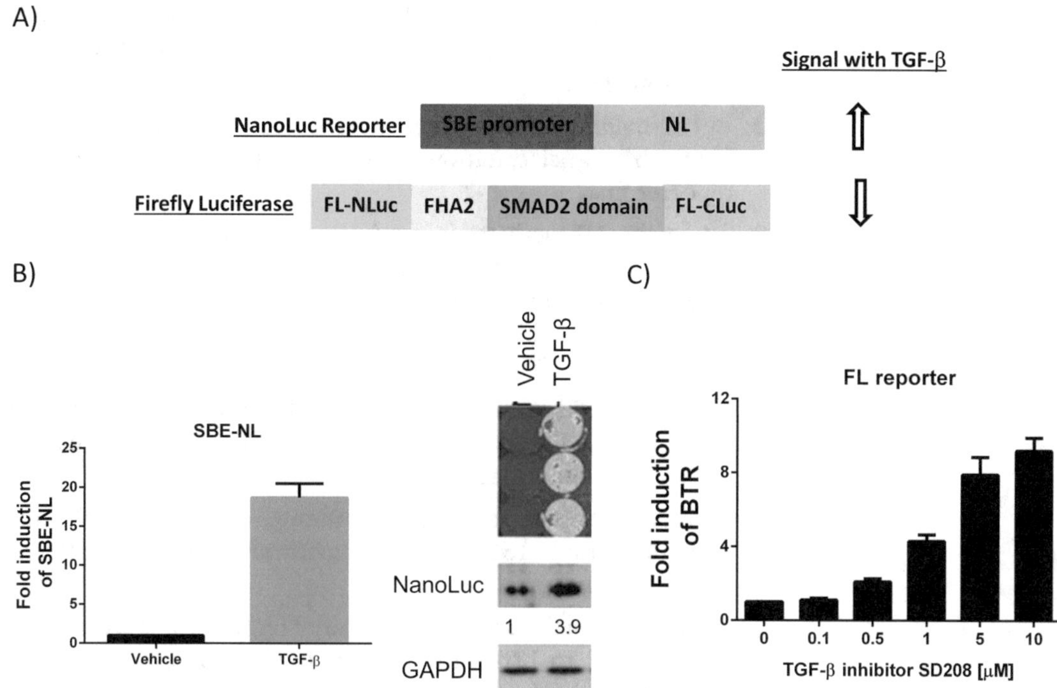

Fig. 1 Dual luciferase imaging of TGF-β signaling in cell-based assays. (**a**) Schematic of NL and FL reporter constructs. Expression of NL is regulated by a promoter with a SMAD binding element (SBE), so typical TGF-β signaling increases bioluminescence. The BTR FL reporter utilizes luciferase complementation to detect phosphorylation of target substrates by the activated receptor, TGF-βR1. TGF-β signaling decreases bioluminescence from this reporter. (**b**) A549 cells expressing both reporters were treated with 10 ng/ml of TGF-β. Graph shows mean values + SEM for fold induction of the NL reporter. Images show bioluminescence imaging and a Western blot of cells treated with vehicle or TGF-β, respectively. (**c**) A549 cells were treated with increasing concentrations of the TGF-β receptor inhibitor SD208. Graph shows mean values + SEM for the activation of the firefly luciferase reporter by inhibition of TGF-βR1 kinase activity

5. Measure NL by adding furimazine at a 1:1000 dilution from the stock solution and mix gently by tapping the side of the well or briefly placing the plate in a shaker (*see* **Notes 12** and **13**).
6. After acquiring NL images, add 10 μl PBS with 150 μg/ml final concentration of D-luciferin (Promega) to each well.
7. Incubate cells for five minutes at 37 °C and then measure bioluminescence from FL with 595 nm long pass filter to exclude light from NL.
8. Measure photon flux values from NL in either culture medium or cells using region-of-interest tools on the IVIS and by subtracting bioluminescence from cells not transfected with the reporter (*see* **Note 14**) (Fig. 1).

3.3 Animal Studies

1. All animal studies should be approved by the institutional committee for care and use of animals prior to performing experiments. For orthotopic breast tumor xenografts, implant

5×10^5 MDA-MB-231 cells co-expressing reporters for NL and FL into fourth inguinal mammary fat pads of NSG mice (*see* **Note 15**).

2. Begin imaging studies when tumors reach 8–10 mm diameter. Since the signal duration is shorter for NL, we image this reporter first.
3. To image NL activity, inject 5 μg (0.25 mg/kg) furimazine (about 40× dilution of Nano-Glo substrate) in 100 μl sterile PBS via tail vein and image mice on an IVIS Spectrum as quickly as possible after injecting the substrate, preferably within 30 s (*see* **Note 16**).
4. Image NL with an open filter, large binning, and acquisition times from 1–60 s depending on size of tumor and relative intensity of bioluminescence.
5. FL imaging can be performed 30 minutes or more after NL. Inject D-luciferin at 150 mg/kg intraperitoneally and wait 10 min before imaging.
6. Image FL signal with open filter, large binning, and acquisition times from 1 to 120 s as determined by tumor size and anticipated strength of signal.
7. To measure serum levels of secreted NL, collect 20 μl blood samples by retro-orbital puncture or other appropriate location for the collection of venous blood. Transfer blood to tubes with 2 μl of 20 mM EDTA to prevent blood clotting (*see* **Note 17**).
8. Centrifuge blood samples at top speed in a microfuge for 10 min and collect 10 μl of plasma for analysis. Analyze amounts of secreted NL as described for measuring this enzyme in culture medium except for adding 40 μl of PBS with NL substrate diluted 1:1000 (*see* **Note 18**). Quantify imaging data using ROI tools on the IVIS software (Fig. 2).

4 Notes

1. NL vectors are available with either secreted or intracellular NL. We use secreted NL because we determined this version of the enzyme produced higher bioluminescence than the intracellular enzyme. Using secreted NL also gives the option to measure levels of the enzyme in blood. NL can be obtained in vectors without or with constitutive mammalian promoters and a variety of different drug selection markers.
2. Vectors for codon optimized firefly luciferase are available in pGL4 vectors with or without different mammalian promoters or drug selection markers.

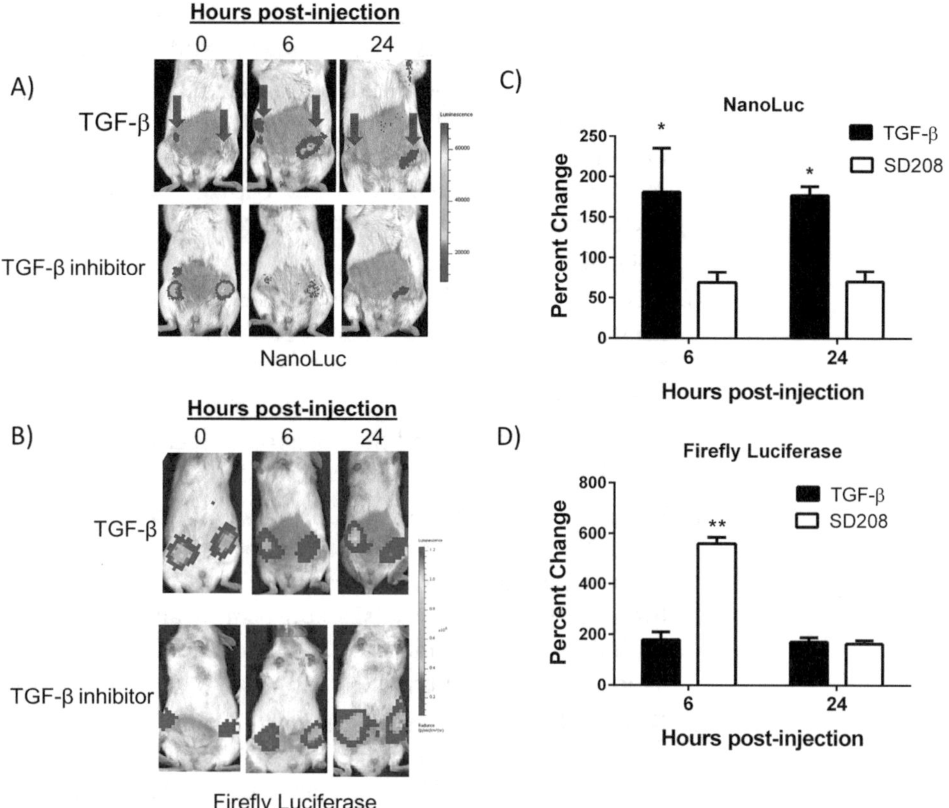

Fig. 2 Imaging TGF-β signaling with NL and FL in living mice. Mice were implanted with A549 lung cancer cells expressing NL and FL reporters for monitoring TGF-β signaling. We treated mice with either 100 ng TGF-β or 50 mg/kg SD208 by intraperitoneal injection ($n = 5$ per group). (**a**) Bioluminescence images of SBE-NL activity show representative mice from each group prior to treatment and at times 6 and 24 h after treatment. Pseudocolor scale shows range of depicted photon flux values. (**b**) Firefly luciferase imaging performed immediately after NL imaging shows induction of signal in mice treated with an inhibitor of TGF-β signaling. (**c**) Graph shows mean values + SEM for NL signal. Data were normalized to values at time 0 prior to treatment. (**d**) Graph shows mean values + SEM for firefly luciferase activity in mice treated with either TGF-β or SD208 normalized to values from the same mice prior to treatment. Note that activation of TGF-β signaling increases the NL reporter, while inhibition of the pathway decreases the NL reporter and increases the FL signal. This strategy allows quantification of two different aspects of the same signaling pathway in vivo. NanoLuc data for 6 and 24 h time points were normalized to corresponding photon flux values prior to treatment. Graph shows mean values + SEM for the percent change in luciferase signal relative to untreated animals in each group at 6 and 24 h time points. $*p < 0.05$; $**p < 0.01$ relative to pretreatment values

3. We describe reagents used for imaging TGF-β signaling at levels of receptor activation and transcription with FL and NL, respectively. FL and NL reporters can be used to image defined components of other signaling pathways of interest to other investigators.
4. We use human MDA-MB-231 breast cancer cells (ATCC) because they form primary and metastatic tumors efficiently in mice, but any desired mammalian cell line will work for cell-

based assays. Using a cancer cell line that forms tumor xenografts in mice is necessary for imaging studies in mice.

5. For cell-based assays, readers may opt to use the Nano-Glo® Dual-Luciferase® Reporter Assay System (Promega), which includes substrates for both NL and FL and a reagent to quench luminescence from FL. Separate stock solutions of each substrate (furimazine and luciferin) are needed for animal imaging studies.
6. Immunocompromised mice are needed for human tumor xenografts. We use NSG mice (The Jackson Laboratory) since these highly immunocompromised mice facilitate growth of human cancer cells.
7. While optional, we find that a restraint device improves success of tail vein injections in mice.
8. We use lentiviral transduction to generate populations of cancer cells expressing imaging reporter genes of interest for cell-based assays and mouse studies. Cell-based assays can be performed by transient transfection using transfection protocols optimized for specific reagents and cell types. Cells stably expressing imaging reporters are needed for animal studies.
9. Black wall plates prevent light emitted by cells in one well from shining into adjacent wells. We typically use cells at 70–90% confluence on the day of imaging, so cell density may need to be optimized for different types of cells. We generally do not starve cells prior to imaging assays because growth factor deprivation can reduce bioluminescence from FL due to depletion of ATP. For experiments regulating the TGF-β signaling pathway, we added varying concentrations of recombinant TGF-β or small molecule inhibitors overnight. If starvation is necessary to activate a signaling pathway with a defined stimulus, we plate cells in normal growth medium and allow cells to adhere to the plate for at least 2 h before changing to starvation medium.
10. Medium from control wells is needed to quantify background luminescence produced by oxidation of furimazine in medium with serum. Background can be reduced by decreasing amounts of serum in medium and/or performing assays with PBS.
11. Acquisition parameters likely will need to be adjusted based on amount of bioluminescence in different samples to avoid saturating the detection camera since saturated pixels cannot be quantified accurately. If an exposure gives saturated pixels, then shorten the acquisition time and/or use smaller binning. For an IVIS, do not use acquisition times less than one second since smaller exposure times are not accurate. Use longer acquisitions and/or larger binning to improve detection of a weak signal.

12. These steps are written for sequential imaging with separate NL and FL substrates added sequentially. Investigators may opt to perform cell-based imaging with the Nano-Glo® Dual-Luciferase® Reporter Assay System, which measures FL signal first and then quenches this signal to allow measurement of NL. The Nano-Glo® Dual-Luciferase® Reporter Assay System should be used according to the manufacturer's specifications.
13. Serum containing medium modestly increases background bioluminescence from the NL substrate. If the imaging signal is dim, NL signal can be measured by removing culture medium and assaying with furimazine diluted in PBS.
14. Investigators optionally may subtract background bioluminescence from control cells not expressing FL. We typically find the background signal for this luciferase to be negligible.
15. Investigators may use separate populations of cells expressing NL or FL reporters, respectively, rather than cells co-expressing both reporters. NL and/or FL reporters may be expressed constitutively for purposes such as tracking cell numbers and localization or regulated reporters to analyze specific signaling pathways. We typically use 6–10 week-old female NSG mice, although other ages, sexes, or mouse strains may be used as appropriate. Other sites for implantation of cancer cells may be selected as appropriate for the experimental question and model system.
16. To reduce time between injection of furimazine and imaging, we anesthetize each mouse prior to intravenous injection and immediately transfer the animal to the stage of the IVIS. The requirement for tail vein injection and immediate imaging means that only one animal is imaged at a time. Maintaining a consistent, short time interval between injection and image acquisition is essential to generate reproducible data since the NL signal decreases over the course of minutes in animals.
17. NL is stable in serum, so samples do not need to be processed immediately after collection but preferably should be analyzed the same day.
18. To control for background signal, it is essential to have plasma from the same strain of mouse without implanted NL cells.

References

1. Luker K, Luker G (2010) Bioluminescence imaging of reporter mice for studies of infection and inflammation. Antivir Res 86 (1):93–100
2. Luker K, Smith M, Luker G et al (2004) Kinetics of regulated protein-protein interactions revealed with firefly luciferase complementation imaging in cells and living animals. Proc Natl Acad Sci U S A 101(33):12288–12293
3. Zhang L, Lee K, Bhojani M et al (2007) Molecular imaging of Akt kinase activity. Nat Med 13(9):1114–1119
4. Wang H, Cao F, De A et al (2009) Trafficking mesenchymal stem cell engraftment and

differentiation in tumor-bearing mice by bioluminescence imaging. Stem Cells 27 (7):1548–1558

5. de Almeida P, van Rappard J, Wu J (2011) In vivo bioluminescence for tracking cell fate and function. Am J Physiol Heart Circ Physiol 301 (3):H663–H671
6. Luker K, Mihalko L, Schmidt B, Lewin S et al (2012) In vivo imaging of ligand receptor binding with Gaussia luciferase complementation. Nat Med 18(1):172–177
7. Zinn K, Chaudhuri T, Szafran A et al (2008) Noninvasive bioluminescence imaging in small animals. ILAR J 49(1):103–115
8. Bhaumik S, Gambhir S (2002) Optical imaging of Renilla luciferase reporter gene expression in living mice. Proc Natl Acad Sci U S A 99 (1):377–382
9. Tannous B, Kim D, Fernandez J et al (2005) Codon-optimized Gaussia luciferase cDNA for mammalian gene expression in culture and in vivo. Mol Ther 11(3):435–443
10. Venisnik K, Olafsen T, Gambhir S (2007) Fusion of Gaussia luciferase to an engineered anti-carcinoembryonic antigen (CEA) antibody for in vivo optical imaging. Mol Imaging Biol 9(5):267–277
11. Hall M, Unch J, Binkowski B et al (2012) Engineered luciferase reporter from a deep sea shrimp utilizing a novel imidazopyrazinone substrate. ACS Chem Biol 7 (11):1848–1857
12. Stacer A, Nyati S, Moudgil P et al (2013) NanoLuc reporter for dual luciferase imaging in living animals. Mol Imaging 12(7):1–13
13. Nyati S, Schinske K, Ray D et al (2011) Molecular imaging of TGFβ-induced Smad2/3 phosphorylation reveals a role for receptor tyrosine kinases in modulating TGFβ signaling. Clin Cancer Res 17(23):7424–7439

Chapter 5

Reporter-Based BRET Sensors for Measuring Biological Functions In Vivo

Maitreyi Rathod, Arijit Mal, and Abhijit De

Abstract

Genetic reporter systems provide a good alternative to monitor cellular functions in vitro and in vivo and are contributing immensely in experimental research. Reporters like fluorescence and bioluminescence genes, which support optical measurements, provide exquisite sensitivity to the assay systems. In recent years several activatable strategies have been developed, which can relay specialized molecular functions from inside the cells. The application of bioluminescence resonance energy transfer (BRET) is one such strategy that has been proved to be extremely valuable as an in vitro or in vivo assay to measure dynamic events such as protein-protein interactions (PPIs).

The BRET assay using RLuc-YFP was introduced in biological research in the late 1990s and demonstrated the interaction of two proteins involved in circadian rhythm. Since then, BRET has become a popular genetic reporter-based assay for PPI studies due to several inherent attributes that facilitate high-throughput assay development such as rapid and fairly sensitive ratio-metric measurement, the assessment of PPI irrespective of protein location in cellular compartment and cost effectiveness. In BRET-based screening, within a defined proximity range of 10–100 Å, the excited energy state of the luminescent molecule excites the acceptor fluorophore in the form of resonance energy transfer, causing it to emit at its characteristic emission wavelength. Based on this principle, several such donor-acceptor pairs, using *Renilla* luciferase or its mutants as donor and either GFP2, YFP, mOrange, TagRFP or TurboFP as acceptor, have been reported for use.

In recent years, the applicability of BRET has been greatly enhanced by the adaptation of the assay to multiple detection devices such as a luminescence plate reader, a bioluminescence microscope and a small animal optical imaging platform. Apart from quantitative measurement studies of PPIs and protein dimerization, molecular spectral imaging has expanded the scope for fast screening of pharmacological compounds that modulate PPIs by unifying in vitro, live cell and in vivo animal/plant measurement, all using one assay. Using examples from the literature, we will describe methods to perform in vitro and in vivo BRET imaging experiments and some of its applications.

Key words Reporter gene, Luciferase, Fluorescent proteins, Optical imaging, Bioluminescence resonance energy transfer, Protein-protein interactions

1 Introduction

Current efforts in the life sciences to dissect protein function have led to tremendous developments in the field of protein interaction analysis. A full understanding of how the proteins function and

Purnima Dubey (ed.), *Reporter Gene Imaging: Methods and Protocols*, Methods in Molecular Biology, vol. 1790, https://doi.org/10.1007/978-1-4939-7860-1_5,

contribute to the signaling network within a cell requires varied approaches to study protein-protein interactions (PPIs). Once the specific and relevant interactions are established, in-depth characterization of the molecular and biophysical parameters such as the kinetic rate constants, formation of oligomer by the interacting partners and their stoichiometric ratio in the complex may be determined, using purified and well-characterized proteins. To identify the protein interaction partners physiological screening techniques are required that can function in living cells.

This chapter will focus on molecular imaging guided in vitro and in vivo technology for PPI. The assay that fulfils the major criteria for determining PPIs both in vitro and in vivo, is bioluminescence resonance energy transfer (BRET), which has been used successfully in various studies. This approach provides simultaneous visual representation and quantification of biological processes involved in cellular signaling and thus can impact a wide variety of biological research, such as drug discovery and molecular medicine (Fig. 1). Signal transduction is a complex chain reaction. The development of multiplexed BRET systems with distinct spectral signatures expands the ability to noninvasively image signal transduction processes.

Imaging strategies can be broadly classified into three main categories:

1. Direct Imaging: detecting a molecular target directly using a labeled probe, e.g., labeled antibody or peptide for a receptor.
2. Surrogate Imaging: visualizing downstream physiological effects of a molecular-genetic process [1], e.g., perfusion imaging for HIF1 (hypoxia inducible factor I).

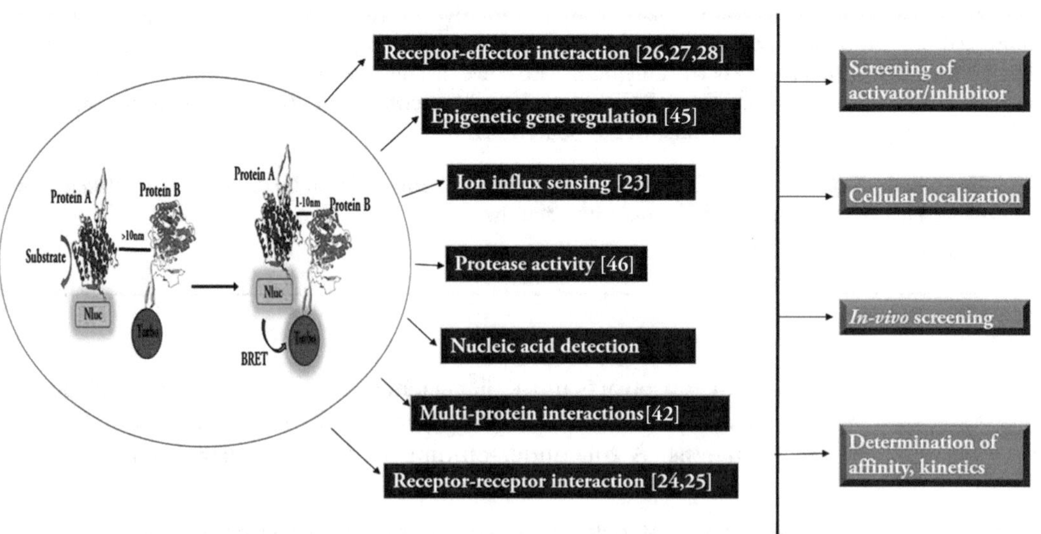

Fig. 1 Schematic diagram showing various applications of BRET for sensing in vivo biological functions

3. Indirect Imaging: the use of reporter gene technology, where accumulation of the reporter protein in cells indirectly indicates the expression level of the target molecule.

This chapter will primarily focus on the third approach where reporter gene-based methods are used to detect gene regulation or signal transduction. The reporter genes include (a) radionuclide reporters such as Herpes Simplex Virus (HSV)-1 Thymidine kinase (TK), Sodium Iodide Symporter (NIS), dopamine 2 receptor, (b) magnetic resonance imaging (MRI) reporters such as the ferritin receptor, (c) fluorescence-based reporters such as Green Fluorescent Protein (GFP) and Yellow Fluorescent Protein (YFP), and (d) bioluminescent reporters such as luciferases [2]. Ideally, the reporter gene should not be endogenously expressed in the host cell and should be amenable to assays that are sensitive, quantitative, rapid, reproducible, and non-toxic. Among these reporter gene options, fluorescent and bioluminescent optical reporters are cost effective, rapid and high throughput, and require little specialized equipment.

Various luminescent proteins have been isolated from natural organisms:

- Firefly luciferase (FLuc) isolated from the North-American firefly *Photinus pyralis*, is an ATP-dependent luciferase that uses D-luciferin as its substrate and requires molecular oxygen and co-factors. Emission maximal wavelength (EmMax) is 611 nm.
- Renilla luciferase (RLuc) isolated from Sea pansy, *Renilla reniformis* is an ATP-independent luciferase that uses coelenterazine as its substrate. EmMax is 480 nm.
- Vargulin luciferase isolated from a marine ostracod *Vargula hilgendorfii* uses vargulin substrate that has an EmMax of 462 nm.
- Gaussia luciferase is a secretory luciferase isolated from *Gaussia princeps*, with EmMax of 480 nm. It is secreted in an active form and requires coelenterazine as a substrate [3].
- Nano luciferase (NanoLuc) is a 19 kDa protein engineered from a naturally occurring 106 kDa luciferase, produced by a deep sea shrimp *Oplophorus gracilirostris*, and shows very bright luminescence with furimazine substrate emitting at (EmMax) 454 nm [4].
- Bacterial luciferase: Luciferase has also been isolated from several bacteria such as *Vibrio harveyi*, *Photorhabdus luminescens*, *Allivibrio fischeri*. Bacterial luciferin is reduced by riboflavin phosphate [5].
- Proteins such as aequorin, having an EmMax at 469 nm, which is isolated from luminous jellyfish *Aequorea victoria*, represent a natural Ca++ ion influx sensor [6].

Mutations of luminescent proteins have been developed that have a spectral shift toward the red wavelength and provide higher stability and greater photon output (e.g., *Photinus pyralis* luciferase Ppy RE8, EmMax 618 nm, Click beetle luciferase CBG99, EmMax 537 nm [7], Renilla luciferase mutants RLuc8, RLuc8.6, that have an EmMax of 540 nm [8]), and thus increase the versatility of this imaging technique.

Bioluminescent reporters are preferred over fluorescent reporters due to background-free signal that provides excellent imaging sensitivity and several humanized versions of these reporters are available for mammalian expression. In contrast, endogenous fluorescent signals may interfere with fluorescent imaging and compromise the resolution [1].

Several sensors have been developed for monitoring dynamic cellular functions such as TGF-B-SMAD signaling sensors [9], Tango assay for measuring GPCR signaling [10], estrogen receptor signaling [11], apoptosis sensors [12, 13], and secondary messenger induced activation sensors [14].

1.1 Noninvasive Imaging of Gene Regulation

Understanding gene dynamic expression provides insight relevant to disease onset and progression. Gene expression is primarily controlled by the promoter and hence capturing promoter modulation in response to various stimuli or disease conditions elucidates gene regulation. Noninvasive, real-time monitoring of promoter modulations can be achieved by cloning a reporter downstream of the promoter of interest. Theoretically, the level of reporter protein expressed mirrors the expression level of that particular gene. Reporter gene constructs can be designed where reporters are under the control of enhancer elements/promoter that possesses transcription factor binding sites. Promoters are activated by the endogenous transcription factor(s) and subsequently associate with specific endogenous genes. This is called a *cis*-promoter/enhancer reporter system. An example of this system is the p53RE-hNIS reporter where the NIS gene was expressed under the control of a p53 response element, and Adriamycin-driven increase in p53 expression resulted in increased ^{125}I uptake in a dose-dependent manner [15].

Other examples of studies that used optical reporters for gene expression analysis include use of the HIF-1α-FLuc reporter to compare HIF-1α expression in normal versus glioma condition [16], effect of MYC inactivation in liver cancer [17], TGF β signaling dynamics by TGFβ expression in vivo [18].

One study used three different luciferases emitting red, orange, and green wavelengths using the same substrate to image multiple genes in the same reaction. The effect of RORa4 (orphan nuclear transcription factor) on expression of the clock gene Bmal1 was monitored in the study [19]. Various approaches have been developed to simultaneously express and monitor multiple reporter genes.

1.2 Noninvasive Imaging of Protein-Protein Interaction

Protein-protein interactions are essential for cellular processes and live cell monitoring provides insight that is useful for the development of new therapies [20]. These interactions are regularly studied by standard biochemical methods [21] that require cell lysis, using detergents and other chaotropic agents that may disrupt native protein interactions. Importantly, these methods do not provide spatio-temporal information and do not permit real-time monitoring of protein-protein interactions in vivo [22].

In the past two decades, new noninvasive techniques have been developed to study resonant energy transfer. One such technique was developed based on a biological phenomenon observed in *Aequorea victoria* jellyfish. In this organism successive activation of the photoprotein aqueorin and green fluorescent protein (GFP) generates green light. Upon sensing calcium ions aqueorin is activated to emit blue light which then excites GFP (which colocalizes) to emit a green light rather than the blue light of aqueorin. This anomalous occurrence was explained as resonance energy transfer (RET) between the aqueorin chromophore and GFP [23]. The event, subsequently named BRET, has evolved as one of the prominent techniques in the field for protein-protein interaction studies. In this method, one of the interacting proteins is tagged to a luminescent photon donor and the other is tagged to an acceptor that fluoresces at a longer wavelength.

Another RET-based method for the detection of protein-protein interaction is Fluorescence Resonance Energy Transfer (FRET) where both donor and acceptor are fluorescent proteins. However, a major limitation of FRET is auto-fluorescence and photo-bleaching created by the excitation of the donor photons. Further, tissue absorbance and tissue attenuation limits the FRET assay for tissue imaging [22]. In contrast, BRET has been extensively used to demonstrate oligomerization of GPCRs [24, 25] to monitor ligand binding kinetics [26], and to elucidate signaling pathways [27, 28]. In recent advances, red-shifted fluorescent proteins are used to minimize tissue attenuation.

Protein-protein interaction may also be studied by the split luciferase assay [29] and bimolecular fluorescent protein complementation (BiFC). Both the methods follow the same basic principle.

The reporter protein fragmented is divided into N-terminal and C-terminal constructs that are each tagged to a reporter gene. As the two proteins interact, the reporter proteins are complemented and recapitulate the reporter function. In small animal imaging, BRET is more sensitive than split luciferase as the split luciferase after complementation exhibits only 20–50% activity of the intact luciferase [30]. Additionally, nonspecific association of the split fragment may result in false positive signals. Thus for imaging protein-protein interaction in small animal, BRET demonstrates clear advantages over all existing techniques.

BRET signals are typically quantified using a luminescence plate reader equipped with suitable bandpass filter sets that allow measurement of donor and acceptor emission peak. The plate reader typically quantifies the two filtered light signals sequentially. Some equipment also provides simultaneous detection capability of donor and acceptor signal using dual head photomultiplier tubes (PMT). With progress in bioluminescent-based imaging technology, one can simultaneously visualize and quantify signals emitted from live cells in a culture dish or implanted in an animal.

1.3 Imaging Protein-Protein Interaction in Single Cells Using Bioluminescence Microscope

Imaging protein interactions has traditionally used advanced fluorescent microscopic techniques. However, the dependence of fluorescent proteins on external illumination, background signal due to autofluorescence, photo-bleaching or photo-sensitizing effects demands alternative approaches that allow imaging over extended time periods under unperturbed conditions.

Bioluminescence imaging overcomes many of these limitations and permits highly sensitive and background-free detection of protein-protein interactions. However, bioluminescent signals from single cells may be weak and hence may require highly sensitive detection devices. The development of short focal length lens and ultra-low light capturing cameras, such as cooled charged couple device (CCD) cameras and electron multiplying CCD (EMCCD) cameras, overcomes some of these limitations [31]. Such technology has also been used to monitor the rhythms of hundreds of individual neurons in the brain slices of transgenic mice expressing luciferase [32].

Protein-protein interactions in single cells can also be resolved using BLI microscopes. Examples include imaging the rapamycin-induced FRB-FKBP12 interaction in single live mammalian or insect cells using the BRET3 (mOrange-RLuc8) platform [33] and monitoring real-time dynamics of β-arrestin recruitment to V2R in single cells at their respective subcellular locations [34]. Single cell imaging may be enhanced by the use of brighter versions of luciferase, such as the use of a variant of click beetle luciferase-Emerald luciferase (Eluc) to monitor Drosophila embryogenesis in real time using a BLI microscope [35].

In this chapter, we discuss detailed methods to perform a BRET imaging assay and applications of this methodology (Fig. 2).

2 Materials

2.1 Cloning

1. An appropriate mammalian expression plasmid vector containing luciferase encoding gene, e.g., firefly luciferase (FLuc), *Renilla* luciferase (RLuc), and a fluorescent protein encoding gene.

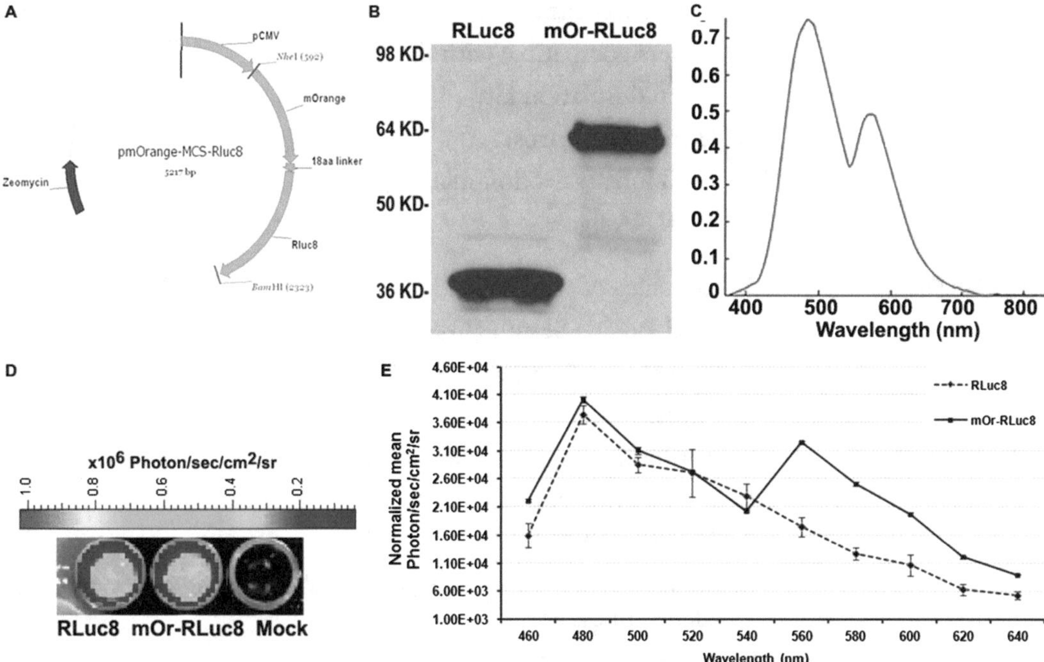

Fig. 2 Basic steps involved in BRET methodology exemplified by mOrange-RLuc8 BRET construct [33]. (**a**) As a first step, an expression plasmid vector of mOrange-RLuc8 fusion BRET constructs was made. (**b**) Next, after DNA transfection, the protein product was verified by Western blotting probed with monoclonal anti-RLuc8 antibody. The size difference between the fusion protein and the donor alone (RLuc8) is used to determine fusion protein expression. (**c**) By producing purified protein using suitable system, the luminescence emission spectra may be verified by the addition of a suitable substrate. In this case a dual pick is shown by adding coelenterazine substrate, one for the donor (RLuc8) and the other for acceptor (mOrange). (**d**) Live cell imaging can be performed by adding substrate to the well plate containing cells expressing only donor or donor-acceptor fusion as well as the mock transfected cells. (**e**) A spectral imaging scan is performed using 20 nm bandpass filter sets and an IVIS imaging system. The BRET ratio is computed by quantitative analysis of the emission maximum for donor and acceptor. Data partially reproduced with permission from reference [33]

- A dual luciferase system is generally used where RLuc is used as a normalization control, which is driven by a constitutive promoter, e.g., Cytomegalovirus (CMV). FLuc is used as a reporter for gene of interest due to its higher emission wavelength (*see* **Note 1**).
- A fluorescent reporter can be included along with luciferase, to monitor transfection efficiency.

2. DH5α strain of *E. coli*.
3. Lysogeny broth (LB) broth.
4. LB agar.
5. Polymerase chain reaction (PCR) amplified promoter fragment.
6. Gel extraction kit.

7. Restriction enzymes.
8. Buffers compatible with the enzymes.
9. Plasmid isolation kit.
10. Ultra-pure agarose.
11. Antibiotic (selection marker).
12. T4 DNA ligase.

2.2 Cell Culture

1. Cell lines of choice.
2. Fetal Bovine Serum (FBS).
3. Suitable medium, e.g., RPMI-1640, DMEM, MEM, IMDM.
4. Trypsin–EDTA.
5. Antibiotic, e.g., penicillin-streptomycin.
6. Transfection reagent.
7. Phosphate-buffered saline (PBS).
8. Tissue culture disposables, e.g., flasks, culture dishes, pipettes, falcon tubes, etc.
9. Passive lysis buffer (PLB).

2.3 Bioluminescence Imaging

1. IVIS spectrum series (or equivalent) small animal imaging system with Living Image analysis software.
2. Compatible substrate to the luciferase.
3. Black well plates with clear bottom.
4. Mice, e.g., NUDE, SCID mice.
5. Anesthesia, e.g., Isoflurane.
6. 26, 30 G needle with 1 cc syringe.
7. Saline (PBS PH 7.4).
8. 70% Alcohol.
9. Substrates.
   - D-Luciferin: Stock concentration—15 mg/ml or 30 mg/ml in PBS. Storage temperature −80 °C. Dilute 1000 times in PBS, add 50 μl/well of 96-well plate (from 30 mg/ml stock).

     Working concentration in vivo—150 mg/kg body weight.
   - Coelenterazine: Stock concentration—1 mg/ml in methanol. Storage temperature is at −80 °C. Dilute 100 times in PBS, add 50 μl in each well of a 96-well plate.

     Working concentration in vivo—1 mg/kg body weight.
   - EnduRen™: Stock concentration—60 mM in DMSO. Storage temperature: −20 °C.

     Working concentration—60 μM (follow the manufacturer's guideline).

- For dissolving EnduRen™, vortex repeatedly for at least 10 min. The solution should be at a temperature of 37 °C, to ensure that it is completely dissolved.

3 Methods

3.1 Visualization of Promoter Modulation

3.1.1 Construction of Reporter Plasmid

1. PCR amplify the promoter of interest by using primers containing the required restriction enzymes (RE) sites at the flanking regions.
2. Run on agarose gel to verify amplification.
3. Purify the amplification product using gel extraction kit.
4. Remove the existing upstream promoter sequence of luciferase (in the vector) by compatible RE digestion.
   - For normalization, use CMV-driven RLuc or another reporter (*see* **Note 1**).
5. Subclone the purified promoter of interest into the vector by ligation of the DNA fragment and the digested vector, using compatible restriction endonuclease (digested vector can be used as control).
6. Amplify plasmid by transformation using DH5α strain of *E. coli* competent cells and plate on LB agar plates, containing selection marker, e.g., ampicillin or kanamycin.
7. Screen colonies either by colony PCR method [36], or grow colonies and isolate the plasmids using a mini-prep plasmid isolation kit, followed by restriction analysis of DNA.
8. Further verify plasmids by PCR or sequencing.

3.1.2 Confirmation of Luciferase Enzyme Function

Check that the luciferase is expressed in the construct. This can be accomplished by Western blot analysis of transfected cells to detect the translated reporter protein. Alternately, as described here, conduct a luciferase reporter assay to detect reporter activity in transiently transfected cells.

1. Seed 5×10^4 cells in a 24-well plate with suitable medium and incubate for 24 h in a humidified incubator, with appropriate level of CO_2 for the cell culture medium used. Cells should reach 70–80% confluence prior to transfection.
2. Aspirate the medium carefully without disturbing the monolayer of cells, and replace with cell culture media containing low serum (1–2% FBS).
   - High serum (5–10%) may interfere with transfection efficiency.
3. Transfect the plasmid using a suitable transfection reagent, following the manufacturer's instructions.

Transfection efficiency is dependent on a number of variables including the cell type, transfection procedure used and confluence of the cells at the time of transfection (maintain the confluency of the cells to 60–70%).

4. Forty-eight hours post transfection, harvest cells by trypsinization and pellet them by centrifugation at 500 × *g* at 4 °C for 5 min.
5. Add 1× PLB and incubate at room temperature for 20 min. Centrifuge for 10 min at room temperature at 500 × *g*.
   - The appropriate volume of buffer depends on the pellet size. A general guideline is to use 3× the volume of buffer to the volume of the pellet. Collect supernatant, which contains the lysate and discard the pellet which contains the cell debris. Quantify protein concentration by Bradford assay using standard procedures.
6. Add lysate (10 μl) and substrate, e.g., LARII for firefly luciferase (50 μl) to a white 96-well plate and immediately read the luciferase activity for 10 s in a luminometer (*see* **Note 2**). The signal of light output (RLU) will confirm that the transfection has worked well.
   - For optimum enzyme activity the substrate should be equilibrated to room temperature prior to use. Activity is reduced by 5–10% if the substrate is cold at the time of use.

3.1.3 Stable Cell Line Preparation

1. Seed a 35 mm tissue culture dish with sufficient cells to reach 70% confluence following incubation for 24 h. This cell number is determined empirically according to the growth rate of the cells, of interest.
2. Transfect the plasmid using a suitable transfection reagent, following the manufacturer's instructions and incubate for 48 h.
3. Trypsinize the cells and seed them in a 10 cm^2 tissue culture plate at 30–50% confluence. If adherent cells are transfected, wait for 3–4 h or overnight to allow cells to attach and spread out. Add complete growth medium containing the drug for selection.
   - Prior to transfection, the appropriate dose of selection should be determined by a kill curve using untransfected cells. The minimum dose that results in 100% death of the untransfected cells within 5–10 days of selection should be used for the selection of transfected cells.
4. Change cell culture medium every 3–4 days. Drug resistant colonies will appear in the culture dish in approximately 2 weeks.

5. To check for expression of a co-linked fluorescent marker, observe cells using a fluorescent microscope. Screen luciferase-expressing cells by adding the luciferase substrate to the dish and imaging in an IVIS system.
6. Spot trypsinize the colonies that express the marker and transfer them to a 96-well plate. Incubate in complete growth medium with drug selection until the well is confluent.
7. Expand the clones by transferring to larger culture dishes. Verify expression as described in Subheading 3.1. The clones that show positive signal for at least three passages are considered stable cells, for the protein of interest (*see* **Note 3**).

3.1.4 Imaging Promoter Modulation in Live Cells

1. Seed the stably transfected cells ($1–3 \times 10^4$ cells per well in triplicate, in a black well plate with clear bottom). Incubate in a humidified CO_2 incubator for 24 h.
   - To accurately quantify promoter modulation it is important that the number of cells plated in each well is consistent
2. Treat the cells with desired stimulus of interest, e.g., hormones, drug inhibitors, transcription factor inducers, signaling pathway ligands, etc., for desired time point.
3. Add suitable luciferase substrate, with appropriate dilution to the wells. Use a multi-channel pipette to quickly add substrate simultaneously to all wells.
4. Immediately capture the light emitted, using IVIS live cell imaging system and quantify light output.
5. Transfected cells treated with buffer alone should be used as negative control, to determine promoter modulation.
6. The relative light signal (RLU) produced from the luciferase driven by the gene specific promoter, is an indirect measure of promoter activity or gene expression. Light output readings are normalized with respective protein concentration and *Renilla* luciferase readings by the following formula:

$$\frac{\text{RLU}/\mu g \text{ protein/s of FLuc}}{\text{RLU}/\mu g \text{ protein/s of RLuc}}$$

3.1.5 Promoter Modulation in Mouse Model

1. To study in vivo promoter modulation, implant cells stably expressing the reporter system into animals. The number of cells implanted for optical imaging can be relatively low (~$1–5 \times 10^6$ cells, determined empirically for each cell line). A maximum of two subcutaneous sites on one animal may be used for implantation. Follow local IACUC guidelines. Transiently transfected cells may be used for short term analysis (maximum 3–7 days). Determine the uniformity of cell implantation by BLI of the control luciferase reporter.

2. Provide stimulus of interest (at predetermined dose and schedule) in one group of mice. Administer buffer alone to a second group of mice that will serve as negative control.
3. Conduct IVIS imaging to detect the luciferase signal. A detailed protocol for image acquisition and analysis is provided in Chapter 3 of this volume.

3.2 Monitoring Protein-Protein Interaction in Small Animal

3.2.1 Construction of Donor and Acceptor Vector

1. Choose an appropriate donor luciferase and its acceptor with suitable substrate (Guidelines for choosing a donor-acceptor pair are listed in Box 1).

Box 1: Selection of a Donor–Acceptor Pair:
While choosing a donor and acceptor one needs to consider R_0 between the given pairs as the maximum distance at which resonance energy transfer (RET) can take place is determined by the R_0. The maximum distance for detecting RET is given by the equation:

$$r = 1.6 \times R_0. \quad (1)$$

while R_0 is calculated by:

$$R_0 = \left(\kappa^2 \times J(\lambda) \times n^{(-4)} \times Q\right)^{1/(6)} \times 9.7 \times 10)^2,$$

where Q = quantum yield of the donor, n = refractive index of the intervening medium, κ^2 = dipole orientation, $J(\lambda)$ = overlap integral of donor acceptor [37].

Different donor-acceptor pairs for BRET, FRET, BiFC are designed keeping the above factors under consideration. From the Eq. 1 it is obvious that the higher the value of R_0 RET will be detected over a longer distance. Even under favorable conditions the R_0 will never cross 7 nm which makes the upper distance limit to ~11 nm.

The donor and acceptor chosen for protein-protein interaction should be spectrally different enough for distinct detection of donor signal. Reporters with red-shifted emission wavelengths result in higher signal intensity [38].

2. To prepare the vector for the expression of the proteins of interest along with the donor or the acceptor, either subclone the cDNA or amplify the cDNA by using PCR (*see* **Notes 4** and **5**). If using PCR, a high fidelity polymerase is preferred to avoid errors in amplification.
3. While making the vectors, multiple combinations of fusion proteins should be tested to optimize appropriate dipole-dipole orientation. Test amino- and carboxy-terminal fusions

of donor and acceptor to determine the optimal combination. Sometimes the absence of a BRET signal may indicate inappropriate dipole orientation of the donor and acceptor, rather than lack of protein-protein interaction [39].

3.2.2 Evaluation of Gene Expression

It is important to assess the reporter gene expression and function as well as the expression and function of the protein of interest after the generation of the fusion construct in cultured cells prior to imaging in animals.

1. Donor function—To check for luminescence output carry out a luciferase enzyme reporter assay. Cells may be transiently transfected with the donor vector for this test.
2. Acceptor function—The fluorescence should be detectable in cell culture under microscopy (inverted fluorescence microscopy or confocal microscopy) using appropriate filter sets.
   - Confirm that the cells are healthy and have expected morphology. The proportion of fluorescent cells indicates transfection efficiency (*see* **Note 6**).
3. Protein function—Check functionality of the fusion protein using an appropriate assay (the fusion tag sometime affects the protein folding (*see* **Note 7**)).
   - Cellular localization may be checked by immunofluorescence/confocal microscopy.

3.2.3 Verification of the BRET Signal

It is important to monitor whether the non-radiative transfer of energy is taking place from the donor luciferase to the complementary fluorophore. Therefore, to verify this energy transfer and proper detection of BRET signal between the donor-acceptor pair, perform the following:

1. Construct a vector in which only the donor and acceptor are fused.
2. Transfect the cells.
3. After 24 h of transfection trypsinize the cells.
4. Suspend the cells in HEPES buffered medium without phenol red and split the cells (in triplicate) at a density of 10,000–30,000 cells/100 μl/well in a 96-well black well plate.
5. The cells to be maintained at 37 °C, 5% CO_2 in a humidified incubator for further 24 h before BRET assay, to allow cell attachment.
   - Initial titration is required to establish cell dilution.
6. Use phenol red-free medium or replace medium with suitable assay buffer such as Dulbecco's phosphate-buffered saline (DPBS) for the BRET assay.

7. Remove medium from the cells and add substrate prepared in the respective assay buffer. The appropriate incubation condition should be maintained for each substrate.
8. Acquire the image using IVIS system as described in Chapter 3 of this volume. The image is acquired in luminescence mode. The emission filters should be set as per EmMax of specific donor and acceptor. Using IVIS, first photograph the plate, then capture the luminescence signal for a set period of time (acquisition time). The acquired image appears as a superimposed image of the plate with pseudo-color representing the luminescence. Alternately, use a luminescence plate reader equipped with donor and acceptor-specific bandpass filters to quantify BRET.
9. For data analysis, draw a region of interest (ROI) on the desired area. The measured luminescence may be in the form of total flux (photon/sec/cm^2) from a specific ROI, or as average radiance, i.e., photons/s/cm^2/steradian (steradian is a measure of solid angle).
10. Analyze the BRET ratio as mentioned in Subheading 3.2.7.

A positive BRET signal indicates that the proteins are in close proximity. Thus, it is necessary to determine the true signal devoid of nonspecific interactions that may result from over-expression of proteins or interaction with other endogenous competitors. This can be monitored by a saturation assay or competition assay (Box 2).

Box 2: Evidence for Specificity:
Specificity of constitutive protein interactions is measured in the following ways:

Saturation assay: Cells co-expressing a constant amount of donor-labeled protein with increasing amount of acceptor-labeled protein are assayed. If the proteins are interacting then increasing the acceptor-labeled protein will result in an increased signal, that will reach a saturation ($BRET^{max}$) level once all the donor molecules are occupied (Hyperbola curve). Beyond $BRET^{max}$ any further increase in acceptor concentration will not enhance the BRET output signal. If the proteins are not interacting and there is random collision between the proteins, then the signal will increase in a quasi-linear fashion with increasing amounts of acceptor labeled protein [40].

Competition assay: In this assay donor-labeled protein and acceptor labeled protein are co-expressed along with unlabeled protein, which competes for interaction at a single concentration (generally excess) or in a dose-dependent manner. If the proteins are interacting, then the signal will decrease with increasing concentrations of unlabeled competing protein. As negative control an unlabeled non-competing protein should be used, where the BRET signal will not be affected [41]. Expression of the competitor may down-regulate the tagged protein, especially in the case of membrane proteins. Thus in order to overcome this issue, a type-3 BRET was developed, in which the BRET signal along with the relative protein expression is considered [42].

3.2.4 BRET Signal in Live Cells

Before visualizing protein-protein interaction in small animals using BRET, it is important to check for a BRET signal in cell culture.

1. Generation of stable cells expressing donor and acceptor labeled proteins and cells expressing donor-labeled protein only. Proper controls should be used (*see* **Note 8**).
2. Same as Subheading 3.2.3, **steps 4–10** (Fig. 3).

3.2.5 To Monitor Protein–Protein Interaction in Small Animal Using BRET

1. Implant the reporter-expressing cells subcutaneously in an appropriate mouse. To study in vivo protein-protein interaction, it is recommended to use stably transduced cells that express the reporter system. Transiently transfected cells may be used for short term analysis (maximum 3–7 days). The number of cells implanted for optical imaging can be relatively low (~1–5 × 10^6 cells). A maximum of two subcutaneous sites on one animal may be used. Follow local Institutional Animal Care and Use Committee (IACUC) guidelines.

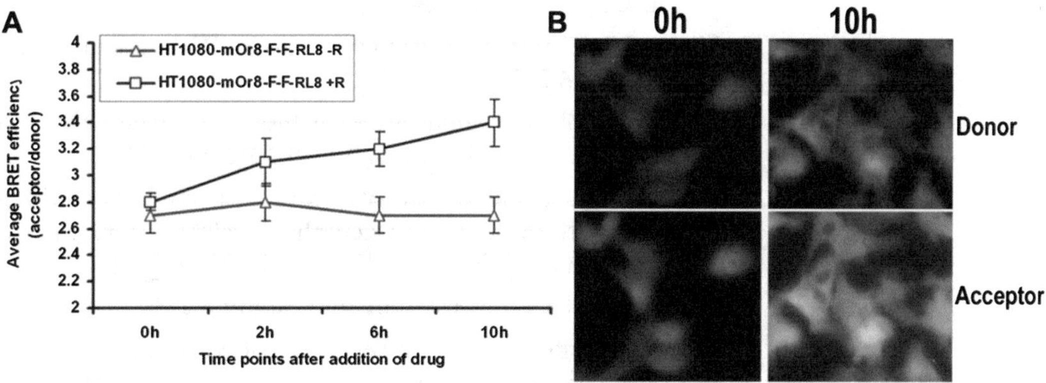

Fig. 3 BRET imaging from live cells expressing mOrange-RLuc8 fusion protein using BLI microscopy [33]. (**a**) Mean BRET ratio of HT1080 stable cells expressing mOrange-FRB-FKBP12-RLuc8 (mOr-F-F-RLuc8) fusion at different time points after exposure to rapamycin. (**b**) Luminescence images captured using BLI microscope of live HT1080 cells overexpressing mOrange-FRB-FKBP12-RLuc8 fusion at 0 and 10 h of incubation with rapamycin. As the two proteins form a heterodimer in the presence of rapamycin, signal on the acceptor channel increases, thus increasing the BRET ratio as in **a**. Data partially reproduced with permission from ref. [33]

2. Injection of substrate: Substrate can be delivered by two ways—intraperitoneal (IP) or intravenous (IV). It is up to the investigator to decide which method is suitable for the injection of substrate, keeping in mind the objective of the experiment. IP injection of substrate leads to over-estimation of tumor size located in IP space [43]. Uptake of IV injection of substrate is slower in peritoneal space than IP. There is lower uptake of D-luciferin in liver, lung, myocardium, and muscle when administered through IP [44].
3. Calculate the BRET ratio as described in Subheading 3.2.7.

3.2.6 BRET Using BLI Microscopy

1. Construct a donor, acceptor plasmid construct by cloning the donor and acceptor in mammalian expression vectors at appropriate orientations (refer to Subheading 3.2.1).
   - For live cell BLI microscopy, usually BRET pairs chosen should be able to generate high light output, e.g., RLuc8-mOrange, NanoLuc-TurboFP, etc.
   - For studying subcellular localization of these interacting proteins, these can be tagged to localization signal peptides, e.g., nuclear localization signal (NLS).
2. Transiently transfect these plasmids into cells and evaluate functional expression of these proteins by luciferase assay using appropriate substrate. For acceptor plasmid, view cells under a fluorescent microscope in suitable filter (refer Subheading 3.1.2 for luciferase assay).
3. Ensure that the fusion proteins generated do not have an altered function as compared to its wild type counterpart, by performing functional assays.
4. Verify BRET signal by imaging cells in IVIS system (refer Subheading 3.2.3 for details).
   - Donor only and donor acceptor fusion constructs are used as control, and only cells as background correction.
   - Generally, it is preferred to perform a spectral scan (with a band width of 20 nm wavelength) initially to capture emission maxima for both the donor and the acceptor.
5. Analyze results as described in Subheading 3.2.7.
6. After the verification of the BRET signal, generate stable cells expressing these donor acceptor constructs. One stable cell generated will have donor only as control and the other set of cells should be stable for both donor and acceptor (refer Subheading 3.1.3 for details of stable cell generation).
7. Culture these stable cells on glass bottom 35 mm tissue culture dishes used for live cell imaging, in complete growth medium for 24 h in a humidified CO_2 incubator.

8. After 24 h, add suitable substrate at predetermined concentration to the cells.
9. Image the cells on a BLI microscope equipped with 5% CO_2 and temperature control of 25–37 °C by sequential acquisitions at set time intervals.
   - The light output is first captured by short focal lens, and then transmitted to the EM-CCD camera.
   - The gain and binning of the camera must be optimized according to the system used and brightness of the luciferase used, e.g., Olympus LV2000 microscope is usually set at binning 1 and gain of 1600, where exposure time for bright luciferases like NanoLuc is as low as 10 s.
   - Emission filters are usually set at 480 and 550 nm.
   - Acquisition software used is Metamorph [34] or the equivalent that is provided on the microscope.
10. Calculate the mean intensity of all pixels from the cell of choice using ImageJ to count pixels. The background values from cell free regions are subtracted from raw intensity values of donor and acceptor emissions.
11. Calculate the pixel by pixel ratios of acceptor to donor emissions.
12. Subtract these values by basal donor/acceptor ratio, i.e., reading with only donor and not acceptor, to minimize the contamination of bleed through signal.
13. Kaleidagraph [34] software is used to calculate median distribution of donor/acceptor ratios of each cell.

3.2.7 Calculation of the BRET Ratio

BRET ratio is defined as the ratio of acceptor and donor bioluminescence from which the ratio of acceptor and donor bioluminescence of donor only cells is subtracted. This is used to correct the bleed through of the donor absorbed in the acceptor filter, which may be a consequence of spectral overlap of donor and acceptor [30].

$$\text{BRET ratio} = \frac{\text{BL emission (Acceptor}\,\lambda) - \text{Cf} \times \text{BL emission (Donor}\,\lambda)}{\text{BL emission (Donor}\,\lambda)},$$

$$\text{where Cf} = \frac{\text{BL emission (Acceptor}\,\lambda)\,\text{donor only}}{\text{BL emission (Donor}\,\lambda)\,\text{donor only}},$$

where BL emission denotes the average radiance measured at donor (Donor λ) and acceptor (Acceptor λ) channel. Cf represents the BRET signal of only donor transfected cells. As the BRET signal quantification is a ratio-metric, any variability in BRET signal due to differences in assay volume, cell number, or time point will become void. But it has been observed that the BRET ratio of cultured cells differs from that in mice [30, 45]. This dissimilarity is due to attenuation, scattering of signal in tissue which is mainly associated with hemoglobin absorption. To confirm that the BRET ratio is the same in cells and mice, the BRET signal is quantified in mice (tissue) by calculating the Double Ratio (DR) which partially corrects for signal attenuation. The DR remains constant independent of tissue depth as the attenuation factors are nullified (assuming the attenuation factor is the same in a particular type of tissue/organ/region and the same in all mice within the experimental group). The DR from different replicates is similar, but not identical due to the assumption made.

$$\mathrm{DR} = \frac{\mathrm{BL\ emission\ (Acceptor\ }\lambda)\ \mathrm{BRET} \times \mu t\ (\mathrm{Acceptor}\lambda)}{\mathrm{BL\ emission\ (Donor\ }\lambda)\ \mathrm{BRET} \times \mu t\ (\mathrm{Donor}\lambda)} \Bigg/ \frac{\mathrm{BL\ emission\ (Acceptor\ }\lambda)\ \mathrm{donoronly} \times \mu t\ (\mathrm{Acceptor}\lambda)}{\mathrm{BL\ emission\ (Donor\ }\lambda)\ \mathrm{donoronly} \times \mu t\ (\mathrm{Donor}\lambda)},$$

where μt is the attenuation coefficient [30].

If the interaction is ligand induced then there is no need for donor only control. The background control can be the BRET signal where the cells expressing acceptor and donor are treated with only the vehicle.

4 Applications of BRET

In this section we discuss strategies to apply BRET technology to investigate different biological functions in cells.

4.1 Monitoring of Cellular Signaling

Cells receive many signals from the environment that are integrated to carry out cellular functions. Upon receiving its specific ligand, the receptor activates its immediate downstream effector molecule. This effector molecule is responsible for carrying out the downstream signaling. BRET technology is extensively used to study this interaction between receptor and effector molecule. This technology is exhaustively used to investigate functional signaling through GPCRs [26] and receptor tyrosine kinases [27].

Here, we discuss a generalized strategy to design a BRET-based biosensor to analyze cellular signaling.

1. *Donor and acceptor construct preparation*: An expression vector coding for the receptor is fused with either donor (luciferase) or acceptor (fluorescence protein). To optimize the dipole orientation factor make fusions on both N- and C-terminus of the molecules.
2. *BRET assessment*: The BRET assay is conducted as described earlier (refer to Subheading 3.2). As the PPI is generally ligand induced in signaling experiments, to follow the time kinetics

the ligand needs to be added after incubating the cells with the live cell substrate of luciferase, e.g., Enduren. Optimize the concentration of the ligand prior to conducting BRET.

3. *Dose response experiment*: Different ligands have varying affinity and specificity for different receptors. Receptor–effector BRET at predetermined optimal concentration of donor plasmid and acceptor plasmid, allows maximal BRET in the presence of the different ligands in a dose-dependent manner. This property is used to deduce the potency of different ligands in the activation of cell signaling. The ligand is increased while the concentration of donor and acceptor plasmids is kept constant. The ligand that reaches BRET saturation at a lower concentration can be considered the more potent signaling molecule.
4. *Time response experiments*: The dissociation and association kinetics of the receptor-effector can also be studied. Use the optimal determined concentration of donor, acceptor plasmid and ligand and perform sequential BRET to study the kinetics of receptor-effector interaction.

4.2 Multiple Protein Interaction

Cellular biochemistry is a highly confound phenomenon, where cells often function through formation of multi-protein complexes. Investigating this ternary complex is needed to understand different biological functions. BRET is limited to investigating interaction between two proteins. Expanding BRET applications toward studying higher order PPIs was achieved with the advancement in RET technology by multiplexing BRET with a third order of measurement by sequential BRET, i.e., SRET [46, 47], BRET-BiFC combinations [48]. Here, we briefly mention about SRET and BRET-BiFC measurement strategies:

1. *SRET*: It involves the use of the bioluminescent energy produced by the catabolism of the substrate by luciferase which is fused to first protein. This excites the first immediate acceptor fluorescence protein fused to second partner protein, and then this acceptor acts like a donor to excite the second RET fluorescence protein fused to the third partner protein, thus sequentially transferring energy. SRET (sequential BRET-FRET) has two known versions, i.e., SRET1 is the RLuc-YFP-DsRed pair, and SRET2 is RLuc–GFP2-YFP pairs. SRET 1 utilizes coelenterazine as substrate whereas SRET2 utilizes DeepBlueC substrate.

   SRET quantification:
   SRET quantification is similar to that of BRET.

$$\text{Net SRET} = \frac{\text{long wavegth emission}}{\text{short wavelength emission}} - \text{Cf},$$

where

$$\text{Cf} = \frac{\text{long wavegth emission}}{\text{short wavelength emission}}.$$

Cf is measured in cells expressing BRET donor luciferase fused to first protein, FRET donor fluorescent protein fused to second partner protein and the third protein not fused to any fluorescence protein.

So for SRET2,

$$\text{net SRET2} = \frac{\text{emission at 530 nm}}{\text{emission at 410 nm}} - \text{Cf},$$

where

$$\text{Cf} = \frac{\text{emission at 530 nm}}{\text{emission at 410 nm}}$$

for cells expressing protein-RLuc, protein-GFP, and other partner protein which is not fused with fluorescence protein.

2. *BRET-BiFC*: It uses combination of BRET and biomolecular fluorescence complementation assay to detect trivalent protein complex. It involves two partner proteins fused to N- and C-terminal fragments of a fluorophore, and the third potential interacting partner fused to a luciferase. When the three proteins interact in the cell at the same time, the fluorophore reconstitutes, which in turn gets excited by bioluminescent energy produced by the luciferase in the presence of its substrate. Generally, RLuc is used as the donor while YFP or Venus is used as the acceptor. The quantification is the same as that of BRET quantification in Subheading 3.2.7. Sometimes, BRET between two complemented luminescent and fluorescent proteins is used for the detection of tetramers.

4.3 Inhibitor/Activator Screening

In human diseases, like cancer and neurodegenerative diseases, there is anomalous regulation of proteins (hyperactivation or inhibition). In disease condition there is abnormal modification of receptor activation, protease activity, and PPI. So target-driven screening assays are needed to identify inhibitor/agonist/antagonist molecules. With development in BRET, it has been used in various screening assays [49]. BRET-based screening assay for identifying ligand binding to membrane receptors has been developed [26]. This technology has also been used to understand the binding kinetics of drugs inside intact cells. Use of this technique is not limited to identifying small molecule. Identification of drugs targeting bromodomain and chromatin can also be carried out using this technique [50]. BRET has also been used to detect protease activity [51] and ion influx assessment [52].

Strategies:

1. *PPI biosensor*: The generation of a biosensor for PPI has been discussed in Subheading 3.2. This biosensor can be used to screen inhibitors which are targeted against interacting proteins of a signaling network. In the presence of the inhibitors the BRET signal will decrease indicating inhibition in interaction. In other cases, a molecule may trigger interaction between protein molecules and thus may show enhanced BRET signal. A similar method is also used to detect agonists and antagonist for receptors. The biosensor is based on interaction between a receptor and its effector molecule. In the presence of agonist the receptor will interact with effector giving BRET signals.
2. *Protease biosensor*: Biosensors for protease activity have the donor and acceptor linked by a substrate peptide sequence while maintaining proximity. Activated protease cleaves the peptide sequence, hence donor-acceptor pair fall apart and loose proximity and thus BRET signal drops. In the presence of inhibitor against this protease, BRET will be detectable. Using appropriate control comparisons, quantified BRET ratio would indicate the potency of the inhibitors.
3. *Ion influx biosensor*: The photoprotein obtained from the jelly fish *Aequorea victoria* is a natural calcium ion (Ca2+) biosensor which has been adopted for research use, where the aequorin (photoprotein) undergoes conformational change upon Ca2+ binding, resulting in the oxidation of coelenterazine that causes release of flash of blue light (465 nm). This light then excites the GFP chromophore in proximity. Thus different levels of Ca2+ in the presence of activators/inhibitors can be monitored using this sensor, where activator would generate BRET signal and inhibitor would cause a loss of signal.

5 Notes

1. Dual reporter assays improve experimental accuracy and efficiency, by reducing variation introduced by experimental conditions such as fluctuations in transfection efficiency.
2. The read time may be shortened, if photon signal output is sufficient. Multiple readings should be taken until maximum photon output is reached. A pilot study should be conducted to monitor the kinetics of different enzymes after the addition of the respective substrate. The length of time that a signal

remains and the time when the photon output peak is reached must be determined. The exposure time should be determined empirically to avoid saturation, as the image that is captured from a saturated image is error prone.

3. A widely used alternative method for stable cell preparation is lentiviral-mediated cell transduction.
4. If the cDNA lacks a translation initiation site then ATG initiation codon should be incorporated in the cDNA. For optimal translation, a Kozak sequence (i.e., GCCACC) is placed in frame just upstream of the initiation codon.
5. For the generation of a fusion protein, the stop codon of the first cDNA must be removed either by site-directed mutagenesis or by PCR amplification. It is recommended to include a flexible amino acid linker sequence between the proteins (*see* Chapter 2 of this volume for details on this method).
6. The expression level of ectopic fusion protein can be checked by Western blot analysis. The cellular localization can be verified by immunofluorescence under confocal microscopy.
7. The fusion tag may disrupt protein function by affecting the protein conformation. To bypass this problem, the tag should be positioned at the N- or C-terminus of the protein, and these constructs should be tested for function. The linker length between the protein of interest and the tag may be increased (but is generally not more than 12–14 amino acids as it may be susceptible to protease cleavage). The linker amino acid sequence is generally glycine or serine type which allows flexibility during protein folding.
8. While performing a BRET measurement the following controls are needed: (a) Background control where substrate is added to un-transfected; (b) Donor alone control to determine donor bleed-through correction on the acceptor channel, and (c) Positive control where donor and acceptor proteins are directly fused using an optimized linker sequence.

References

1. Blasberg RG, Tjuvajev JG (2003) Molecular-genetic imaging: current and future perspectives. J Clin Invest 111(11):1620–1629
2. Ray P et al (2001) Monitoring gene therapy with reporter gene imaging. Semin Nucl Med 31(4):312–320
3. Tannous BA (2009) Gaussia luciferase reporter assay for monitoring biological processes in culture and in vivo. Nat Protoc 4(4):582–591
4. Hall MP et al (2012) Engineered luciferase reporter from a deep sea shrimp utilizing a novel imidazopyrazinone substrate. ACS Chem Biol 7(11):1848–1857
5. Greer LF III, Szalay AA (2002) Imaging of light emission from the expression of luciferases in living cells and organisms: a review. Luminescence 17(1):43–74
6. Kelkar M, De A (2012) Bioluminescence based in vivo screening technologies. Curr Opin Pharmacol 12(5):592–600
7. Mezzanotte L et al (2011) Sensitive dual color in vivo bioluminescence imaging using a new red codon optimized firefly luciferase and a

green click beetle luciferase. PLoS One 6(4): e19277

8. Loening AM et al (2006) Consensus guided mutagenesis of Renilla luciferase yields enhanced stability and light output. Protein Eng Des Sel 19(9):391–400
9. Nyati S et al (2011) Molecular imaging of TGFbeta-induced Smad2/3 phosphorylation reveals a role for receptor tyrosine kinases in modulating TGFbeta signaling. Clin Cancer Res 17(23):7424–7439
10. Dogra S et al (2016) Tango assay for ligand-induced GPCR-beta-arrestin2 interaction: application in drug discovery. Methods Cell Biol 132:233–254
11. Barnea G et al (2008) The genetic design of signaling cascades to record receptor activation. Proc Natl Acad Sci U S A 105(1):64–69
12. Pogmore JP et al (2016) Using forster-resonance energy transfer to measure protein interactions between Bcl-2 family proteins on mitochondrial membranes. Methods Mol Biol 1419:197–212
13. Ray P et al (2008) Monitoring caspase-3 activation with a multimodality imaging sensor in living subjects. Clin Cancer Res 14 (18):5801–5809
14. Prinz A et al (2006) Novel, isotype-specific sensors for protein kinase A subunit interaction based on bioluminescence resonance energy transfer (BRET). Cell Signal 18 (10):1616–1625
15. Kang JH, Chung JK (2008) Molecular-genetic imaging based on reporter gene expression. J Nucl Med 49(Suppl 2):164S–179S
16. Moroz E et al (2009) Real-time imaging of HIF-1alpha stabilization and degradation. PLoS One 4(4):e5077
17. Shachaf CM et al (2004) MYC inactivation uncovers pluripotent differentiation and tumour dormancy in hepatocellular cancer. Nature 431(7012):1112–1117
18. Korpal M et al (2009) Imaging transforming growth factor-beta signaling dynamics and therapeutic response in breast cancer bone metastasis. Nat Med 15(8):960–966
19. Nakajima Y et al (2005) Multicolor luciferase assay system: one-step monitoring of multiple gene expressions with a single substrate. BioTechniques 38(6):891–894
20. Arkin MR, Wells JA (2004) Small-molecule inhibitors of protein-protein interactions: progressing towards the dream. Nat Rev Drug Discov 3(4):301–317
21. Phizicky EM, Fields S (1995) Protein-protein interactions: methods for detection and analysis. Microbiol Rev 59(1):94–123
22. Ciruela F (2008) Fluorescence-based methods in the study of protein-protein interactions in living cells. Curr Opin Biotechnol 19 (4):338–343
23. Gorokhovatsky AY et al (2004) Fusion of Aequorea victoria GFP and aequorin provides their Ca(2+)-induced interaction that results in red shift of GFP absorption and efficient bioluminescence energy transfer. Biochem Biophys Res Commun 320(3):703–711
24. Canals M et al (2004) Homodimerization of adenosine A2A receptors: qualitative and quantitative assessment by fluorescence and bioluminescence energy transfer. J Neurochem 88 (3):726–734
25. Terrillon S et al (2003) Oxytocin and vasopressin V1a and V2 receptors form constitutive homo- and heterodimers during biosynthesis. Mol Endocrinol 17(4):677–691
26. Stoddart LA et al (2015) Application of BRET to monitor ligand binding to GPCRs. Nat Methods 12(7):661–663
27. Siddiqui S et al (2013) BRET biosensor analysis of receptor tyrosine kinase functionality. Front Endocrinol (Lausanne) 4:46
28. Kaczor AA et al (2014) Application of BRET for studying G protein-coupled receptors. Mini Rev Med Chem 14(5):411–425
29. Paulmurugan R, Umezawa Y, Gambhir SS (2002) Noninvasive imaging of protein-protein interactions in living subjects by using reporter protein complementation and reconstitution strategies. Proc Natl Acad Sci U S A 99(24):15608–15613
30. Dragulescu-Andrasi A et al (2011) Bioluminescence resonance energy transfer (BRET) imaging of protein-protein interactions within deep tissues of living subjects. Proc Natl Acad Sci U S A 108(29):12060–12065
31. Ogoh K et al (2014) Bioluminescence microscopy using a short focal-length imaging lens. J Microsc 253(3):191–197
32. Yamaguchi S et al (2003) Synchronization of cellular clocks in the suprachiasmatic nucleus. Science 302(5649):1408–1412
33. De A et al (2009) BRET3: a red-shifted bioluminescence resonance energy transfer (BRET)-based integrated platform for imaging protein-protein interactions from single live cells and living animals. FASEB J 23(8):2702–2709
34. Coulon V et al (2008) Subcellular imaging of dynamic protein interactions by bioluminescence resonance energy transfer. Biophys J 94 (3):1001–1009
35. Akiyoshi R et al (2014) Bioluminescence imaging to track real-time armadillo promoter

activity in live Drosophila embryos. Anal Bioanal Chem 406(23):5703–5713

36. Bergkessel M, Guthrie C (2014) Colony PCR. Methods Enzymol 529:299–309
37. Verveer PJ et al (2006) Imaging protein interactions by FRET microscopy: FRET measurements by acceptor photobleaching. CSH Protoc 2006(6):pii:pdb.prot4598. https://doi.org/10.1101/pdb.prot4598
38. Close DM et al (2011) In vivo bioluminescent imaging (BLI): noninvasive visualization and interrogation of biological processes in living animals. Sensors (Basel) 11(1):180–206
39. De A, Arora R, Jasani A (2014) Engineering aspects of bioluminescence resonance energy transfer systems. In: Cai W (ed) Engineering in translational medicine. Springer, London, pp 257–300
40. Mercier JF et al (2002) Quantitative assessment of beta 1- and beta 2-adrenergic receptor homo- and heterodimerization by bioluminescence resonance energy transfer. J Biol Chem 277(47):44925–44931
41. Kroeger KM et al (2001) Constitutive and agonist-dependent homo-oligomerization of the thyrotropin-releasing hormone receptor. Detection in living cells using bioluminescence resonance energy transfer. J Biol Chem 276 (16):12736–12743
42. Felce JH, Knox RG, Davis SJ (2014) Type-3 BRET, an improved competition-based bioluminescence resonance energy transfer assay. Biophys J 106(12):L41–L43
43. Inoue Y et al (2009) Comparison of subcutaneous and intraperitoneal injection of D-luciferin for in vivo bioluminescence imaging. Eur J Nucl Med Mol Imaging 36 (5):771–779
44. Lee KH et al (2003) Cell uptake and tissue distribution of radioiodine labelled D-luciferin: implications for luciferase based gene imaging. Nucl Med Commun 24 (9):1003–1009
45. De A et al (2013) Evolution of BRET biosensors from live cell to tissue-scale in vivo imaging. Front Endocrinol (Lausanne) 4:131
46. Carriba P et al (2008) Detection of heteromerization of more than two proteins by sequential BRET-FRET. Nat Methods 5(8):727–733
47. Branchini BR et al (2011) Sequential bioluminescence resonance energy transfer-fluorescence resonance energy transfer-based ratiometric protease assays with fusion proteins of firefly luciferase and red fluorescent protein. Anal Biochem 414(2):239–245
48. Vidi PA, Watts VJ (2009) Fluorescent and bioluminescent protein-fragment complementation assays in the study of G protein-coupled receptor oligomerization and signaling. Mol Pharmacol 75(4):733–739
49. Bacart J et al (2008) The BRET technology and its application to screening assays. Biotechnol J 3(3):311–324
50. Machleidt T et al (2015) NanoBRET—a Novel BRET platform for the analysis of protein-protein interactions. ACS Chem Biol 10 (8):1797–1804
51. Kim GB, Kim YP (2012) Analysis of protease activity using quantum dots and resonance energy transfer. Theranostics 2(2):127–138
52. Bakayan A et al (2011) Red fluorescent protein-aequorin fusions as improved bioluminescent Ca2+ reporters in single cells and mice. PLoS One 6(5):e19520

Chapter 6

Fluorescence Imaging of Mycobacterial Infection in Live Mice Using Fluorescent Protein-Expressing Strains

Ying Kong and Jeffrey D. Cirillo

Abstract

Fluorescence imaging has been applied to various areas of biological research, including studies of physiological, neurological, oncological, cell biological, molecular, developmental, immunological, and infectious processes. In this chapter, we describe methods of fluorescent imaging applied to examination of subcutaneous and pulmonary mycobacterial infections in an animal model. Since slow growth of *Mycobacterium tuberculosis* (*Mtb*) hinders development of new diagnostics, therapeutics, and vaccines for tuberculosis (TB), we developed fluorescent protein (FP) expressing mycobacterial strains for in vivo imaging, which can be used to track bacterial location and to quantitate bacterial load directly in living animals. After comparison of imaging data using strains expressing different fluorescent proteins, we found that strains expressing L5-tdTomato display the greatest fluorescence. Here, we describe detailed protocols for tdTomato-labeled *M. bovis BCG* imaging in real time for subcutaneous and pulmonary infections in living mice. These procedures allow rapid and accurate determination of bacterial numbers in live mice.

Key words Mycobacteria, Fluorescent proteins, Noninvasive imaging, tdTomato

1 Introduction

Tuberculosis (TB) is a major public health threat, with approximately nine million new cases and 1.5 million deaths each year [1]. TB is caused by *Mycobacterium tuberculosis* complex that includes *M. tuberculosis*, *M. bovis*, *M. africanum*, and *M. microti*. Most human TB cases are caused by *M. tuberculosis. M. tuberculosis* replicates slowly and divides once every 15–20 h. Research on TB has been impeded by the slow growth rate of *M. tuberculosis.* Conventionally, quantitation of *M. tuberculosis* in vitro and in vivo relies on counting bacterial colony forming units (CFU) on agar plates. It takes 4 weeks for *M. tuberculosis* to form visible colonies on solid agar plates [2–4]. Imaging technologies that are capable of rapidly quantitating tubercle bacilli in vitro and in vivo would greatly accelerate TB research.

Purnima Dubey (ed.), *Reporter Gene Imaging: Methods and Protocols*, Methods in Molecular Biology, vol. 1790,
https://doi.org/10.1007/978-1-4939-7860-1_6,

Fluorescent proteins (FPs) have been applied to various areas of biological research, such as in vitro cell imaging [5, 6] and in vivo tracking organisms or specific cells in real time [7–10]. Recently, fluorescent imaging as a powerful tool is emerging in studies of infectious diseases. In vivo fluorescent imaging with FPs requires the FP has an emission wavelength within or at least close to the near-infrared (NIR) window, which is 650–900 nm, because hemoglobin and water have their lowest absorption coefficients in the NIR window [11]. Several FPs including Tdtomato have red or far-red emissions ranging from 581 nm to 655 nm [12]. Brightness of the mature protein and photostability also impact in vivo fluorescence imaging. TdTomato has high photostability and is the brightest FP among the variants of DsRFP developed by Dr. Roger Tsien's group [13]. We cloned the tdTomato gene into mycobacteria under the control of either a mycobacterial L5 or Hsp60 promoter, and compared the in vivo imaging results. We found that the strain expressing L5-tdTomato displayed the highest fluorescence signal in vivo [14]. In this chapter, we describe the methods for in vivo imaging of mycobacteria infected mice using the L5-tdTomato-expressing strain. The first section of this chapter focuses on in vivo imaging using a mycobacterial subcutaneous infection model, and the second section describes procedures for in vivo imaging of a lung infection model using the same strain.

2 Materials

2.1 Bacterial Preparation

1. *M. bovis* BCG-tdTomato frozen stock.
2. 7H9 broth supplemented with 0.5% glycerol, 10% OAD (oleic acid dextrose complex without catalase) and 0.05% Tween-80 (M-OAD-TW broth).
3. Kanamycin (stock solution at 50 mg/mL in H_2O).
4. Middlebrook 7H9 supplemented with 10% OAD and 15 g/l Bacto agar (M-OAD agar) or on 7H11 selective agar. Add 25 μg/ml kanamycin into the medium.
5. Phosphate-buffered saline (PBS), adjust pH to 7.4.
6. Tween-80 (20%).

2.2 Mouse Subcutaneous Infection

1. BALB/c female mice 7-weeks old.
2. Isoflurane for mouse anesthesia.
3. Oxygen tank for mouse anesthesia.
4. Electric hair trimmer for shaving mouse fur.
5. 1 ml syringe with 26 G needles.

2.3 Mouse Intratracheal Infection

1. BALB/c female mice 7-weeks old.
2. Mixture of Ketamine 10 mg/ml and Xylazine 1 mg/ml for intratracheal infection (Ketamine 100 μg + 10 μg Xylazine per 1 ml ddH_2O, store at −4 °C), working dose: 10 μl per gram of mouse body weight.
3. Otoscope with intubation speculum.
4. 22 G catheter for intra-tracheal infection.
5. Guide wire for 22 G catheter.
6. Forceps.
7. Tape.
8. 1 ml syringe, with 26 G needles.

2.4 IVIS Imaging

1. Xenogen IVIS 200 with nose cone manifold.
2. XGI-8 gas anesthesia system.
3. Activated charcoal scavenger filters connected to the isoflurane out-flow tube.

3 Methods

3.1 Bacterial Preparation

1. Thaw frozen stocked *M. bovis* BCG-tdTomato strain.
2. Inoculate 50 μl of *M. bovis* BCG from frozen seed-lots to 5 ml of MOAD with kanamycin in 25 cm^2 tissue culture flasks.
3. Keep the flasks horizontal with the caps tightly closed.
4. Grow the bacteria at 37 °C with occasional agitation until an $OD_{600} = 0.5–1$, which usually takes 5–7 days.
5. Make PBS-Tween by mix 1 L PBS with 2.5 ml 20% Tween-80.
6. Take cultured bacteria from the flasks and add them into conical microfuge tubes.
7. Centrifuge bacteria at 10,000 rpm (9.6 × *g*) for 5 min to remove culture medium.
8. Wash bacteria with PBS-Tween twice, and resuspend bacteria into PBS.

3.2 Mouse Subcutaneous Infection

Follow institutional Animal Care and Use Committee guidelines for all animal work.

1. House mice in polycarbonate micro-isolator cages in a controlled environment with 12 h light and 12 h dark cycle, ~18–23 °C, and 40–60% humidity.
2. Allow mice to acclimate to the facilities for one week and feed commercial chow with low chlorophyll content and autoclaved tap water ad libitum.

3. Prepare the isoflurane gas anesthesia system that is attached to the IVIS imaging system before beginning an anesthetic procedure. Make sure that the gas delivery and evacuation return hoses are not obstructed or leaking. Fill the isoflurane chamber if needed.
4. Slowly turn on the oxygen cylinder.
5. Put mice into the anesthesia induction chamber that is attached to the XGI-8 system. Close the chamber.
6. Set the vaporizer value to 2.5–3%.
7. Turn ON the "Induction Chamber" toggle valve on the XGI-8 system.
8. Turn ON the gas flow to the XGI-8 System (oxygen on/off valve at left-lower corner of XGI-8), and anesthetize mice with isoflurane using the induction.
9. When mice are anesthetized, take a mouse out of the chamber one at a time and shave the back of the mouse with an electric hair trimmer (necessary for subcutaneous infection). Put mice back into the chamber after shaving. Turn off the "Induction Chamber" toggle valve whenever the lid of the induction chamber is open.
10. Take 50 μl of bacterial suspension with a 1 ml syringe.
11. Take out a mouse from the induction chamber, and inject 3–4 different concentrations of bacteria and the negative control under the skin at separated spots on the back of each mouse.
12. Put the infected mice back into the anesthesia induction chamber.
13. Titrate the bacteria on MOAD agar plates for CFU enumeration to confirm the number of bacteria injected under the skin.

3.3 IVIS Imaging of Mice with Subcutaneous Infection

1. When mice are anesthetized, turn ON the "IVIS Flow on/off" valve on the XGI-8 System (anesthesia gas flow into the manifold inside the imaging chamber of IVIS). Set the flow as 0.25 LPM using the manifold rotameter on the XGI-8 System.
2. Turn OFF the "CHAMBER on/off" toggle valve before removing animals from the Induction Chamber.
3. Quickly take mice out of the Induction Chamber and place them into the nose cones inside the IVIS imaging chamber. Place mice in the dorsal position. Close the door of the imaging chamber. Mice are ready to be imaged now.
4. Start the Living Image software on the computer connected to the IVIS.
5. Initialize the IVIS System and wait for the CCD camera temperature to lock by clicking "Initialize" on the pop-up control panel. (Temperature bar will turn green).

6. Choose the "Fluorescence" option on the control panel, and set the Fluorescent Lamp Level as "High."
7. Select Excitation and Emission Filters. For tdTomato, the excitation wavelength is 535 nm and emission is collected in 20 nm increments from 580 to 660 nm to allow subsequent spectral unmixing [15]. If "Transillumination" is not selected, epi-illumination is the default selection. For imaging subcutaneous infection, we used epi-illumination.
8. Set the binning as "Medium," and "F/Stop = 2." Set the "Exposure Time" as "1–300 seconds" or "Auto." Set the "Field of View (FOV) "by selecting from the FOV drop-down list. A "FOV" of "B" is selected for imaging one mouse, "C" is selected when imaging three mice, and "D" for imaging 4–5 mice.
9. As soon as the IVIS imaging chamber door is closed, a picture of the mice inside of the chamber is taken and shown in the "Alignment Grid" box on the imaging acquisition panel. Check if mice are positioned properly. Adjust mouse position if necessary.
10. Click "Acquire" to collect fluorescent images.
11. Save the images into a folder.
12. Use Living Image software to analyze the acquired images.
13. Load images with different emission wavelengths by clicking "File." Click "Browse" from the menu to select the folder with stored images.
14. From the "Living Image Browser," select the image set to analyze (Fig. 1a).
15. Click "Spectral Unmixing" on the "Tool Palette" window.
16. Check the boxes of all wavelengths in "Analyze."
17. In the list of "Methods" on "Spectral Unmixing," select "Automatic," and then click "Start Unmixing" (Fig. 1b).
18. In the pop-up window, there are two view options: "Sequence view," and "Auto Unmix." In the "Auto Unmix" view, select "Imaging Subject" as "Mouse," and "Probe Information" as "Proteins" and "tdTomato." Click "Finish" will show two panels on the pop-up window: the left one is a chart with two curves of emission and the right one contains mouse images. In the right panel, find the image labeled with "tdTomato" (Fig. 1c). The other two images are labeled as "AF tissue" and "Composite," respectively.
19. Double click the tdTomato image on the right panel (Fig. 1d). Use "ROI Tools" on the pop-up "Tool Palette" to do the quantitative analysis. The ROI measurement has various shapes. We selected circle shape for mice with subcutaneous

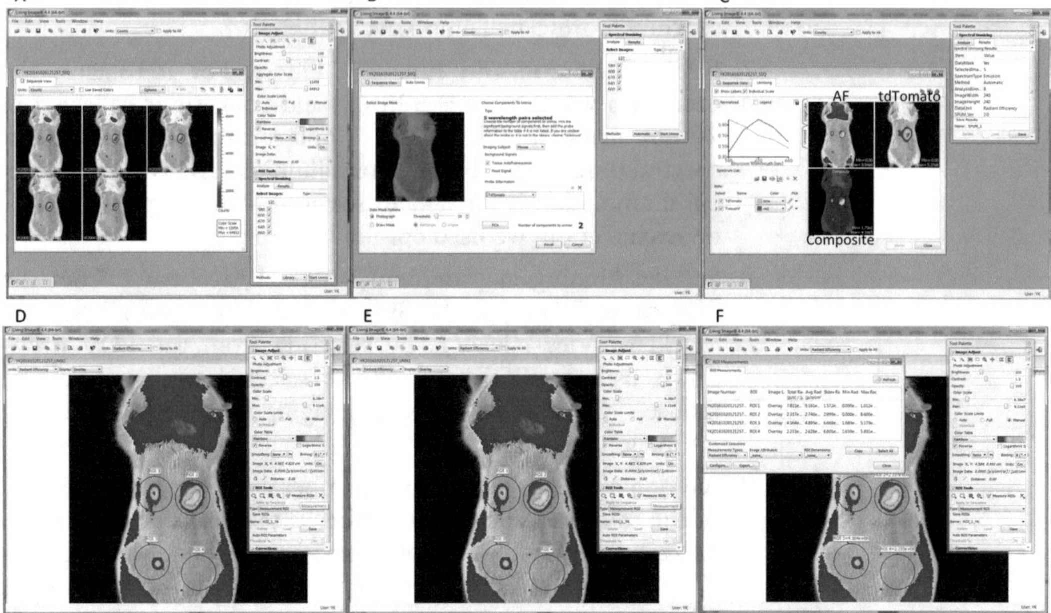

Fig. 1 Procedure for quantitation of fluorescent signal from mice subcutaneously infected with tdTomato-expressing *M. bovis* BCG. (**a**) Load the image set to analyze; (**b**) Open Spectral Unmixing window; (**c**) Finished spectral unmixing images; (**d**) Images with tdTomato-specific fluorescence signal; (**e**) Quantitate fluorescence with "ROI Tools"; and (**f**) Measure ROIs

infection. Try to cover the fluorescence source with the right size ROI circles (Fig. 1e). The sizes of circles for all sites of infection on all imaged mice should be kept the same for comparison of fluorescence between different sites and different groups.

20. Click "Measure ROIs." A "ROI Measurement" window will pop-up and show all values of ROIs. The unit of ROI for data analysis is "Total Radiant Efficiency" (equals to [p/s]/[μW/cm^2]) (Fig. 1f).

3.4 Mouse Intra-Tracheal Inoculation to Image Lung Infections

1. House mice in polycarbonate micro-isolator cages in a controlled environment with 12 h light/12 h dark cycle, ~18–23 °C, and 40–60% humidity.
2. Allow mice to acclimate to the facilities for one week and fed commercial chow with low chlorophyll content and tap water ad libitum.
3. Weigh each mouse for anesthesia dosage.
4. I.P. inject Ketamine 10 mg/ml and Xylazine 1 mg/ml mixture into the mice with 10 μl per gram of mouse body weight to anesthetize the mice.
5. Put an anesthetized mouse in a ventral position on a stand and tape the legs to the stand.

6. Pull the mouse tongue out of the mouth with a forceps to expose the larynx opening.
7. Run the guide wire through a catheter and carefully insert the catheter into the larynx by monitoring the process through an otoscope.
8. Leave the catheter in the larynx and remove the guide wire.
9. Pipet 50 μl of the bacterial solution to the hub of the catheter. Take a 1 ml syringe to pull 50 μl air in it, connect the syringe with the catheter hub, and flush the bacteria into mouse lungs with the 50 μl of air. Place the infected mouse back into the cage. Wait for the mouse to recover from anesthesia. It usually takes 20–30 min.
10. Titrate the left-over bacteria on M-OAD agar plates for CFU enumeration.

3.5 IVIS Imaging of Mice with Lung Infections Following Intra-Tracheal Inoculation

1. When mice are anesthetized in the induction chamber, put one mouse into the imaging chamber of IVIS.
2. To image mice with trans-illumination excitation, the glass bottom panel of the imaging chamber is used so that the excitation light can run though the mouse body from bottom of the glass panel.
3. Turn on the "Live Imaging" software, initialize the acquire image function by click the "Initialize" button, and wait until the control bar color changes from red into green.
4. Mouse images are acquired by selecting "Photo."
5. When "Photo" is selected, photographic images will be directly overlaid onto the fluorescent images to be acquired.
6. Select "Transillumination" on the control panel. The photo of the mouse to be imaged is overlaid with a map of spots where excitation light will pass through. Select the spots wherever you want the excitation light to be by clicking the spots. For lung imaging, we usually select two spots in central chest area of the mouse. (*Transillumination: the excitation light from the bottom of the chamber goes through a glass or mesh panel and the mouse is placed on the panel. Light is transmitted to the site of infection, excites the fluorescence source, generates emission which is captured by the CCD camera on top of the chamber*).
7. Select appropriate "Excitation wavelength," "Emission wavelength," "Exposure time," "F-stop," "Binning," and "FOV."
8. In the case of tdTomato, the excitation wavelength is 535 nm and emission is collected in 20 nm increments from 560 to 640 nm. Multiple emission wavelengths are selected for later spectral unmixing analysis.
9. Set exposure time as "Auto," "F-stop = 2," and binning as "Medium."

10. Select "FOV" as level "B" to take transillumination images for a single mouse.
11. Click "Add Sequence" to add all the imaging conditions into the window of image acquiring.
12. Click "Acquire" to collect images.
13. Use Living Image software to analyze the acquired images.
14. Load images with different emission wavelengths by clicking "File." Click "Browse" from the menu to select the folder with stored images.
15. From the "Living Image Browser," select the image set to analyze (Fig. 2a).

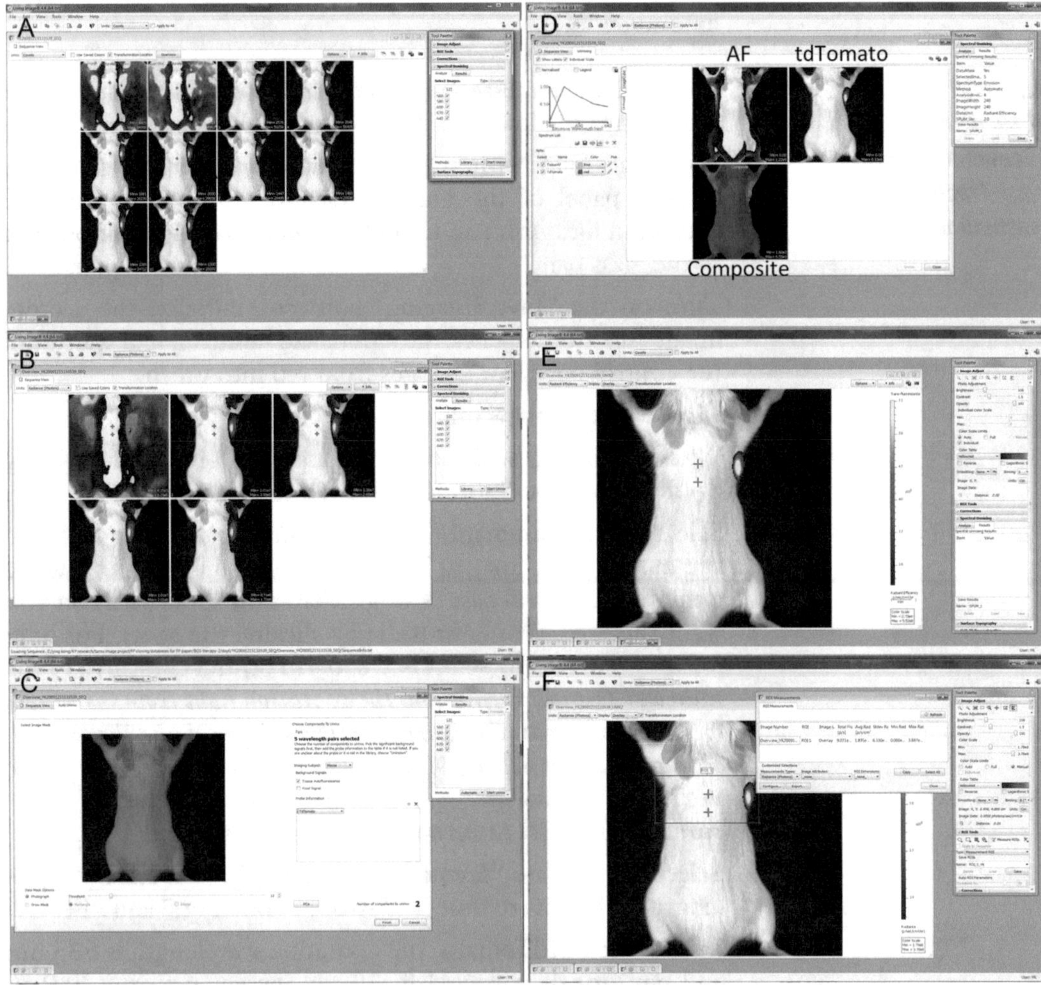

Fig. 2 Procedure for quantitation of fluorescent signal from mice intra-tracheally infected with the tdTomato-expressing *M. bovis* BCG. (**a**) Load the image set to analyze; (**b**) Use "Transillumination overview" to combine images taken with the same excitation and emission wavelengths. (**c**) Open Spectral Unmixing window; (**d**) Finished spectral unmixing images; (**e**) Images with tdTomato-specific fluorescence signal; (**f**) Quantitation fluorescence with "ROI Tools" and measurement of ROIs

16. Click "Tools" on the top bar of Living Image, and then click "Transillumination overview for XXX seq." The function of this button is to merge images that have been taken with the same excitation and emission wavelengths but with different locations of excitation into a single image (Fig. 2b).
17. Click "Spectral Unmixing" on the "Tool Palette" window (Fig. 2c).
18. Check the boxes of all desired wavelengths in "Analyze."
19. In the list of "Methods" on "Spectral Unmixing," select "Automatic," and then click "Start Unmixing" (Fig. 2c).
20. In the pop-up window, there are two view options: "Sequence View," and "Auto Unmix." On the "Auto Unmix" view, select "Imaging Subject" as "Mouse," and "Probe Information" as "Proteins" and "tdTomato." Click "Finish" will show two panels on the pop-up window: the left is a chart with two curves of emission and the right contains three mouse images. In the right panel, find the image labeled with "tdTomato" (Fig. 2d).
21. Double click the tdTomato image on the right panel. Use "ROI Tools" to do the quantitative analysis. We select a rectangle shape for mice with lung infection. Try to cover the fluorescence source with the right size ROI rectangle. The sizes of rectangles for all sites of infection on all mice should be the same, so that the quantitative data are comparable between groups of mice.
22. Click "Measure ROIs." A "ROI Measurement" window will pop-up and show all values of ROIs. The unit of ROI for data analysis is "Total Radiant Efficiency."

4 Notes

In vivo imaging works best with near-infrared excitation and emission wavelengths due to improved penetration through mammalian tissues [11]. Some mutant derivatives of DsRed have longer excitation and emission wavelengths, including tdTomato [13], mCherry [13], mKate [16], mPlum [17], Katushka [16], mRuby [18], mNeptune [19], and Cardinal [20]. Mycobacteria expressing mCherry and tdTomato have been used to image mycobacterial infection in vivo [14, 21, 22]. Background autofluorescence is a confounding factor in in vivo fluorescence imaging. Spectral unmixing is very helpful for reducing autofluorescence. Spectral unmixing is carried out by first imaging using several sets of excitation and emission wavelengths around the known optimal wavelengths of the FP and then using the emission data to subtract autofluorescence signal from signal matching the FP. In this way, optimal conditions for spectral unmixing can be determined during the analysis. Autofluorescence from mice can be also controlled by imaging of uninfected mice, and then subtracting the background autofluorescence signal of uninfected mice from the fluorescence signal of infected mice during data analysis. Signal from uninfected mice should be quantitated in the same way as the infected mice. To accurately estimate bacterial load in mice, we always conduct spectral unmixing with both infected and uninfected mice, and then subtract the final signal of uninfected mice from the infected ones. Trans-illumination imaging usually requires longer exposure times than epi-illumination imaging. It is important to carefully choose trans-illumination locations so the fluorescent protein is optimally excited to obtain optimal emission signal. All of the mice to be imaged should be carefully aligned using the laser cross as a reference, so that the mice share the same trans-illumination locations. Exposure time can be approximated by running an "Auto" exposure to explore how long it takes to get a good quality image, and then choose an exposure time accordingly. If 3-D images are planned to be collected, "Structure" should be selected on the control panel, which allows molecular tomography to be acquired. The detailed methods of collecting 3-D fluorescent images have been described elsewhere [23]. In summary, we describe the protocols that we used in our recently published studies using in vivo imaging for mycobacterial infection with FP-expressing mycobacterial strains [14]. More detailed information regarding the IVIS and Living Image Software can be obtained from the PerkinElmer website, which also offers technical support (http://www.perkinelmer.com/product/ivis-instrument-spectrum-120v-andor-c-124262).

References

1. WHO (2015) Global tuberculosis control 2014. WHO, Geneva
2. Glickman MS, Jacobs WR Jr (2001) Microbial pathogenesis of *Mycobacterium tuberculosis*: dawn of a discipline. Cell 104(4):477–485
3. Smith I (2003) Mycobacterium tuberculosis pathogenesis and molecular determinants of virulence. Clin Microbiol Rev 16(3):463–496
4. Zumla A, Raviglione M, Hafner R, von Reyn CF (2013) Tuberculosis. N Engl J Med 368 (8):745–755. https://doi.org/10.1056/NEJMra1200894
5. Passamaneck YJ, Di Gregorio A, Papaioannou VE, Hadjantonakis AK (2006) Live imaging of fluorescent proteins in chordate embryos: from ascidians to mice. Microsc Res Tech 69 (3):160–167. https://doi.org/10.1002/jemt.20284
6. Wacker SA, Oswald F, Wiedenmann J, Knochel W (2007) A green to red photoconvertible protein as an analyzing tool for early vertebrate development. Dev Dynam 236(2):473–480. https://doi.org/10.1002/dvdy.20955
7. Hoffman RM (2005) Advantages of multi-color fluorescent proteins for whole-body and in vivo cellular imaging. J Biomed Opt 10 (4):41202. https://doi.org/10.1117/1.1992485
8. Stewart CN Jr (2006) Go with the glow: fluorescent proteins to light transgenic organisms. Trends Biotechnol 24(4):155–162. doi: S0167-7799(06)00030-8 [pii]10.1016/j.tibtech.2006.02.002
9. Seitz G, Warmann SW, Fuchs J, Mau-Holzmann UA, Ruck P, Heitmann H, Hoffman RM, Mahrt J, Muller GA, Wessels JT (2006) Visualization of xenotransplanted

human rhabdomyosarcoma after transfection with red fluorescent protein. J Pediatr Surg 41(8):1369–1376. https://doi.org/10.1016/j.jpedsurg.2006.04.039

10. Winnard PT Jr, Kluth JB, Raman V (2006) Noninvasive optical tracking of red fluorescent protein-expressing cancer cells in a model of metastatic breast cancer. Neoplasia 8 (10):796–806
11. Weissleder R (2001) A clearer vision for in vivo imaging. Nat Biotechnol 19(4):316–317
12. Muller-Taubenberger A, Anderson KI (2007) Recent advances using green and red fluorescent protein variants. Appl Microbiol Biotechnol 77(1):1–12. https://doi.org/10.1007/s00253-007-1131-5
13. Shaner NC, Steinbach PA, Tsien RY (2005) A guide to choosing fluorescent proteins. Nat Methods 2(12):905–909
14. Kong Y, Yang D, Cirillo SL, Li S, Akin A, Francis KP, Maloney T, Cirillo JD (2016) Application of fluorescent protein expressing strains to evaluation of anti-tuberculosis therapeutic efficacy in vitro and in vivo. PLoS One 11(3):e0149972. https://doi.org/10.1371/journal.pone.0149972
15. Xu H, Rice BW (2009) In-vivo fluorescence imaging with a multivariate curve resolution spectral unmixing technique. J Biomed Opt 14(6):064011. https://doi.org/10.1117/1.3258838
16. Shcherbo D, Merzlyak EM, Chepurnykh TV, Fradkov AF, Ermakova GV, Solovieva EA, Lukyanov KA, Bogdanova EA, Zaraisky AG, Lukyanov S, Chudakov DM (2007) Bright far-red fluorescent protein for whole-body imaging. Nat Methods 4(9):741–746
17. Wang L, Jackson WC, Steinbach PA, Tsien RY (2004) Evolution of new nonantibody proteins via iterative somatic hypermutation. Proc Natl Acad Sci U S A 101(48):16745–16749. https://doi.org/10.1073/pnas.0407752101
18. Kredel S, Oswald F, Nienhaus K, Deuschle K, Rocker C, Wolff M, Heilker R, Nienhaus GU, Wiedenmann J (2009) mRuby, a bright monomeric red fluorescent protein for labeling of subcellular structures. PLoS One 4(2):e4391. https://doi.org/10.1371/journal.pone.0004391
19. Lin MZ, McKeown MR, Ng HL, Aguilera TA, Shaner NC, Campbell RE, Adams SR, Gross LA, Ma W, Alber T, Tsien RY (2009) Autofluorescent proteins with excitation in the optical window for intravital imaging in mammals. Chem Biol 16(11):1169–1179. https://doi.org/10.1016/j.chembiol.2009.10.009
20. Chu J, Haynes RD, Corbel SY, Li P, Gonzalez-Gonzalez E, Burg JS, Ataie NJ, Lam AJ, Cranfill PJ, Baird MA, Davidson MW, Ng HL, Garcia KC, Contag CH, Shen K, Blau HM, Lin MZ (2014) Non-invasive intravital imaging of cellular differentiation with a bright red-excitable fluorescent protein. Nat Methods 11(5):572–578. https://doi.org/10.1038/nmeth.2888
21. Carroll P, Schreuder LJ, Muwanguzi-Karugaba J, Wiles S, Robertson BD, Ripoll J, Ward TH, Bancroft GJ, Schaible UE, Parish T (2010) Sensitive detection of gene expression in mycobacteria under replicating and non-replicating conditions using optimized far-red reporters. PLoS One 5(3):e9823. https://doi.org/10.1371/journal.pone.0009823
22. Zelmer A, Carroll P, Andreu N, Hagens K, Mahlo J, Redinger N, Robertson BD, Wiles S, Ward TH, Parish T, Ripoll J, Bancroft GJ, Schaible UE (2012) A new in vivo model to test anti-tuberculosis drugs using fluorescence imaging. J Antimicrob Chemother 67 (8):1948–1960. https://doi.org/10.1093/jac/dks161
23. Kong Y, Akin AR, Francis KP, Zhang N, Troy TL, Xie H, Rao J, Cirillo SLG, Cirillo JD (2011) Whole-body imaging of infection using fluorescence. Curr Protoc Microbiol Chapter 2:Unit 2C.3. https://doi.org/10.1002/9780471729259.mc02c03s21

Chapter 7

In Vivo Bacterial Imaging Using Bioluminescence

Mariette Barbier, Justin Bevere, and F. Heath Damron

Abstract

Bacterial luminescence allows for noninvasive continuous monitoring of promoter activity in a wide range of model systems. This chapter details various examples of use of the *lux* reporter system to measure promoter activity in bacteria using the vector pUC18T-mini-Tn7T-*lux*-Tp. Here, we describe the construction of promoter fusions with bacterial luciferase, and how to quantify promoter activity in real time in vitro and in vivo in plant, insect, and murine infection models.

Key words Bacteria, Bioluminescence, In vivo imaging, Reporter system, Promoter activity, Bacterial pathogenesis, Pathogen-host interaction

1 Introduction

Bioluminescence is a naturally occurring phenomenon in marine and soil Gram-negative bacteria from the genera *Photobacterium*, *Vibrio*, and *Photorhabdus* (*Xenorhabdus*). In these bacteria, bioluminescence is produced though the activity of bacterial luciferase which catalyzes the oxidation of a reduced flavin mononucleotide ($FMNH_2$) with the reduction of molecular oxygen (Fig. 1).

The excess energy from this reaction is released as blue/green light emission. The genes essential for luminescence are encoded on the *luxCDABE* operon, also called *lux*. *luxA* and *luxB* encode the subunits A and B of bacterial luciferase [1], while *luxC*, *luxD*, and *luxE* encode the subunits of a fatty acid reductase that provides fatty aldehydes to the luciferase. While most bacterial luciferases are active at temperatures such as those found in marine environments, *Photorhabdus luminescens* encodes a bacterial luciferase active at temperatures encountered in mammals. For this reason, the *lux* operon from *P. luminescens* has been used extensively as a reporter system to study bacterial gene expression, function, and virulence.

Numerous genetic tools have been created to facilitate the use of bacterial luciferase. For the purpose of this protocol chapter, we will describe ways to use luminescence as a reporter of promoter

Purnima Dubey (ed.), *Reporter Gene Imaging: Methods and Protocols*, Methods in Molecular Biology, vol. 1790,
https://doi.org/10.1007/978-1-4939-7860-1_7,

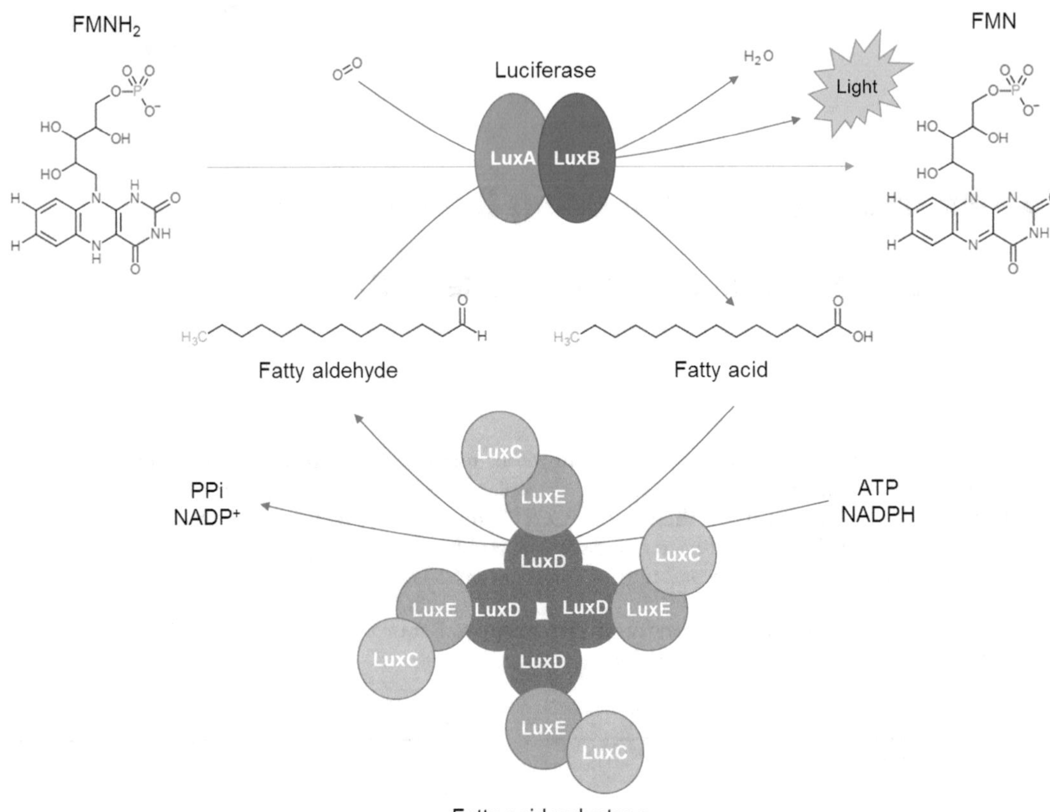

Fig. 1 Chemical reactions catalyzed by bacterial luciferase and fatty acid reductase complexes. Bacterial luciferase (LuxAB complex) catalyzes the oxidation of a reduced flavin mononucleotide ($FMNH_2$) with the reduction of molecular oxygen to generate FMN and water. Fatty acids are then reduced to fatty aldehydes by the LuxCDE complex

activity, or as a way to localize and determine relative amount of bacteria in infection models. While *in trans* reporters encoded on plasmids have been extensively used, there are many advantages of encoding reporter genes on vectors that can shuttle the constructs to the chromosome of the bacteria of interest. Upon the insertion of a reporter construct into the chromosome, antibiotic selection is no longer needed which may be helpful in the experimental design, especially if the goal is to study gene expression during infection or localize bacteria in a host. The mini-Tn7 transposon system is possibly the most versatile and frequently used genetic tool for this application, and many reporters have been cloned into this system. The mini-Tn7 vectors have been described elsewhere [2, 3]. In this chapter, we will describe uses of one of the available mini-Tn7 plasmids: pUC18T-mini-Tn7T-*lux*-Tp [4]. This vector can be used directly for stable integration of the *lux* operon on the chromosome of a wide range of Gram-negative bacteria for bioluminescence labeling or engineered to detect the expression of a promoter of interest in single copy. We will first describe how to generate a promoter fusion in this plasmid using molecular cloning methods, and how to test its function in bacteria such as *Pseudomonas aeruginosa* using in vitro techniques. We will then describe infection and imaging procedures for measuring promoter activity using in vivo imaging technologies in hosts such as the wax worm (*Galleria mellonella*), the lettuce (*Lactua romana*), and the mouse (*Mus musclus*). This protocol has been designed for use in *P. aeruginosa* but can be readily adapted to numerous Gram-negative microorganisms.

2 Materials

All solutions should be prepared in ultrapure distilled water, using analytical grade reagents, and sterilized as indicated. All work with recombinant DNA should be performed using DNAse-free tubes and filter pipette tips. Recombinant DNA and biohazardous materials should be handled and disposed in accordance with institutional regulations.

2.1 Promoter Amplification and Cloning to Generate a Reporter System

1. Design PCR primers for the amplification of the promoter region of interest. For restriction digestion and directional cloning of the fragment, add a BamHI restriction site to the 5′ end of the forward primer, and an EcoRI restriction site to the 5′ end of the reverse primer. Adding four additional random nucleotides on the 5′ end of each primer will also facilitate restriction enzyme binding and cleavage. Primers should therefore have the following sequence: NNNN-GGATCC binding region (forward primer) and NNNN-GAATTC binding region (reverse primer).
2. Agarose gel electrophoresis buffer (TAE buffer): 40 mM Tris acetate, 1 mM EDTA, pH 8.3.
3. Prepare 1% agarose electrophoresis gel by mixing 0.5 g of low-melt agarose with 50 mL of TAE buffer. Bring to a boil and add ethidium bromide (2 μg/mL). Cast the gel in a gel electrophoresis cassette.
4. Lysogeny broth and agar media: to prepare Lysogeny broth (LB), mix 10 g tryptone, 5 g yeast extract, and 10 g of sodium chloride in 1 L of distilled water. For Lysogeny agar (LA), add 15 g of bacterial agar. Adjust the pH at 7.4 and sterilize by autoclaving. For supplementation with antibiotics, bring the sterilized molten medium to 56 °C and add 100 μg/mL carbenicillin (use in *E. coli*) or 1,500 μg/mL trimethoprim (use in *P. aeruginosa*) of the antibiotic. To prepare trimethoprim stock, dissolve 75 mg/mL in DMSO. Pour the medium into Petri dishes and store at 4 °C for a maximum of 7 days.

5. Additional materials and buffers required: High-fidelity *taq* polymerase, BamHI, and EcoRI enzymes, DNA ligase, and their respective restriction buffers; 3 M sodium acetate solution, isopropanol. The plasmid pUC18T-mini-Tn7T-*lux*-Tp is also necessary to perform the cloning procedure [4]; however, other lux plasmids could also be adapted for this same protocol.

2.2 In Vivo Detection of Promoter Activity in G. mellonella

1. Pseudomonas isolation broth and agar media: to prepare Pseudomonas isolation broth (PIB), mix 20 g of peptone, 1.4 g of magnesium chloride, 10 g of potassium sulfate, 25 mg of Irgasan, and 20 mL of glycerol in 1 L of distilled water. For Pseudomonas isolation agar (PIA), add 13.6 g of bacterial agar. Sterilize by autoclaving. Pour the medium into Petri dishes and store at 4 °C for a maximum of 7 days.
2. A minimum of 10 *G. mellonella* wax worms should be used for each condition and strain tested. The worms should be used within 14 days of their purchase to avoid differences in age and weight between experiments. All dead worms and cocoons should be removed (*see* **Note 1**).
3. 10 mM $MgSO_4/H_2O$ (autoclaved).
4. 70% ethanol/H_2O.

2.3 In Vivo Detection of Promoter Activity in L. romana

1. *L. romana* lettuce can be obtained from grocery stores. The leaves must be as similar as possible between the different samples. Do not use the leaves on the exterior or at the center of the lettuce.
2. For this protocol, prepare 5 L of a solution of 0.1% bleach and a solution of 10 mM $MgSO_4$ (autoclave). Additionally, sterilize 5 L of distilled water by autoclaving.

2.4 Detection of Bioluminescence in Murine Models of Infection

1. Prepare phosphate-buffered saline (PBS) by mixing 7.65 g of NaCl, 0.72 g of Na_2HPO_4 and 0.21 g of K_2HPO_4 in 1 L of distilled water and sterilize by autoclaving.
2. Prepare the anesthetic solution by following institutionally approved protocols and guidelines.

3 Methods

Carry out all procedures at ambient temperature unless otherwise indicated. Follow regulations for handling and discarding biohazardous agents and carcinogenic chemicals such as ethidium bromide.

3.1 Promoter Amplification and Cloning to Generate a Reporter System

In this section, we describe how to generate a reporter system to study the activity of a promoter of interest using standard molecular methods. However, it is important to note that the vector pUC18T-mini-Tn7T-*lux*-Tp can also be used directly without additional modifications for direct bacterial labeling.

1. Amplify the promoter region of interest using standard PCR methods (*see* **Note 2**). Verify the length of the amplification product by running it on a 1% agarose gel.
2. Clean 100 μL of the amplification product by adding 20 μL of 3 M sodium acetate and 80 μL of isopropanol. Place at −80 °C for a minimum of 15 min. Centrifuge at 13,000 rpm (10,000 × *g*) on a table top centrifuge for 20 min. Carefully pipette off the supernatant and wash the pellet with 70% ethanol and repeat the centrifugation step. Remove the supernatant and resuspend the pellet in DNAse-free water. Alternatively, commercially available DNA cleanup kits can also be used.
3. Digest the purified PCR product and the plasmid pUC18T-mini-Tn7T-*lux*-Tp [4] with EcoRI and BamHI following the enzyme manufacturer's instructions (*see* **Note 3**). Run the plasmid on a 1% agarose gel. Restriction digestion of the plasmid pUC18T-mini-Tn7T-*lux*-Tp with EcoRI and BamHI should generate three bands: 11,324 kb (backbone, band of interest), 391 bp (excised P1 promoter), and 35 bp (difficult to visualize on a gel). Excise the band corresponding to the size of the backbone and purify it using a commercial kit and the manufacturer's instructions.
4. Ligate the digested PCR product and plasmid following the manufacturer's instructions. Electroporate 1–3 μL of ligation reaction into *Escherichia coli* electrocompetent cells (*see* **Note 4**). Allow the cells to recover and plate various dilutions on LA supplemented with carbenicillin at 100 μg/mL. Incubate overnight to allow recombinant colonies to grow.
5. Using standard molecular microbiology methodologies (restriction digestion, PCR, or sequencing), verify the correct insertion of the promoter of interest in the plasmid. This plasmid will be referred in the remainder of this chapter as pUC18T-mini-Tn7T-*lux*-Tp*.
6. Integrate pUC18T-mini-Tn7T-*lux*-Tp* onto the chromosome of the strain of interest (here, *P. aeruginosa* type strain PAO1) using tri-parental mating. To do so, grow overnight *E. coli* strains carrying pUC18T-mini-Tn7T-*lux*-Tp* and pTNS3 [5] and *P. aeruginosa* PAO1 in Lysogeny broth in the presence of antibiotics (*see* **Note 5**). Centrifuge 1 mL of each culture at 13,000 rpm (10,000 × *g*) and pour the supernatants out. Combine the pellets and plate the cells in the center of an LA plate. Incubate overnight at 37 °C. Using a swab,

resuspend the cells in 1 mL of LB and plate various dilutions on LA supplemented with trimethoprim at 1500 μg/mL. Incubate overnight to allow recombinant colonies to grow (*see* **Note 6**).

7. Bioluminescence 96-well plate growth and stimulation assays can be used to accurately measure the activity of the promoter of interest in vitro (*see* **Note 7**). This high-throughput assay can be used to screen for numerous conditions potentially affecting promotor activity in a single assay. Grow the bacterial strains overnight, dilute them in a fresh medium, and place them into promoter-inducing conditions. Place 100 to 200 μL of culture in triplicate in a 96-well plate with white walls and incubate at the temperature of interest under constant shaking. Measure luminescence and absorbance (600 nm) at regular intervals using a bioluminescence microplate reader (Fig. 2b).
8. To determine promoter activity, divide the number of counts per second (measurement of light emitted) by the absorbance at 600 nm to correct for relative differences in cell number between strains and growth phases.

3.2 In Vivo Detection of Promoter Activity in *G. mellonella*

In this section, we describe how promoter activity can be tested in an in vivo model of infection of the wax worm *G. mellonella* with *P. aeruginosa* bacteria.

1. Grow overnight cultures of *P. aeruginosa* with the *lux* reporter on the chromosome in LB. Dilute the suspension 1:100 in the same culture medium and grow until the bacteria reach mid-exponential phase (e.g., $OD_{600} = 0.4$).
2. Pellet the cultures and resuspend the pellets in 10 mM $MgSO_4$. Using a spectrophotometer, adjust bacterial concentration to a final OD_{600} of 0.1 in 10 mM $MgSO_4$ (*see* **Note 8**). Prepare serial dilutions in 10 mM $MgSO_4$ (10-fold dilutions). Plate 5 μL of each dilution on PIA plates to count the number of CFU injected in each worm.
3. Place the insect between the thumb and forefinger. Using a sterile swab soaked in 70% ethanol, swab the skin of the worm around the site of infection. Allow the ethanol to dry and inject 5 μL of bacterial suspension into the larvae via the hindmost left proleg. Inject a minimum of 10 worms per dilution for each strain. Include 5–10 larvae injected with 10 mM $MgSO_4$ only as a negative control.
4. Larvae infected should be left to incubate at 37 °C on a 9 cm petri dish without food (10 larvae/dish). Worms should be monitored as soon as 12 h and up to 48 h post infection.
5. Measure bacterial luciferase activity using bioluminescence imaging equipment such as ChemiDoc XRS or Touch (Biorad) at regular intervals (Fig. 3).

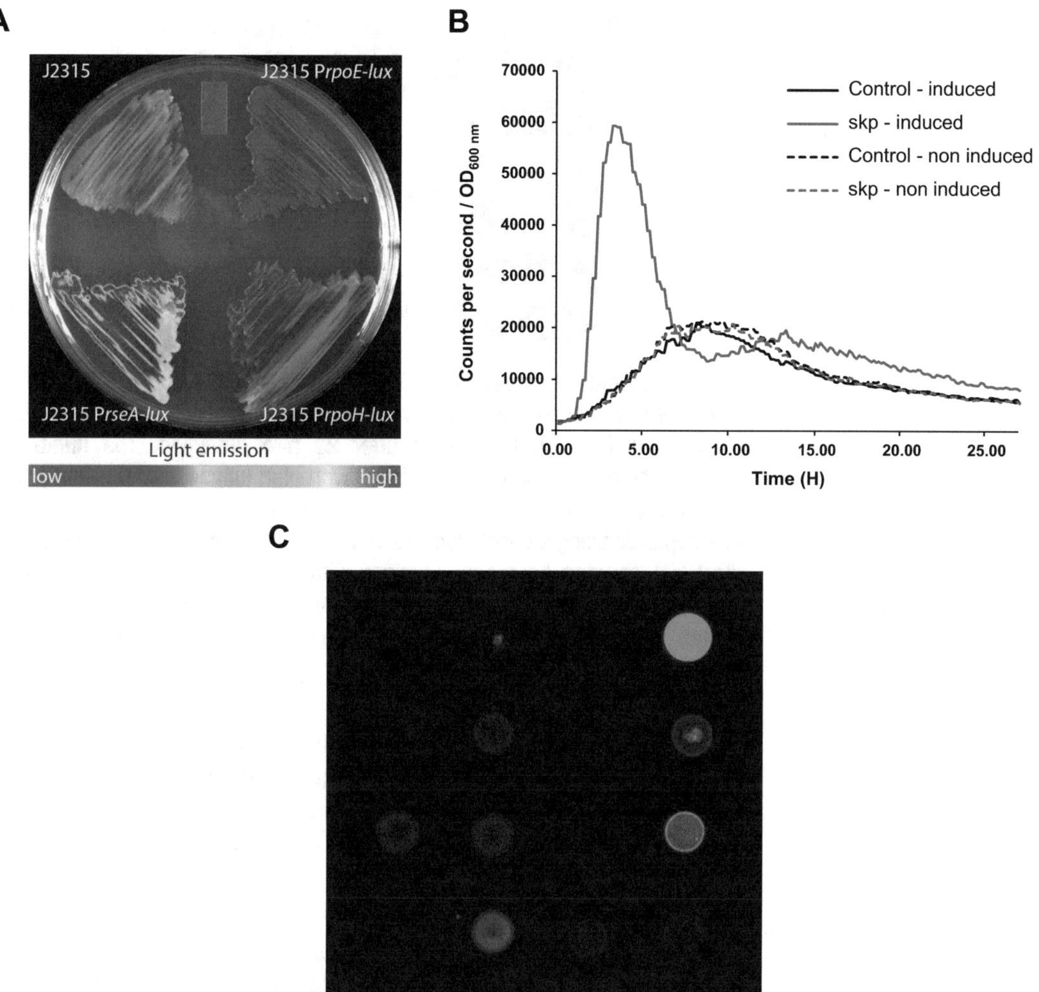

Fig. 2 Detection of luciferase activity in vitro. (**a**) Detection of *Burkholderia cenocepacia* promoters P_{rpoE}, P_{rseA}, and P_{rpoH} fusions with *lux* constructed using pUC18T-mini-Tn7T-*lux*-Tp integrated on the chromosome of the strain J2315. Colonies were grown on LA for 24 h at 37 °C and imaged using a ChemiDoc XRS+ (Biorad). (**b**) Bacterial luminescence measured in counts per second and divided by optical density at 600 nm measured in cultures of *P. aeruginosa* grown at 29 °C in Pseudomonas isolation broth. The amount of bioluminescence reflects the activity of the *P. aeruginosa* P_{algD} promoter (reflecting alginate expression) driving expression of *lux* in conditions where the expression of the gene *skp*, encoding a chaperone, was induced *in trans* (continuous lines, induction with 0.5% arabinose) or not (dashed lines, no arabinose). Measurements were taken every 15 min using a Spectramax I3 (Molecular Devices). (**c**) Detection of the activity of the *P. aeruginosa* P*algD* promoter in response to the induction of various genes of interests *in trans*. Overnight bacterial culture was diluted 1:50 in a fresh medium and 5 μL were inoculated for each strain on PIA plates containing 300 μg/mL carbenicillin and 0.5% arabinose. Bioluminescence was detected using a ChemiDoc Touch (Biorad) and false colored. Bioluminescence and white light images were then superimposed using Photoshop (Adobe) (http:/tinyurl.com/clzy830) [4]

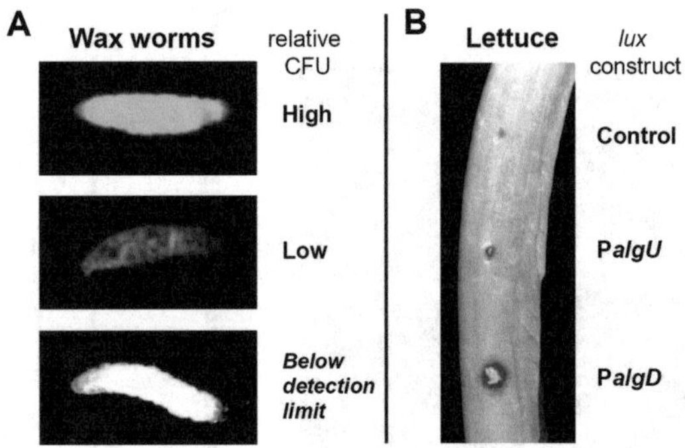

Fig. 3 Bacterial luciferase detection in *G. mellonella* and *L. romana*. (**a**) *G. mellonella* worms harboring various amounts of *P. aeruginosa* PA01 pUC18T-mini-Tn7T-*lux*-Tp imaged after 22 h of infection. The number of colony forming units (CFU) in the picture with high luminescence levels (top) is equivalent to 6×10^9 CFU/g of worm. White light and bioluminescence images were captured using a ChemiDoc Touch (Biorad). (**b**) Lettuce mid-ribs inoculated with PA01 carrying *lux* reporter fusions with the P*algD* and P*algU* promoters. White light and bioluminescence signals were detected using a ChemiDoc XRS+ (Biorad). In A and C, images were superimposed in Photoshop (Adobe) (http:/tinyurl.com/clzy830) [4]

6. After counting the number of dead worms for each dose, the LD_{50} of each strain can be determined using the method of Reed-Muench [6]. At time points of interest, euthanize the worms and homogenize in $MgSO_4$. Plate serial dilutions of the homogenates on PIA to enumerate the number of viable bacteria in each worm (*see* **Note 9**).
7. Measure promoter activity by analyzing luminescence intensity (densitometry) on the picture of each worm using software such as ImageJ [7].

3.3 In Vivo Detection of Promoter Activity in *L. romana*

1. Wash the leaves of a *L. romana* lettuce for 1 min with 0.1% bleach, then rinse them in sterile distilled water. Cut the sides and the top to leave only the rib. Cut fragments of the same size for each sample and allow them dry for 30 min.
2. Grow *P. aeruginosa* PAO1 pUC18T-mini-Tn7T-*lux*-Tp overnight in Lysogeny broth. Dilute the suspension 1:100 in fresh Lysogeny broth and grow the bacteria until mid-exponential phase. Pellet the cells and wash the pellet twice using sterile 10 mM $MgSO_4$. Resuspend the cells at an absorbance of 0.1 at OD_{600} (*see* **Note 8**).
3. Inject 10 μL of bacterial suspension in the top of the midrib in triplicate and incubate it in closed containers with absorbent paper soaked with sterile 10 mM $MgSO_4$ at the desired temperature. Monitor the size of the rotten area around the inoculation point daily.

4. Detect bacterial luminescence in the lettuce using bioluminescent imaging equipment such as the ChemiDoc Touch (Biorad) (Fig. 3b).

3.4 Detection of Bioluminescence in Murine Models of Infection

This section describes how luminescent reporter systems can be used to image bacteria in murine hosts. Here, we use an intranasal infection model as an example of detection of luciferase expression in the lung during acute respiratory infection. However, this method can also be used with other types of infections [8]. All the animal experiments must receive prior approval from institutional committees and be conducted following institutional regulations.

1. Grow *P. aeruginosa* strains harboring the *lux* reporter on PIA overnight. Transfer the cells to PBS and adjust the optical density to $OD_{600} = 1$ in sterile PBS (*see* **Note 10**). Plate serial dilutions of the suspension on PIA to enumerate the number of viable bacteria in the suspension.
2. Anesthetize the mice following institutional guidelines.
3. Once mice are fully unconscious, administer 10 μL of bacterial suspension in each nostril using a pipette tip. Monitor the mouse to ensure complete inhalation of the dose and stable breathing after administration. Mice should then be placed on their dorsal side in their cages and monitored until regaining consciousness.
4. Twenty four hours post-infection, image mice using In Vivo Imaging Systems (IVIS, Perkin Elmer) for noninvasive analysis (Fig. 4a). Create regions of interest and calculate luminescence

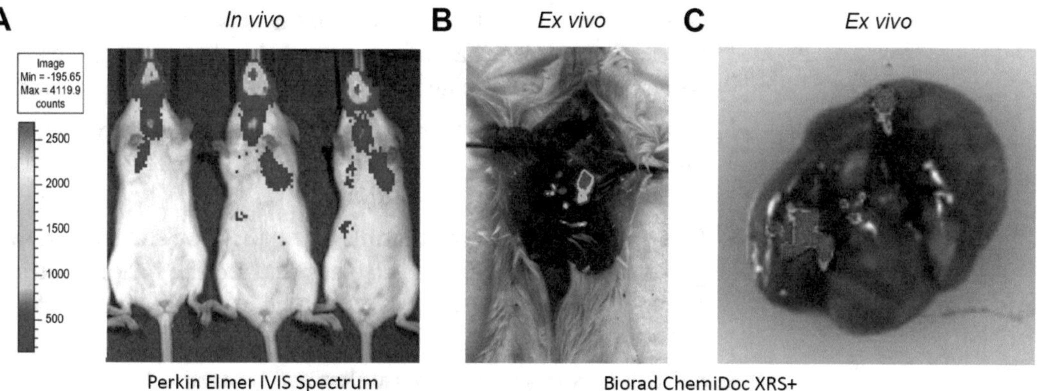

Fig. 4 In vivo and ex vivo bacterial luminescence imaging in murine models of infection. (**a**) CD1 mice 24 h post intranasal infection with *Bordetella pertussis* carrying the P1 *lux* fusion on the chromosome imaged using the IVIS Spectrum imaging system (Perkin Elmer). (**b**) BALBc mouse infected intranasally with *P. aeruginosa* PA01 carrying the P1 *lux* fusion on the chromosome. (**c**) Lung of a Gp91phox- (B6.129S-Cybbtm1Din/J) mouse infected intranasally with *B. cenocepacia* carrying the P1 *lux* fusion on the chromosome. In B and C, mice and tissue were imaged using a ChemiDoc XRS+ (Biorad). Luminescence and white light image were superimposed using Photoshop (Adobe) (http:/tinyurl.com/clzy830) [4]

to determine changes in luciferase activity over time, as described in Chapter XX of this volume. To determine luminescence in tissues ex vivo, euthanize the animal per IACUC guidelines. Harvest tissues and analyze luminescence using non-specialized equipment such as the ChemiDoc XRS or Touch (Biorad) (Fig. 4b, c). Promoter activity is measured by counting the counts per second on an area/tissue of interest compared to background signal. Images of luminescence signals and white light images can then be overlaid using programs such as Photoshop (Adobe) and published scripts (http://tinyurl.com/clzy830) [4] for visual representation of the data (Fig. 4).

4 Notes

1. *G. mellonella* wax worms can be obtained from numerous vendors. Maintain the worms in a dry and cool place. Humidity and low temperatures (i.e., 4 °C) will significantly affect worm viability. Do not store the worms for more than 14 days after purchase as the worms have reached a life stage in which they do not feed and their weight decreases over time.
2. Amplification can be optimized by designing two sets of primers. A first set with perfect annealing can be used for a first round of amplification. PCR product can then be purified and a second round of PCR performed using the primers indicated in Subheading 2.1, **item 1**.
3. pUC18T-mini-Tn*7*T-*lux*-Tp contain the robust P1 promoter which drives constitutive *luxCDBAE* gene expression. Digestion with EcoRI and BamHI removes this promoter and creates cohesive ends for the ligation with the promoter of interest.
4. Electrocompetent *Escherichia coli* cells can be prepared following previously described methodologies [9, 10] or purchased directly from numerous vendors.
5. If the strains used in the mating do not encode the *tra* and *mob* genes required to transfer the plasmids into the recipient strain, a helper strain carrying a plasmid such as pRK2013 should be added to the mating [11].
6. pTNS3 encodes a transposase that will transpose mini-Tn7 containing the *lux* operon to the chromosome of *P. aeruginosa*. During this process, the carbenicillin resistance cassette is lost. However, the trimethoprim resistance cassette will be transferred to the chromosome with mini-Tn7 and can therefore be used for the selection of transposon insertions. Additionally, auxotrophic *E. coli* strains such as RHO3 can be used to facilitate counter selection when using selective media is not possible [12].

7. Other methodologies can be used to test the activity of a promoter. For example, bacterial colonies or suspensions can be exposed to photographic film to capture the emission of photons from the cultures, or imaged with instruments such as the GelTouch imaging system (Biorad) (Fig. 2a, c). Strong promoter activity may be visible with the naked eye in a dark room.
8. A suspension prepared at that optical density should correspond to around 10^7 CFU/mL for PAO1. This density may require adjustment for other strains or species.
9. One significant advantage of using *lux* expressing bacteria is that the bacteria infecting the worm can easily be differentiated from contaminating microflora using bioluminescence imaging. This technique also facilitates automated colony counting.
10. A suspension at an $OD_{600} = 1$ prepared in these conditions has a final concentration of approximately 2.5×10^9 CFU/mL. Administration of 10 μL of this suspension in each nostril is therefore equivalent to the administration of 5×10^7 CFU/mouse. This dose is sub-lethal in outbred mice and should be cleared within 48–72 h.

References

1. Baldwin TO, Christopher JA, Raushel FM et al (1995) Structure of bacterial luciferase. Curr Opin Struct Biol 5:798–809
2. Choi K-H, Schweizer HP (2006) Mini-Tn7 insertion in bacteria with single attTn7 sites: example *Pseudomonas aeruginosa*. Nat Protoc 1:153–161. https://doi.org/10.1038/nprot.2006.24
3. Choi K-H, Gaynor JB, White KG et al (2005) A Tn7-based broad-range bacterial cloning and expression system. Nat Methods 2:443–448. https://doi.org/10.1038/nmeth765
4. Damron FH, McKenney ES, Barbier M et al (2013) Construction of mobilizable mini-Tn7 vectors for bioluminescent detection of gram-negative bacteria and single-copy promoter lux reporter analysis. Appl Environ Microbiol 79:4149–4153. https://doi.org/10.1128/AEM.00640-13
5. Choi K-H, Mima T, Casart Y et al (2008) Genetic tools for select-agent-compliant manipulation of *Burkholderia pseudomallei*. Appl Environ Microbiol 74:1064–1075. https://doi.org/10.1128/AEM.02430-07
6. Reed LJ, Muench H (1938) A simple method of estimating fifty per cent endpoints. Am J Epidemiol 27:493–497
7. Schneider CA, Rasband WS, Eliceiri KW (2012) NIH image to ImageJ: 25 years of image analysis. Nat Methods 9:671–675
8. Weiner ZP, Ernst SM, Boyer AE et al (2014) Circulating lethal toxin decreases the ability of neutrophils to respond to *Bacillus anthracis*. Cell Microbiol 16:504–518. https://doi.org/10.1111/cmi.12232
9. Choi KH, Kumar A, Schweizer HP (2006) A 10-min method for preparation of highly electrocompetent *Pseudomonas aeruginosa* cells: application for DNA fragment transfer between chromosomes and plasmid transformation. J Microbiol Methods 64:391–397. https://doi.org/10.1016/j.mimet.2005.06.001
10. Sambrook DWJR (2001) Molecular cloning: a laboratory manual, 3rd edn. Cold Spring Harbor Laboratory Press, Cold Spring Harbor
11. Figurski DH, Helinski DR (1979) Replication of an origin-containing derivative of plasmid RK2 dependent on a plasmid function provided in trans. Proc Natl Acad Sci U S A 76:1648–1652
12. López CM, Rholl DA, Trunck LA, Schweizer HP (2009) Versatile dual-technology system for markerless allele replacement in *Burkholderia pseudomallei*. Appl Environ Microbiol 75:6496–6503. https://doi.org/10.1128/AEM.01669-09

Chapter 8

Production of GFP and Luciferase-Expressing Reporter Macrophages for In Vivo Bioluminescence Imaging

Jukka Pajarinen, Tzu-Hua Lin, and Stuart B. Goodman

Abstract

Macrophages have emerged as crucial regulators of tissue homeostasis, inflammation, and tissue regeneration. In vivo bioluminescence imaging could offer a powerful tool to study many poorly understood aspects of macrophage biology. Thus, we recently developed a straightforward method for the production of large numbers of green fluorescent protein (GFP) and firefly luciferase (fLUC)-expressing reporter macrophages for various in vivo bioluminescence imaging applications. Lentivirus vector containing the GFP/fLUC reporter gene is produced and mouse bone marrow macrophages are isolated following established protocols. Macrophages are then exposed to the lentivirus in the presence of 10 μM cyclosporine for 24 h. After a 24-h recovery period, the transduction is repeated. Three days after the second infection the cells are ready to be used in vivo. Following this cyclosporine-mediated double infection strategy up to 60% of the macrophages express GFP in flow cytometry. The macrophages maintain their ability to polarize to M1 and M2 phenotypes and, when injected to the systemic circulation of a mouse model, reporter cells are both easily detectable with BLI and migrate to a local site of inflammation. These GFP/fLUC-expressing reporter macrophages could prove to be useful tools to study the role of macrophages in health and disease.

Key words Macrophage, Lentivirus, Bioluminescence imaging, Firefly luciferase, Green fluorescent protein

1 Introduction

Macrophages have emerged as key regulators of tissue homeostasis, inflammation, and tissue regeneration [1]. Aberrant macrophage function has been implicated in a wide variety of conditions including arthritis, atherosclerosis, cancer, metabolic syndrome, etc. [2–4]. In the field of biomaterial science, macrophages play a key role in successful implant integration, and modulation of their function has emerged as one effective means to counter adverse foreign body response [5, 6]. Similarly, harnessing macrophages' potential for tissue regeneration and tissue engineering has attracted growing interest [7, 8].

Despite the recent advances made in understanding macrophage biology, many aspects of macrophage in vivo behavior and

Purnima Dubey (ed.), *Reporter Gene Imaging: Methods and Protocols*, Methods in Molecular Biology, vol. 1790,
https://doi.org/10.1007/978-1-4939-7860-1_8,

properties remain poorly understood. Green fluorescent protein (GFP) and firefly luciferase (fLUC)-expressing reporter macrophages offer a useful tool to study many of these poorly understood aspects of macrophages including systemic recruitment, chemotaxis, and survival. Furthermore, the ability to follow and quantify the recruitment and local survival of macrophages in various disease models could be useful to identify pathophysiological mechanisms and to develop novel treatments.

Production of such cells has however been hindered by the relative difficulty of successful reporter gene transfer into mouse primary macrophages [9, 10]. Alternately, direct isolation of macrophages from fLUC transgenic mice would be an elegant way to obtain reporter macrophages [11, 12]. However, variable and stain-dependent expression of the reporter gene with the time laborious process of backcrossing the GFP/fLUC reporter gene into new mouse strains limit the usefulness of this otherwise elegant approach [13].

Following the initial discovery that cyclosporine is highly effective agent in facilitating lentivirus-mediated gene transfer into mouse primary cells, we recently developed an effective and straightforward method for the production of large numbers of GFP/fLUC-expressing reporter macrophages for various in vivo bioluminescence imaging (BLI) applications [9, 13]. Lentivirus vector containing the reporter gene is produced and mouse bone marrow macrophages isolated following established protocols [14–16]. Purified macrophage cultures are then subjected to the lentivirus vector in the presence of 10 μM cyclosporine for 24 h. After the first transduction the cells are allowed to recover for 24 h after which the 24-h lentivirus infection is repeated. 72 h after the second infection the reporter gene expression is analyzed and the cells are ready to be used in vivo.

Following this cyclosporine-mediated double infection strategy up to 60% of the macrophages express GFP in flow cytometry, with a correspondingly strong signal detectable from cell lysates using a luminometer [13]. The reporter macrophages are not activated by the transduction and maintain their ability to polarize to M1 and M2 phenotypes. When injected to the systemic circulation of a mouse model, reporter cells are both easily detectable with BLI and migrate to a local site of inflammation [13]. These GFP/fLUC-expressing reporter macrophages could prove to be useful tools to study the role of macrophages in health and disease.

2 Materials

2.1 Lentiviral Production

1. The lentiviral vector plasmids including pFU-Luc-GFP, psPAX2, and pMD2G (*see* **Note 1**) are kept at −20 °C. For long-term storage and plasmid amplification, the plasmid is

transformed into Stbl3 competent cells (*see* **Note 2**) and stored at −80 °C with glycerol (>12 months).

2. Human embryonic kidney (HEK) 293 cell line (CRL-1573™, ATCC).
3. HEK 293 growth media: Dulbecco's modified Eagle medium (DMEM, high glucose, pyruvate,) supplied with 10% fetal bovine serum (FBS) and antibiotic-antimycotic solution (100 units of penicillin, 100 mg of streptomycin, and 0.25 mg of amphotericin B per mL is stored at 4 °C (>2 months).
4. Trypsin-EDTA 0.25%.
5. CalPhos™ mammalian transfection kit (Clontech), or similar reagent. 2× HEPES-buffered saline (HBS, pH 7.05) is dispensed into small aliquots for one-time transfection and stored at −20 °C (>6 months, avoid multiple freeze-thaw cycles). Calcium solution (2 M $CaCl_2$) and sterile water is stored at 4 °C (*see* **Note 3**).
6. 10 mM Chloroquine is stored at −20 °C (>6 months).
7. T175 tissue culture flask.
8. 6 mg/mL polybrene (hexadimethrine bromide) is stored at −20 °C (>6 months).
9. Flow cytometry buffer: Phosphate-buffered saline (PBS) supplied with 2% FBS and 5 mM Ethylenediaminetetraacetic acid (EDTA) is stored at 4 °C (>2 months).
10. 5 mL polystyrene round-bottom tubes.
11. FFlow cytometer.

2.2 Isolation and Culture of Mouse Bone Marrow Macrophages

1. BALB/cByJ mice aged 6–8 weeks (The Jackson Laboratory) (*see* **Note 4**).
2. Ethanol.
3. Sterile surgical instruments.
4. Basal media: RPMI 1640 medium supplemented with 10% heat inactivated FBS and 100 mg of streptomycin, and 0.25 mg of amphotericin B per mL. Stored at 4 °C (>2 months).
5. 10 cm cell culture dishes.
6. 6 mL Syringes.
7. 25-gauge needles.
8. 50 mL conical centrifuge tubes.
9. 100 μm pore size cell strainers.
10. Red blood cell lysis buffer.
11. Complete macrophage culture media: RPMI 1640 with 10% FBS, 30% L929 cell-conditioned medium (see **Note 5**), 10 ng/mL macrophage colony-stimulating factor (M-CSF,)

and 100 mg of streptomycin and 0.25 mg of amphotericin B per mL. Store at 4 °C (>2 months).

12. T175 tissue culture flasks.
13. Trypsin-EDTA 0.25%.
14. Cell scrapers.

2.3 Macrophage Transduction

1. Lentivirus containing HEK 293 cell supernatant.
2. Complete macrophage culture media.
3. Cyclosporine dissolved at 50 mM in DMSO and stored at −20 °C.

2.4 Analysis of Successful Transduction

1. Flow cytometry buffer is stored at 4 °C (>2 months).
2. Fixable viability dye eFluo® 506 (eBioscience) or similar reagent.
3. 5 mL polystyrene round bottom tubes.
4. Flow cytometer.
5. Luciferase assay system with reporter lysis buffer (Promega).
6. Protein assay reagent.
7. Luminometer.

2.5 In Vivo Bioluminescence Imaging

1. Trypsin-EDTA 0.25%.
2. Cell scrapers.
3. 50 mL conical centrifuge tubes.
4. 1.5 mL microcentrifuge tubes.
5. Ice-cold HBSS.
6. 0.5 mL insulin syringes.
7. Luciferin (30 mg/mL in PBS), stored at −20 °C.
8. IVIS 100 in vivo imaging system with Living image analysis software (Perkin Elmer) or a similar machine.

3 Methods

3.1 Lentiviral Production

1. HEK 293 cells are cultured in DMEM growth media to 80–90% confluence.
2. The growth media is removed and the cells are detached by trypsin solution a day before transfection. The cells are counted and 1.5×10^7 (in 25 mL growth media) cells are plated in T175 tissue culture flask.
3. Before transfection, the growth media is replaced by 25 mL of media supplemented with 40 μM Chloroquine immediately prior to preparing the solutions A and B.

4. Prepare solution A in a 50 mL tube containing 15 μg pFU--Luc-EGFP, 10 μg psPAX2, 5 μg pMD2G, and 133 μL of 2 M CaCl2 solution. Bring the total volume to 1110 μL by adding sterile water.
5. Vortex the solution A well, and then incubate on ice for 5 min.
6. Slowly add 1110 μL Solution B (2× HBS) dropwise to Solution A by using 1000 μL pipette. Vortex the tube while adding solution B. This step should take approximately 1–2 min.
7. Incubate the solution mixture (A plus B) on ice for 15–30 min (*see* **Note 6**).
8. After the incubation, add the solution mixture (A plus B) dropwise with a 5 mL pipette to the chloroquine containing media in the cell culture flask.
9. Swirl the mixture around gently and then tilt the flask to cover all the cells with the medium.
10. Incubate the flask in the incubator at 37 °C for 6–8 h (*see* **Note 6**).
11. Remove transfection media and replace with 40 mL warm medium.
12. Harvest the supernatant for 48 h after transfection. The GFP expression should be observed in >99% of transfected HEK 293 cells.
13. Centrifuge the collected media at 600 × *g* for 5 min, and collect the supernatant containing the virus. Filter the supernatant through the 0.45 μm membrane.
14. Aliquot the virus into the desired volume and store at −80 °C (>6 months). Keep a smaller amount (0.5–1 mL) of virus for titration.
15. For virus titration, plate 20,000 HEK 293 cells per well in a 24-well plate one day before the infection.
16. On the day of infection, prepare serial diluted virus in HEK 293 cell growth media supplied with 6 μg/mL polybrene at 2× (300 μL virus supernatant plus 300 μL media), 20× (30 μL supernatant plus 570 μL media), 200× (3 μL supernatant plus 597 μL media), and media control.
17. Remove the media from HEK 293 cells, and add 500 μL of diluted samples. Incubate the cells overnight in the incubator at 37 °C. Replace with warm media containing no virus and polybrene.
18. Harvest the cells 72 h post-infection. Resuspend the cells in flow cytometry buffer and analysis the GFP expression using a flow cytometer.

19. The virus titer = cell amount * (GFP + %) × dilution factor / media volume. For example, 20,000 cells * 50% GFP (+) * 200× dilution / 0.5 mL media = 4 × 10^6 infection unit per mL (*see* **Note 7**).

3.2 Isolation and Culture of Mouse Bone Marrow Macrophages

1. Euthanize the mice with CO_2 followed by cervical dislocation immediately prior to the cell isolation (*see* **Note 4**).
2. Sterilize the mice by immerging in 70% ethanol for 2 × 2 min.
3. Using surgical instruments and aseptic technique dissect the femora end tibia free of all the soft tissues (*see* **Note 8**). Place the cleaned bones in basal media in 10 cm cell culture dishes.
4. Cut off the proximal and distal ends of the bone exposing the medullary canal. Be careful not to remove too much of the bone marrow rich metaphyseal trabecular bone region.
5. Flush out the bone marrow into 50 mL centrifuge tube using a 25-gauge needle, 6 mL syringe, and 5 mL of basal media per bone (*see* **Note 9**).
6. Gently mix the cell suspension by pipetting. Filter the bone marrow cells through a 100 μm cell strainer into another 50 mL tube and centrifuge 400 × *g* for 10 min.
7. Remove the supernatant and resuspend the cells with 1 mL of ice-cold red blood cell lysis buffer and incubate for 2 min on ice.
8. Add 20 mL of basal media to stop the cell lysis and centrifuge 400 × *g* for 10 min.
9. Remove the supernatant and resuspend the cells in 10 mL of complete macrophage culture media. Count and plate a total of 5 × 10^7 bone marrow cells per T175 flask in 25 mL of complete macrophage culture media.
10. Change the media at days 2 and 4 to remove the non-adherent bone marrow cells. The adherent cells are bone marrow macrophages. The cultures should be confluent by day 6 (Fig. 1a) (*see* **Note 10**).
11. After reaching confluence split the cells 1:2. Lift with 0.25% Trypsin-EDTA and gentle scraping (*see* **Note 11**). Centrifuge 175 × *g* for 6 min, remove the supernatant, and resuspend in complete macrophage culture media (*see* **Note 12**). Count (*see* **Note 13**) and plate into 175 cm^2 culture flasks or 10cm^2 culture dishes in 25 or 10 mL of culture media respectively.
12. Culture for ~5 days changing media every other day. Allow it to reach 50–80% confluence (5–8 × 10^6 cells/T175 flask) prior to starting the transduction (Fig. 1b).

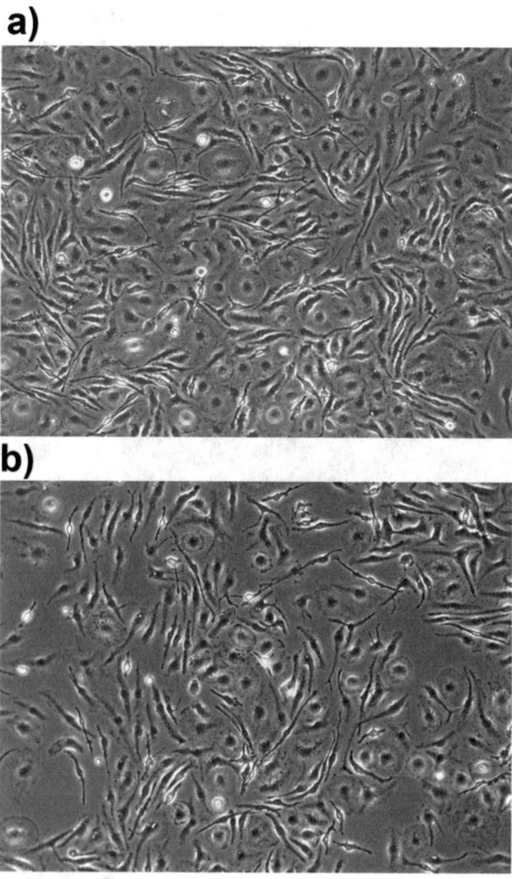

Fig. 1 Phase contrast images of bone marrow macrophages (**a**) Confluent culture 6 days after cell isolation. (**b**) Culture 5 days after subculture ready for transduction at ~70% density

3.3 Macrophage Transduction

1. Prepare macrophage transduction media by mixing a volume of HEK 293 cell supernatant containing the lentivirus with complete macrophage culture media at an approximate ratio of 2:1 and supplement with cyclosporine to a final concentration of 10 μM (*see* **Note 14**). The exact media composition is determined by virus titer and the amount of macrophages transduced with at least 10 infective units per macrophage needed (*see* **Notes 15** and **16**).
2. Remove the media from the macrophage cultures and add a correct volume of transduction media. Incubate in the tissue culture incubator for 24 h.
3. Remove the transduction media and add 25 mL of complete macrophage culture media per flask. Incubate in the tissue culture incubator for 24 h.

4. Remove the media from the macrophage cultures and repeat the transduction by adding a correct volume of transduction media. Incubate in the tissue culture incubator for 24 h.
5. Remove the transduction media and add 25 mL of complete macrophage culture media. Incubate in the tissue culture incubator for 72 h.
6. 72 h after the second transduction GFP positive cells should be visible under fluorescence microscope with ~50% cells showing a weak but detectable signal (Fig. 2a) (*see* **Note 17**).

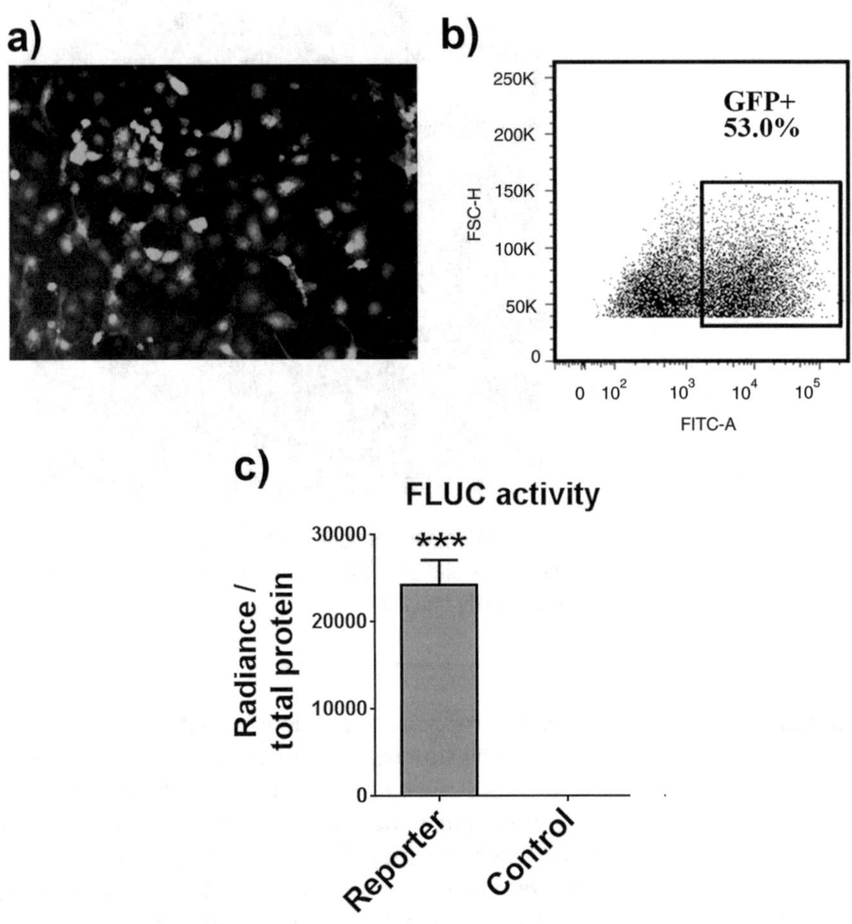

Fig. 2 Reporter gene expression in macrophages 3 days after the second transduction. (**a**) GFP^+ macrophages can be seen in fluorescence microscopy. (**b**) Typical flow cytometry dot blot of the reporter macrophages showing a successful reporter gene transfer in 50–60% of cells. (**c**) Typical luciferase activity observed in reporter macrophages with luminometer. *** $p < 0.001$ Student's T test. Modified from ref. 13 under the Creative Commons Attribution (CC BY) license

3.4 Analysis of Successful Transduction

1. The infected macrophages are detached 72 h post-infection with 0.25% Trypsin-EDTA and gentle scraping. For GFP expression analysis, 5×10^5 cells are washed by PBS and resuspended in 150 μL flow cytometry buffer. For luciferase activity assay, spin down 5×10^5 cells and resuspend in 450 μL reporter lysis buffer.
2. Analyze GFP expression in infected macrophages by flow cytometry. r. Exclude nonviable cells using afixable viability dye. The percentage of GFP positive cells should be around 45–55% of viable macrophages (Fig. 2b). The percentage of nonviable cells should be low, less than 5%.
3. Analyze luciferase activity using a luciferase assay system (Promega) following the manufacturer's protocol. Use a luminometer (to quantify the luminescence signal). Determine total protein concentration using a protein assay kit following the manufacturer's protocol. Normalize luciferase activity to total protein concentration (RLU/μg) (Fig. 2c).

3.5 In Vivo Bioluminescence Imaging

1. Lift the GFP-luciferase-expressing macrophages with 0.25% Trypsin-EDTA and gentle scraping avoiding extended exposure to trypsin. Count the cells and centrifuge at 175 × *g* for 6 min.
2. Remove the supernatant and carefully resuspend in ice-cold HBSS, ~150 μL per 6×10^6 cells (*see* **Notes 18** and **19**).
3. Draw ~200 μL of reporter cell suspension into a 0.5 mL insulin syringe and inject i.v. into the systemic circulation of the desired mouse model via tail vein.
4. Inject luciferin (0.15 mg/gram of body weight) intraperitoneally 10 min prior to in vivo bioluminescence imaging and perform the imaging in two planes (*see* **Note 20**).

4 Notes

1. The lentiviral vector pFu-Luc-EGFP with the expression of luciferase and GFP reporter gene was a gift from Dr. Gambhir's laboratory (Stanford University). The dual reporter lentiviral expression vectors are also commercially available. The packaging vectors of psPAX2 and pMD2G are the 2nd generation of lentiviral vector system developed by the Trono Laboratory. Additional information regarding the lentiviral vector system is available at http://tronolab.epfl.ch/LVG.
2. Stbl3 competent *E. coli* cells have reduced frequency of homologous recombination in long terminal repeats (LTRs) found in lentiviral or retroviral vectors. Please refer to the molecular

cloning protocol or manufacturer's webpages for more information about plasmid transformation, amplification, and preparation.

3. The reagents for calcium phosphate transfection can also be prepared in the laboratory but extreme caution should be taken when adjusting the pH. The pH value in HBS may change during freeze-thaw cycles or storage at 4 °C. Inaccurate pH value in HBS will largely reduce the transfection efficiency in HEK 293 cells.
4. In our hands the isolated bone marrow from the long bones of one mouse yields one confluent flask of macrophages that will produce enough GFP-luciferase-expressing reporter macrophages for injection in one mouse (6×10^6 cells). Thus to image 10 mice, macrophages from 10 donor mice are needed.
5. The L929 conditioned media is produced by culturing L929 cell line in 25 mL of DMEM supplemented with 10% FBS as well as 100 mg of streptomycin and 0.25 mg of amphotericin B per mL in T175 flasks. Collect the media once a week to 50 mL centrifuge tubes. Centrifuge the collected media $400 \times g$ for 10 min to remove any cell debris and store the supernatant (now called L929 conditioned media) in −80 °C (6 months). After media collection, split the cells 1/10 by trypsin-EDTA and repeat the media harvest once a week as needed until passage 4.
6. The incubation time of the solution mixture on ice can also affect the transfection efficiency significantly. The researcher should observe that the transfected cells are covered by black spots at **step 10** with the optimal incubation time. Our optimized condition is to incubate on ice for 20 min. However, the times period may be adjusted depending on the technique of mixing solutions.
7. The virus titer can be up to $1–5 \times 10^6$ per mL. The titer can be enriched up to $1–5 \times 10^8$ by the ultracentrifugation method or by using the filtration-based lentiviral purification kit.
8. 10 cm or 25 cm cell culture dishes are convenient sterile surfaces for the dissection. It is often useful to dissect bones in two stages: first harvest the long bones with the attached soft tissues from the animal and then thoroughly remove soft tissues in the culture dish.
9. The bone should turn white with successful collection of the bone marrow.
10. In the first 24 h after the isolation the number of adherent cells can appear alarmingly low but typically rapidly increase within the first 48–72 h after isolation.

11. Depending on the mouse strain the bone marrow macrophages can be very sensitive to trypsin. Incubate in pre-warmed Trypsin-EDTA for maximum 5 min in +37 °C followed by the addition of at least 2 volumes of complete macrophage media to neutralize the trypsin before scraping.
12. The cell pellet should resuspend easily with gentle pipetting. Difficulty in resuspending the cells indicates extensive cell death due to prolonged exposure to trypsin and/or too harsh scraping. Reduce the time the cells are exposed to trypsin and minimize the time intervals between scraping, spinning, and resuspending the cells.
13. One confluent T175 flask should yield ~1×10^7 macrophages.
14. Vigorous mixing might be required to dissolve the cyclosporine that will first appear as white aggregate when added to the media.
15. For example, with the typically obtained virus titer of ~5×10^6 IU / mL and the typical amount of macrophages in a T175 flask (~5×10^6) at this stage, combine 10 mL of HEK 293 cell supernatant and 5 mL of complete macrophage culture media to achieve sufficient volume (15 mL) and virus amount (multiplicity of infection, MOI 10:1) to transduce macrophages in a one T175 flask. For 10 cm culture dish with about 1×10^6 macrophages use 4 mL of HEK 293 cell supernatant and 2 mL of complete macrophage culture media.
16. Increasing MOI might result in higher transduction efficiency.
17. After the transduction cells can polarized into M1 or M2 phenotype following standard procedures, e.g., exposure to interferon gamma 20 ng/mL or interleukin-4 20 ng/mL for 24 h. However, the GFP-luciferase expression might be altered by the polarization treatment [13].
18. The end volume of the cell suspension will be larger than the added 150 μL due to residual fluid in the cell pellet, typically closer to 200 μL.
19. Be careful to avoid any cell clumps as these can cause significant pulmonary embolism when injected to the venous circulation. Working with injected volumes of 150–200 μL reduced the risk of cell clumping.
20. At the day of the systemic reporter cell injection a clear signal originating from the lungs should be visible followed by migration of cells to the site of inflammation during the subsequent days (Fig. 3a, b). The signal decreases progressively indicating reduction in the reporter cell population; typically the signal is detectable 10–20 days post injection.

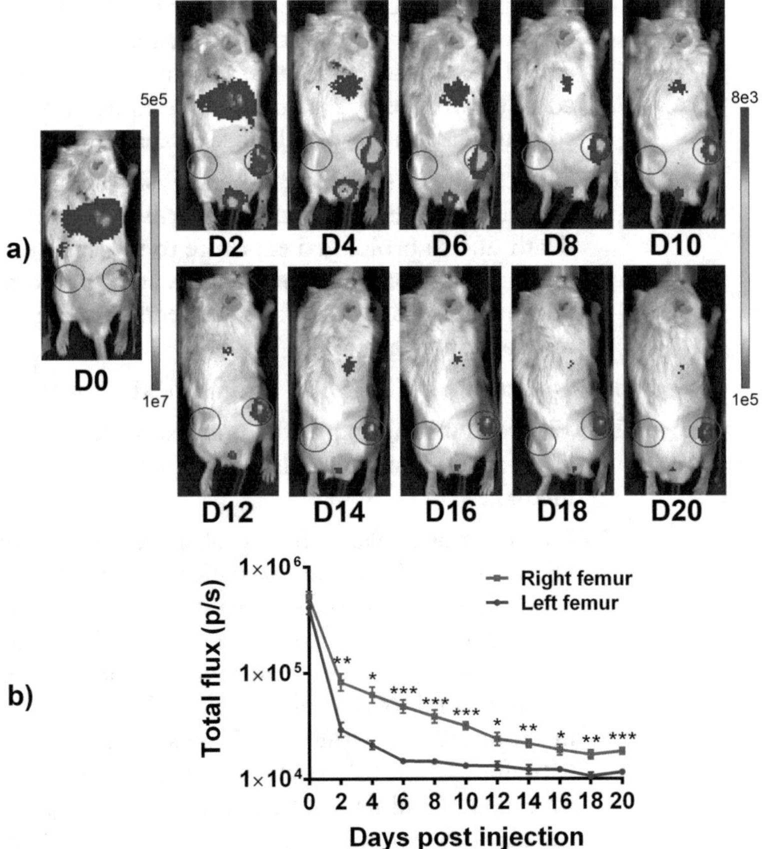

Fig. 3 Reporter macrophages in in vivo bioluminescence imaging. Reporter macrophages were injected into the tail vein of mouse model of biomaterial-induced local inflammation at right distal femur [17]. The cell trafficking was followed by bioluminescence imaging. Luminescence emanating from the local area of inflammation in the right distal femur as well as left distal femur serving as a control was determined from images obtained every other day up to 20 days post injection. (**a**) Bioluminescence images showing the accumulation of reporter cells to the right distal femur starting on the day 2 after the systemic injection of the reporter cells and persisting over the 20 day imaging period. (**b**) XY-blot showing the total flux from regions of interest over the right and left distal femurs. * = $p > 0.05$; ** = $p > 0.01$, *** = $p > 0.001$. Modified from ref. 13 under Creative Commons Attribution (CC BY) license

Acknowledgments

Work was supported by NIH grants 2R01 AR055650 and 1R01AR063717 and the Ellenburg Chair in Surgery in Stanford University. J.P. thanks Jane and Aatos Erkko foundation for postdoctoral fellowship.

References

1. Mosser DM, Edwards JP (2008) Exploring the full spectrum of macrophage activation. Nat Rev Immunol 8:958–969
2. Solinas G, Germano G, Mantovani A et al (2009) Tumor-associated macrophages (TAM) as major players of the cancer-related inflammation. J Leukoc Biol 86:1065–1073
3. Chawla A, Nguyen KD, Goh YP (2011) Macrophage-mediated inflammation in metabolic disease. Nat Rev Immunol 11:738–749
4. Murray PJ, Wynn TA (2011) Protective and pathogenic functions of macrophage subsets. Nat Rev Immunol 11:723–737
5. Nich C, Takakubo Y, Pajarinen J et al (2013) Macrophages-key cells in the response to wear debris from joint replacements. J Biomed Mater Res A 101:3033–3045
6. Goodman SB, Gibon E, Pajarinen J et al (2014) Novel biological strategies for treatment of wear particle-induced periprosthetic osteolysis of orthopaedic implants for joint replacement. J R Soc Interface 11:20130962
7. Brown BN, Sicari BM, Badylak SF (2014) Rethinking regenerative medicine: a macrophage-centered approach. Front Immunol 5:510
8. Nassiri S, Graney P, Spiller KL (2014) Manipulation of macropahges to enhance bone repair and regeneration. In: Zreiqat H, Dunstan CR, Rosen V (eds) A tissue regeneration approach to bone and cartilage repair. Springer, New York. ISBN: 978-3-319-13265-5
9. Noser JA, Towers GJ, Sakuma R et al (2006) Cyclosporine increases human immunodeficiency virus type 1 vector transduction of primary mouse cells. J Virol 80(15):7769–7774
10. Zhang X, Edwards J, Mosser D (2009) The expression of exogenous genes in macrophages: obstacles and opportunities. In: Reiner N (ed) Macrophages and dendritic cells, methods in molecular biology. Springer Protocols, New York, pp 123–143
11. Cao YA, Wagers AJ, Beilhack A et al (2004) Shifting foci of hematopoiesis during reconstitution from single stem cells. Proc Natl Acad Sci U S A 101:221–226
12. Cao YA, Bachmann MH, Beilhack A et al (2005) Molecular imaging using labeled donor tissues reveals patterns of engraftment, rejection, and survival in transplantation. Transplantation 80:134–139
13. Pajarinen J, Lin TH, Sato T et al (2015) Establishment of green fluorescent protein and firefly luciferase expressing mouse primary macrophages for bioluminescence imaging. PLoS One 10:e0142736
14. Zufferey R, Nagy D, Mandel RJ et al (1997) Multiply attenuated lentiviral vector achieves efficient gene delivery in vivo. Nat Biotechnol 15:871–875
15. Weischenfeldt J, Porse B (2008) Bone marrow-derived macrophages (BMM): isolation and applications. CSH Protoc 2008:pdb.prot5080
16. Martinez FO, Helming L, Milde R et al (2013) Genetic programs expressed in resting and IL-4 alternatively activated mouse and human macrophages: similarities and differences. Blood 121:e57–e69
17. Ren PG, Irani A, Huang Z et al (2011) Continuous infusion of UHMWPE particles induces increased bone macrophages and osteolysis. Clin Orthop Relat Res 469:113–122

Chapter 9

Hypoxia-Induced Reporter Genes with Different Half-Lives

Balaji Krishnamachary, Pierre Danhier, Samata Kakkad, Santosh K. Bharti, and Zaver M. Bhujwalla

Abstract

The utility of reporter genes has gained significant momentum over the last three decades. Reporter genes are used to understand the transcriptional activity of a gene both in vitro and in vivo, and in pathway analysis and drug screening for diseases involving protozoan parasites, and in anti-cancer drug developments. Here, using a human prostate cancer xenograft model (PC3), we describe a method to construct and validate hypoxia reporter genes with different half-lives. Using molecular biology and optical imaging techniques, we have validated the expression of long half-life enhanced green fluorescence protein (EGFP) expression and short half-life luciferase gene expression to report on the spatial and temporal evolution of hypoxia in vivo.

Key words Bioluminescence, Lentivirus, Luciferase assay, Hypoxia, Hypoxia response elements (HRE), Reporter gene

1 Introduction

Our understanding of gene function has primarily come from the successful introduction and transfer of genes into cells. Detecting and screening the transformants for phenotypic changes in the transformed cells has advanced from the first use of chloramphenicol acetyltransferase (CAT) as a reporter of enzyme activity [1]. Reporter genes reliably measure gene expression and help in understanding the transcriptional activity of genes in response to a specific signaling event. Subsequently, reporter genes such as acid phosphatase and alkaline phosphatase detected by colorimetry [2, 3] and firefly and renilla luciferase detected by bioluminescence imaging (BLI) have been successfully used as reporters [4–7]. Visualization and localization of successful gene transfer, and corresponding reporter activity has become less challenging since the purification and cloning of green fluorescent protein (GFP) [8, 9]. Colorimetric, BLI, and fluorescence-based reporter genes have both advantages and disadvantages. The GFP protein is a

Purnima Dubey (ed.), *Reporter Gene Imaging: Methods and Protocols*, Methods in Molecular Biology, vol. 1790,
https://doi.org/10.1007/978-1-4939-7860-1_9,

single chain 238 amino acid polypeptide with a compact structure that is stable under various conditions. GFP is minimally toxic and can be noninvasively detected in live cells without cell disruption or addition of an external co-factor, such as luciferin required for BLI. Modifications in the GFP protein to encode a destabilized red-shift variant (d2EGFP) led to brighter fluorescence signals in mammalian cells (excitation max = 488 nm, emission max = 507 nm) and fusion of a sequence rich in proline (P), glutamic acid (E), serine (S), threonine (T) (PEST sequence) on the C-terminus region enabled the degradation of the protein decreasing its half-life in mammalian cells to 9.8 h [10].

Luciferase has been used as a reporter since it was cloned in 1985 [7]. This 550 amino acid, 62 kDa single polypeptide chain enzyme catalyzes the substrate D-luciferin, to emit bioluminescence that is visualized at 562 nm. The disadvantage of luciferase is the need for an additional substrate/co-factor, as well as oxygen and ATP, to detect the reporter. The need to destroy the cell/tissue to determine luciferase reporter activity was considered a disadvantage. However, with the advent of sensitive imaging instruments, bioluminescence can be detected noninvasively. Although the half-life of luciferase is only 2 h, the quantum yield is very high compared to fluorescent reporters, making it a useful reporter gene.

The transcription factor hypoxia inducible factor (HIF) is a heterodimer formed by a constitutively expressed protein subunit HIF-1β and an oxygen regulated protein subunit HIF-1α. In response to hypoxia, HIF binds to response element on the promoter regions of many genes to activate transcription [11]. In a proof-of-principle study, we have cloned five tandem repeats of hypoxia response elements (HREs) to create an artificial promoter and drive the transcription of EGFP and luciferase [12]. This chapter provides in-depth details on the construction, detection, and validation of short and long half-life reporters that are activated in response to hypoxia both in vitro and in vivo.

2 Materials

2.1 Antibodies

EGFP, GAPDH.

2.2 Antibiotics

Neomycin (G418-400 μg/mL from a 50 mg/mL stock).

Puromycin (1 μg/mL from a stock of 10 mg/mL).

2.3 Cell Culture Related Materials

Fetal bovine serum (FBS).

Hanks balanced salt solution (HBSS).

OPTI-MEM medium.

RPMI medium.

PBS/DPBS- Dulbecco's phosphate-buffered saline (Calcium and Magnesium free).

Petri dishes (60 mm and 100 mm).

Tissue culture Flasks (175 mm).

2.4 Cells

293 T cells for virus generation.

PC3 cells.

2.5 Chemicals

D-Luciferin (150 μg/mL for in vitro, 3 mg/mouse).

Dithiothreitol (DTT)—1 μL of DTT (1 M) per 1 mL of RIPA buffer.

Luciferase assay reagent (Promega) diluted according to the manufacturer's instructions.

Orthovanadate (0.2 M stock).

Passive lysis buffer (1×)—Dilute 5× stock to 1× working stock with water.

Poly-D-lysine.

Phenylmethylsulfonyl fluoride (PMSF, 0.2 M).

Polybrene—8 μg/mL (Stock-8 mg/mL).

Protease Inhibitor mixture.

Radioimmunoprecipitation assay buffer (RIPA).

Tween 20–0.05%.

2.6 Instruments

PCR—polymerase chain reaction machine.

Plate reader.

2.7 Plasmids

EGFP plasmid with minimal Cytomegalovirus (CMV) promoter.

Lentiviral packaging plasmids (deltaR8.2 for accessory proteins, VSV-G for envelope protein).

2.8 Transfection Reagent

Lipofectamine 2000 or similar.

3 Construction of Hypoxia Regulated Long-Life EGFP Reporter Expression Plasmid Vector

Five tandem copies of hypoxia response element (5XHRE) generation obtained by polymerase chain reaction (PCR) amplification from vascular endothelial growth factor (VEGF) promoter and their cloning into an expression vector are described by Shibata et al. [13]. PCR amplified 5XHRE promoter was cloned in frame on the 5′-end of the CMV-EGFP sequence to obtain the plasmid

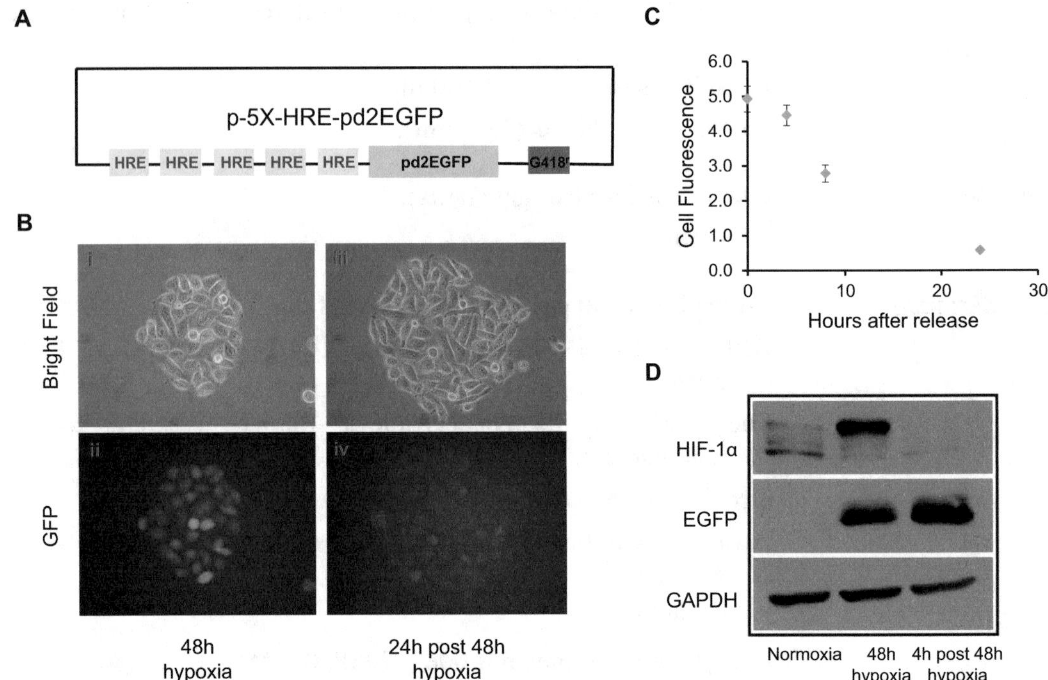

Fig. 1 Long half-life reporter gene activity. (**a**) Box and line schematic showing the long half-life GFP reporter construct under the control of five tandem repeats of HRE. (**b**) Representative photomicrograph of PC3 cells stably expressing the plasmid containing the long half-life GFP reporter construct. Bright field and fluorescent images of a colony of PC3 cells stably expressing the HRE-GFP construct exposed to hypoxia for 48 h (i and ii). The same colony was photographed 24 h post hypoxia release (iii and iv). (**c**) Graph showing decrease in fluorescence intensity following incubation at various times after hypoxia release. Using ImageJ software, fluorescence intensity was calculated from photographs taken on a microscope equipped with a camera, from at least 3 to 5 colonies for each time point. Values represent mean ± S.E from three biological replicates. (**d**) Representative immunoblots showing expression of HIF-1α and EGFP in PC3 cells expressing HRE-GFP culture under normoxia, exposed to hypoxia for 48 h or maintained under normoxia for 4 h after 48 h hypoxia treatment

pd2-5X-HRE-CMV min-EGFP (HRE-EGFP) as shown in Fig. 1a. This mammalian expression vector also contains a geneticin resistant gene as a selection marker. By adding antibiotic G418, which is titrated depending upon the cell line used, cells expressing HRE-EGFP are selected as detailed below.

3.1 Establishing Stable Cell Line-Expressing HRE-EGFP

Prior to transduction, perform a "kill curve" to determine sensitivity of the cell line to G418. The example below uses PC-3 cells, a human prostate cancer cell line [14].

1. Plate 5 × 10^5 PC3 prostate cancer cells in a 60 mm dish 24 h before transfection.
2. In an eppendorf tube, dilute 1 μg of 5 × HRE-EGFP in 250 μL of OPTI-MEM medium In a second eppendorf tube with

250 μL of optimum medium, add 2 μL lipofectamine 2000 (Invitrogen, Carlsbad, CA) and mix well.

3. Add diluted plasmid DNA to diluted lipofectamine dropwise and incubate the complex for 20 min. Meanwhile, replace the media on the plate containing PC3 cells with low serum (1% FBS) containing RPM1640. At the end of incubation time, add the plasmid-lipofectamine complex dropwise on the cells and gently swirl the plate to evenly mix with the medium on the plate and distribute the complex evenly.
4. Twenty-four hours post transfection, change the media on the plate and replace with RPMI-1640 containing 10% FBS. For selecting PC-3 cells expressing the expression plasmid, add G418 (500 μg/mL).
5. Change the media on the plate every 4 days with fresh G418-containing medium till most of the non-transfected cells die. Once cells form colonies on the plate, pick healthy colonies with a sterile pipet tip, and transfer them to a 6-well culture dish (**Note 1**). Expand each colony separately and test the cells for GFP expression.

3.1.1 Detection and Validation of Hypoxia Regulated GFP Reporter Gene Expression

Reporter gene expression can be detected optically and validated for protein expression by western blot analysis of various PC3-HRE-GFP clones as follows.

1. Plate 300,000 PC3-HRE-GFP cells in three 60 mm petri dish.
2. Twenty-four hours later, change the media in both the plates. Place one plate in a 37 °C CO_2 incubator. Place the other two plate in a modular incubator chamber (hypoxia chamber) and flush at 2 psi for 3 min with a gas mixture composition of 1% O_2/5% CO_2 and 94%N_2, close the chamber and place it in the 37 °C CO_2 incubator for 48 h (**Note 2**).
3. At the end of the 48-h period, using a 20× objective, EGFP expression can be detected using a fluorescence microscope equipped with a digital camera and a broadband halogen source (Fig. 1b, image ii). The excitation filter to detect EGFP is set to 500 nm and the emission filter for the detection at 500–540 nm.
4. To determine the half-life of EGFP expression, incubate the EGFP-expressing PC3 cells to normoxia and detect green fluorescence at various time points. As shown in Fig. 1b (image iv), GFP fluorescence is detected at low levels even after 24 h of reoxygenation and diminishes after 30 h (Fig. 1c).
5. To further validate reporter gene expression, perform immunoblotting for GFP and HIF-1α protein using antibodies specific for each component (Fig. 1d).

6. Briefly, seed 1 × 10^6 PC3-HRE-GFP cells in three 100 mm petri dish. On day 2, change media on the plates and place two plates (Plate #2, #3) in the hypoxia chamber and flush with a gas mixture as mentioned above to create hypoxia. Seal the incubator and place it in a 37 °C CO_2 incubator for 48 h. Place the 100 mm petri dish (plate #1) under normoxic condition in a 37 °C CO_2 incubator. At the end of incubation time, open the hypoxia chamber and place one dish (Plate #3) in the CO_2 incubator to reoxygenate the cells for an additional 4 h. Place plate #1 and #2 on ice and aspirate the media. Wash the cells once with ice-cold DPBS and add 1 mL of ice-cold PBS and scrape the cells from the plate using a cell scraper. Collect the cells in an eppendorf tube and spin the tube in a centrifuge at 0.2 × *g* for 5 min at 4 °C to pellet. Aspirate the PBS and resuspend the pellet in radio immuno precipitation assay buffer (RIPA) fortified with protease inhibitor mixture, serine protease inhibitor-phenylmethylsulfonyl fluoride (PMSF, 0.2 M), 1 μL/mL of 1 M DTT, 0.2 M of sodium orthovanadate and 0.5 M sodium fluoride and incubate at 4 °C on ice for 30 min. Spin the contents at 16.1 × *g* for 30 min in a centrifuge set at 4 °C. Collect the supernatant and measure the concentration of the protein.
7. To detect the reporter activity, resolve the 100 μg of protein by polyacrylamide gel electrophoresis (PAGE) and transfer the separated protein to a nitrocellulose membrane by applying 40 mA of current overnight at 4 °C (**Note 3**).
8. Once the transfer of protein is complete, cut the membrane around 80–130 kDa and 32–50 kDa. Block the membrane with 5% nonfat dry milk in tris-buffered saline with Tween-20 (TBST) for 2 h. Probe for HIF-1α and EGFP expression using monoclonal antibodies against HIF-1α (1:1000 dilution, HIF-1α-67, Novus Biological, Littleton, Co) and anti-EGFP (1:2000 dilution, BD Biosciences, San Jose, CA). After the incubation with the primary antibody, wash the membranes three times with TBST and add horseradish peroxidase (HRP) conjugated goat anti-mouse secondary (1:2000). Once EGFP is detected, strip the EGFP bound antibody signal by soaking the membrane in stripping buffer at room temperature for 5 min and wash with phosphate-buffered saline (PBS), and probe for a loading control protein such as GAPDH (Fig. 1d).

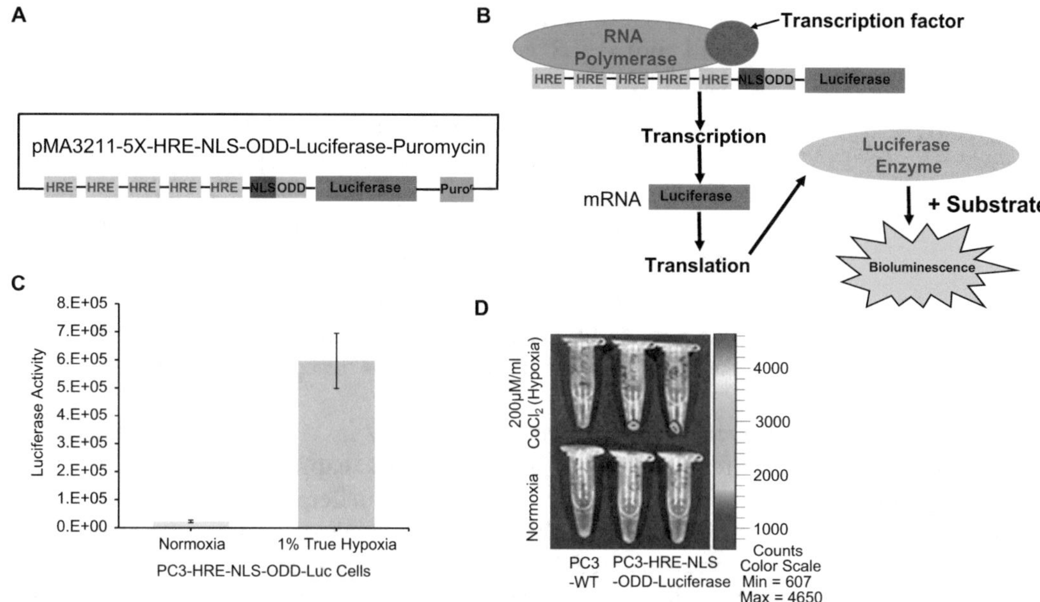

Fig. 2 Short half-life reporter gene activity. (**a**) Box and line schematic showing the short half-life luciferase reporter construct under the control of five tandem repeats of HRE. (**b**) Schematic showing binding of the transcription factor to the HRE and activating luciferase gene transcription that can be visualized as bioluminescence when the supplied substrate is converted by luciferase. (**c**) Luciferase assay quantifying the activity of the enzyme in PC3-HRE-NLC-ODD-Luc cells in response to 48 h of true hypoxia (1% oxygen). Values represent mean $\pm$ SEM from three independent experiments. *** $p < 0.0005$. (**d**) Representative image showing bioluminescence in PC3-HRE-NLS-ODD-Luc cells in response to 48 h treatment with hypoxia mimetic $CoCl_2$. Images were captured using IVIS Spectrum Xenogen system

3.2 Construction of Hypoxia Regulated Short Half-Life Luciferase Reporter Expression Plasmid Vector:

A plasmid containing five tandem copies of hypoxia response element (5×HRE) with oxygen-dependent degradation domain (ODD), nuclear localization signal (NLS), and firefly luciferase gene was kindly provided by Dr. Harada [15]. 5×HRE-NLS-ODD-Luc insert was later sub-cloned into a lentiviral vector as shown in Fig. 2a. This lentiviral vector also has the puromycin resistant gene as a selection marker.

3.3 Generation of Virions-Expressing 5XHRE-NLS-ODD-Luciferase

1. To generate lentiviral particles plate 5×10^6 HEK 293-T cells on a 100 mm petri dish that has previously been coated with polylysine-D (Sigma, St. Louis, MO).
2. Twenty-four hours later, (day 2) change the medium to DMEM with 1% fetal bovine serum and transfect 293-T cells with a combination of lentiviral vector-expressing gene of interest, a packaging construct (ΔR8.2) and plasmid construct to pseudo type the envelop express vesicular stomatitis virus-G protein (VSVG) in the ratio of 12 μg:6 μg:1.5 μg using lipofectamine 2000, or similar reagent.

3. Forty-eight hours post transfection, collect the supernatant, and spin at 0.8 × *g* for 30 min. Transfer the viral supernatant carefully to a new tube (**Note 4**).
4. Seed PC3-HRE-GFP cells at 0.3 × 10^6 in a 60 mm dish. Twenty-four hours later, add 2 μL of polybrene to 2 mL of viral supernatant-expressing HRE-NLS-ODD-Luc virions, gently mix, and add it on to PC3-HRE-GFP cells. Allow the transduction to occur for 24 h and repeat this process again.
5. After a two-time infection, start selecting for clones that express both HRE-GFP and HRE-NLS-ODD-Luciferase by adding G418 and puromycin as described in the earlier section.

3.4 Detection and Validation of Hypoxia Regulated Luciferase Reporter Activity

Quantification of reporter activity in vitro can be performed by luciferase assay of various clones expressing HRE-NLS-ODD-Luciferase gene (Fig. 2). In the luciferase assay, firefly luciferase, the monomeric 61 kDa enzyme, catalyzes luciferin (substrate) oxidation by using ATP-Mg2+ as a cosubstrate. During this process a flash of light is generated that decays rapidly after the enzyme and substrate is combined and the bioluminescence is read at peak emission of 560 nm (yellow-green light) (Fig. 2b).

Briefly, plate PC3-HRE-NLS-ODD-Luc-expressing cells in two 100 mm petri dishes.

1. Twenty-four hours later, change the media in both the plates. Place one plate in a 37 °C CO_2 incubator. Place the other plate in a modular incubator chamber and flush at 2 psi for 3 min with a gas mixture composition of 1% O_2/5% CO_2 and 94% N_2. Close the chamber and place in the 37 °C CO_2 incubator for 48 h.
2. At the end of the 48-h period, wash the cells with ice-cold PBS. Add 100 μL of 1× lysis buffer to lyse the cells. For the assay, add 10 μL of lysate in a 96-well plate with a solid bottom. Place the plate on a plate reader and pump 100 μL of luciferase assay reagent. The amount of light emitted reflects luciferase activity (Fig. 2c).
3. Short half-life luciferase reporter activity can also be detected optically and validated for protein expression in vitro conditions qualitatively by measuring BLI using optical instruments such as the Xenogen IVIS® series (Perkin Elmer).
4. To detect reporter activity in vitro, plate 300,000 HRE-NLS-ODD-Luciferase-expressing cells in two 60 mm petri dishes.
5. Twenty-four hours later, change the media in both the plates. In one set, add 200 μM cobalt chloride which is a hypoxia mimetic. Place both the plates in the 37 °C CO_2 incubator for 48 h.

6. At the end of incubation, wash the cells with ice-cold phosphate-buffered saline (PBS), and scrape the cells in a small volume of buffer. Spin the content to pellet the cells and place them on ice. Switch on the optical imaging equipment (IVIS spectrum) and adjust the setting as follows: exposure is set to 30 s, field of view (FOV) to position (C): 12.8×12.8 cm, F at 1 and binning to 8, add 50 μL of the substrate D-luciferin to the pellet and mix and place the tubes on the stage inside the detection unit and acquire the image. Figure 2d clearly shows increase in bioluminescence in response to hypoxia in PC3 cells expressing HRE-NLS-ODD-Luciferase reporter cells and not in the control cells.

For the in vivo detection of reporter activity, appropriate mouse models should be used depending upon the cell line you choose to study. In the present example, for the in vivo detection of reporter gene activity, PC3 clones expressing both HRE-GFP and HRE-NLS-ODD-Luc construct were validated for EGFP expression and luciferase activity as mentioned above. We used 4–6 weeks old severely combined immunodeficient (SCID) male mice for this study (**Note 5**).

3.5 Tumor Implantation, Monitoring, and Imaging of Reporter Gene Activity

1. Grow PC3-HRE-GFP + HRE-NLS-ODD-Luciferase cells in T175 flasks till they reach 80–90% confluence. Trypsinize the cells and resuspend in Hanks balanced salt solution (HBSS) such that the concentration is 2×10^6 cells per 50 μL. Prepare enough for at least twice the number of animals that one is planning to inject. Monitor the tumor growth by measuring the tumor size with a caliper.
2. Prepare anesthetic according to the guidelines formulated by respective institutional Animal Care and Use Committee to temporarily immobilize the animal and minimize any pain.
3. Once the animal is anesthetized, mix the cell suspension and inject 50 μL of cell suspension subcutaneously in the flank.
4. Monitor tumor growth regularly. Once the tumor reaches 200 mm^3, prepare for in vivo optical imaging using In Vivo Imaging System (IVIS)-Xenogen (Perkin Elmer) or a similar imaging instrument.
5. Place the mice into a clear plexiglass anesthesia box and pass gas-based anesthetic (2.5–3.5% isofluorane) through the tubing until anesthetized (**Note 6**).
6. Once anesthetized, transfer the animals from anesthesia box to the imaging chamber, and place with the nose inserted into the nose cones attached to the manifold in the imaging chamber. Continue to pass anesthetic at 2.5% isoflurane/O2.

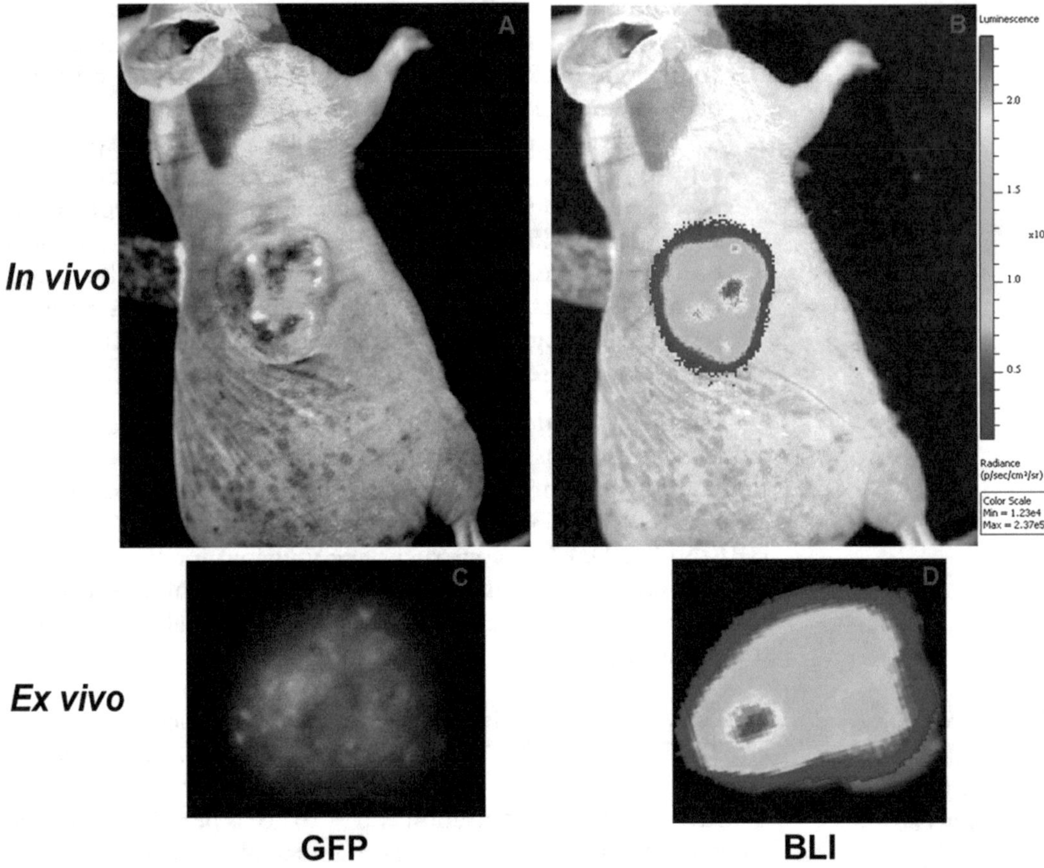

Fig. 3 Hypoxia reporter gene activity in tumors. Representative fluorescence image of a tumor derived from PC3 cells stably expressing both long half-life GFP and short half-life luciferase reporter under HRE control in vivo (**a**, **b**) and ex vivo (**c**, **d**)

7. For reporter activity of long half-life protein, i.e., HRE-GFP, the following parameters are set for the GFP detection. Set the Channel to: 465/520, 465/540, 500/540 (excitation/emission) (**Note 7**). Set the exposure time to 1 s and FOV to (B): 12.8 × 12.8 cm. Set the f-stop to position 2 and binning to 8. Acquire the GFP image and save it (Fig. 3a).
8. Without moving the animal, inject D-luciferin and wait for 15 min before imaging the short half-life reporter using the following parameter: Exposure 30 seconds, FOV set to position (C): 12.8 × 12.8 cm, F = 1 and binning at 8 (Fig. 3b). (**Note 8**)
9. To minimize autofluorescence in the GFP channel and accurately detect both long half-life GFP and short half-life luciferase reporter activity, ex vivo imaging of the tumor slice can be performed.

10. Remove the tumor from the euthanized mouse. Make sure to remove the skin from the tumor.
11. Place the tumor on a tissue slicer to make 1 mm thick slices and place on a glass slide.
12. Place the glass slide with tissue slices on the imaging stage of the Xenogen scanner and capture GFP images using the parameters mentioned before.
13. Without changing the orientation, perform bioluminescence (BLI) imaging using the previously mentioned parameters.

4 Notes

1. Alternatively, cells can be plated in a 100 mm petri dish and subjected to selection pressure as described previously. As a precaution, dislodge single colonies one at a time and do not mix them if you want to select a clone with highest GFP expression. Before you start the antibiotic selection, it is advisable to perform a survival curve with different concentrations of antibiotics using wild-type cells.
2. The maximum psi (pounds per square inch) the modular incubator can hold/withstand is 2 psi. Therefore, do not increase the force gas mixture above 2 psi. This can be monitored and regulated by adjusting the knob on the regulator attached to the gas tank. When the knob is released at the end of the hypoxia treatment, the sound of gas escaping from the chamber will be heard.
3. Acrylamide is a hazardous chemical. Avoid contact with skin. Precast gels may also be used. However, make sure a large volume can be loaded into the wells, especially if the protein concentration is very low. When performing wet transfer of proteins on the gel to nitrocellulose membrane, make sure that there are no air bubbles.
4. Production and handling of lentiviral vectors and viral particles need prior approval from the institutional biosafety committee and environmental health and safety officials. All tissue culture laminar cabinets should comply with BSL 2 certification. The laboratory should be equipped for handling and storing viral particles. Always wear double gloves with sleeves covering the forearm. Have 10% bleach ready in the event of any spill. Clean the bench and all equipment used for viral production with 10% bleach. Dispose used tips and pipettes after soaking them in a bottle containing 10% bleach. 293 T cells are weakly adherent to tissue culture plates. Make sure that the plates are well coated with poly-D-lysine before plating 293 T cells.

5. All surgical procedures and animal handling should be carried out in accordance with protocols approved by the Institutional Animal Care and Use Committee.
6. Ensure the vaporizer is filled with the specific anesthetic agent for which it is designed and certified for use by the manufacturer. Fill the vaporizer using an anti-spill bottle adaptor. Check for leaks, defects, and damage in anesthesia equipment (including hoses and valves) and scavenging system. Always use a sealed chamber. Any isoflurane waste should be disposed of as hazardous waste.
7. Choose the best excitation/emission combination for your study depending upon the expression of the fluorescent protein.
8. Incubation with D-Luciferin and BLI must be standardized for each separate experiment. Conditions may vary depending upon the tumor type and tumor model.

Acknowledgments

This work was supported by National Institutes of Health R01 CA73850, R01 CA82337, and P50 CA103175.

References

1. Gorman CM, Moffat LF, Howard BH (1982) Recombinant genomes which express chloramphenicol acetyltransferase in mammalian cells. Mol Cell Biol 2:1044–1051
2. Reddy SV, Takahashi S, Haipek C, Chirgwin JM, Roodman GD (1993) Tartrate-resistant acid phosphatase gene expression as a facile reporter gene for screening transfection efficiency in mammalian cell cultures. BioTechniques 15:444–447
3. Henthorn P, Zervos P, Raducha M, Harris H, Kadesch T (1988) Expression of a human placental alkaline phosphatase gene in transfected cells: use as a reporter for studies of gene expression. Proc Natl Acad Sci U S A 85:6342–6346
4. de Wet JR, Wood KV, DeLuca M et al (1987) Firefly luciferase gene: structure and expression in mammalian cells. Mol Cell Biol 7:725–737
5. Gould SJ, Subramani S (1988) Firefly luciferase as a tool in molecular and cell biology. Anal Biochem 175:5–13
6. de Wet JR, Wood KV, Helinski DR et al (1986) Cloning firefly luciferase. Methods Enzymol 133:3–14
7. de Wet JR, Wood KV, Helinski DR et al (1985) Cloning of firefly luciferase cDNA and the expression of active luciferase in Escherichia coli. Proc Natl Acad Sci U S A 82:7870–7873
8. Prasher D, McCann RO, Cormier MJ (1985) Cloning and expression of the cDNA coding for aequorin, a bioluminescent calcium-binding protein. Biochem Biophys Res Commun 126:1259–1268
9. Shimomura O, Johnson FH, Saiga Y (1962) Extraction, purification and properties of aequorin, a bioluminescent protein from the luminous hydromedusan, Aequorea. J Cell Comp Physiol 59:223–239
10. Li X, Zhao X, Fang Y et al (1998) Generation of destabilized green fluorescent protein as a transcription reporter. J Biol Chem 273:34970–34975
11. Wang GL, Jiang BH, Rue EA et al (1995) Hypoxia-inducible factor 1 is a basic-helix-loop-helix-PAS heterodimer regulated by cellular O2 tension. Proc Natl Acad Sci 92:5510–5514
12. Danhier P, Krishnamachary B, Bharti S et al (2015) Combining optical reporter proteins with different half-lives to detect temporal

evolution of hypoxia and reoxygenation in tumors. Neoplasia 17:871–881

13. Shibata T, Giaccia AJ, Brown JM (2000) Development of a hypoxia-responsive vector for tumor-specific gene therapy. Gene Ther 7:493–498

14. Kaighn ME, Narayan KS, Ohnuki Y et al (1979) Establishment and characterization of a human prostatic carcinoma cell line (PC-3). Investig Urol 17:16–23

15. Harada H, Kizaka-Kondoh S, Itasaka S et al (2007) The combination of hypoxia-response enhancers and an oxygen-dependent proteolytic motif enables real-time imaging of absolute HIF-1 activity in tumor xenografts. Biochem Biophys Res Commun 360:791–796

Chapter 10

Visualization of Immune Cell Reconstitution by Bioluminescent Imaging

Purnima Dubey

Abstract

Reporter gene-based molecular imaging is a powerful means to detect the movement and function of diverse cell populations in vivo. Reconstitution of an immune system marked with molecular imaging reporter genes permits tracking of primary immune responses to pathogens and cancer in experimental systems. This chapter describes the methods to isolate bone marrow stem/progenitors, transduce them with imaging reporter genes, and track the reconstitution of the peripheral immune system by bioluminescent imaging.

Key words Luciferase, Bone marrow, Lymphocytes, Imaging

1 Introduction

Reporter gene-based molecular imaging techniques have been used to monitor hematopoietic reconstitution [1] and the movement and function of various immune cell populations [2] in the whole animal. This powerful technology permits visualization of immune responses to disease states such as cancer [3, 4] and infectious diseases. Most studies isolate the cell population of interest and use transfection or viral transduction to mark the cells with reporter genes in vitro. The cells are then injected into animal model systems to follow responses to the pathogen or cancer cell of interest. In contrast, reconstitution of the peripheral immune system through adoptive transfer of reporter gene labeled bone marrow stem/progenitor cells permits tracking of primary and secondary immune responses within an intact immune system. Both bioluminescent and PET-based reporter gene marked animals have been used to study responses to autoimmune disease and cancer, demonstrating the power of this methodology to facilitate the study primary responses in an animal with an intact immune system.

To track cell subsets, the reporter gene must be expressed behind a tissue-specific promoter. However, it is difficult to

Purnima Dubey (ed.), *Reporter Gene Imaging: Methods and Protocols*, Methods in Molecular Biology, vol. 1790,
https://doi.org/10.1007/978-1-4939-7860-1_10,

maintain the tissue specificity of gene regulatory elements removed from the chromosome. Thus, the goal of marking individual cell subsets by marking the bone marrow stem/progenitor cells has not been achieved to date, and is a limitation of the approach described here. The discovery of genome editing techniques such as CRISPR/Cas9 [5] that enables gene manipulation in situ may soon permit marking and tracking of individual cell subsets.

Here, we describe the methods to transduce bone marrow stem/progenitor cells with imaging reporter genes, and demonstrate that immune reconstitution can be tracked using Firefly luciferase-based noninvasive imaging. The reporter gene used here is a fusion of enhanced GFP with Firefly luciferase (GFPLuc) expressed behind the murine minimal CD8a promoter and enhancer [6]. Luciferase expression is detected in CD8+ and CD4+ T cells, and B cells and permits tracking of adaptive immune responses.

2 Materials

1. Immunocompetent mice, 6–12 weeks of age (*see* **Note 1**).
2. 5-fluorouracil (200 mg/mL in H_2O).
3. 70% ethanol.
4. Disposable 1 cc insulin syringes.
5. Heat lamp to dilate tail veins.
6. Iscove's Modified Dulbecco's Medium (IMDM).
7. Heat-inactivated fetal bovine serum (HI-FBS).
8. Penicillin-Streptomycin (P/S, 100×).
9. Gentamicin (1000×).
10. L-Glutamine (L-Glut, 100×).
11. 2-ME, 5×10^{-2}M (1000× stock).
12. IL-3 (working concentration, 6 ng/mL).
13. IL-6 (working concentration 10 ng/mL).
14. Stem Cell Factor (SCF, working concentration 100 ng/mL).
15. WEHI cell conditioned medium (WEHI-CM) [PMID 309775].
16. Polybrene, 8 mg/mL in H_2O (1000×).
17. 1× HEPES buffer.
18. 1× HBSS buffer.
19. 1× DPBS (without Ca^{2+}, Mg^{2+}).
20. Concentrated lentiviral supernatant (at least 5×10^8 IU/mL).
21. Cesium source for irradiation.
22. Table top centrifuge.

23. Flow cytometer for detection of fluorescent proteins.
24. D-luciferin (100 mg/mL in H_2O), stored in aliquots at −80 °C.
25. Luminometer.
26. Disposable plastic cuvettes (12 × 50 mm) for measuring luminescence.
27. Passive lysis buffer (PLB, Promega), dilute to 1× following the manufacturer's instructions.
28. Tissue culture-treated 6-well plates.
29. Isoflurane.
30. Oxygen tank for imaging system.
31. IVIS Lumina® imaging system or equivalent equipment to record bioluminescent signals.
32. Living Image® analysis software.
33. Fluorescently labeled antibodies specific for mouse B220, CD4, CD8.
34. Disposable, non-sterile, polystyrene culture tubes 12 × 75 mm (FACS tubes).
35. 70–100 μm cell strainers.
36. 50 mL conical tubes.
37. 15 mL conical tubes.
38. Disposable 3 cc syringes.
39. Red blood cell lysis buffer.

3 Methods

3.1 *In Vitro* Transduction of Bone Marrow Stem/Progenitor Cells

3.1.1 All Animal Experiments Should Be Carried Out After IACUC Approval and in Accordance with Institutional Guidelines

1. To isolate stem/progenitor cells from mouse bone marrow, inject 125 μL of 5-FU solution (25 mg for a 20 g mouse) i.v. through the tail vein into mouse strain of choice on day 0 (*see* **Note 2**).
2. On day 4, euthanize mice as per approved IACUC protocol.
3. Spray animal with 70% ethanol and pin to dissection board.
4. Using sharp scissors and curved forceps, cut away skin from arms and legs and pin back.
5. Remove muscle surrounding bones. Remove bones and place in petri dish with complete medium (IMDM+ 10% HI-FBS, P/S, L-Glut, Gentamicin, 2-ME).
6. Make a small cut at each end of the bone. Fill a 5 cc syringe with complete medium. Insert a 30-gauge needle onto the syringe.

7. Hold the bone over an open 50 mL conical tube and insert needle of 5 cc syringe into one end of the bone. Flush marrow into the tube. Repeat the process with each piece of bone (*see* **Note 3**).
8. Attach an 18-gauge needle to a 10 cc syringe, and pull the marrow-containing medium through the syringe 3–5 times to dissociate the marrow.
9. Strain the marrow through a 70–100 μm screen into a new 50 mL conical tube.
10. Centrifuge solution at 500 × *g* at 4 °C for 5 min to pellet marrow.
11. Resuspend marrow in 5 mL complete medium containing IL-3, IL-6, SCF and 5% WEHI-CM. Count cells.
12. Plate 3 mL ($7.5 \times 10^5 - 1 \times 10^6$ cells/mL) per well of a 6-well plate.
13. Place in 37 °C, 5% CO_2, humidified incubator.
14. On day 3 carefully remove 1.5 mL of the culture medium, taking care to avoid disturbing the cell layer.
15. Add a maximum of 150 μL (10% of the total well volume) of concentrated lentivirus supernatant containing reporter gene of interest (ideally, MOI 10:1 bone marrow cells: virus). Add 8 μg/mL of polybrene and 10 mM HEPES.
16. Culture one well of bone marrow cells without lentivirus transduction.
17. Seal the plate with parafilm to retain optimal pH of the medium.
18. Centrifuge the plate at 1273 × *g*, 30 °C for 90 min. Remove parafilm, add 1.5 mL complete medium containing IL-3, IL-6, SCF, 10% WEHI-CM, and place the plate in an incubator overnight.
19. The next day, remove as much of the supernatant as possible (~2.3–2.5 mL) without disturbing the cell layer.
20. Add 1.5 mL of complete medium, a maximum of 150 μL of concentrated lentivirus and 8 μg/mL polybrene. Seal the plate with parafilm and centrifuge as in **step 18**.
21. Following centrifugation, collect cells from infected wells into a 15 mL conical tube.
22. Pellet cells (500 × *g*, 5 min, 4 °C) and remove the supernatant.
23. Wash cells once with complete medium (without growth factors).
24. Count cells.

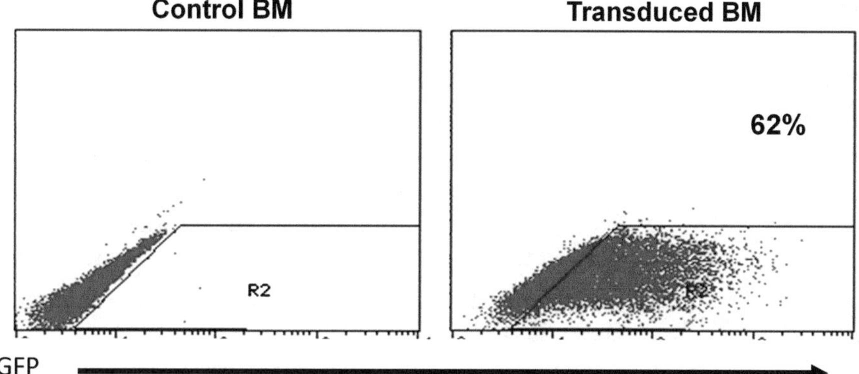

Fig. 1 Analysis of bone marrow transduction by flow cytometry. Following lentiviral transduction, control and transduced bone marrow is checked for expression of GFP by flow cytometry. A representative sample is shown where >60% of the bone marrow is expressing the marker

25. Pellet cells as in **step 22**. Remove the supernatant and resuspend cells in 1× HBSS at a concentration of 5×10^6 cells/mL. Place cells on ice until injection into recipient mice.
26. Transfer 5×10^5 cells from the transduced pool and the control well into FACS tubes.
27. Check expression of GFP by flow cytometry. To achieve marking of all immune cell populations, at least 50% of the bone marrow cells should be transduced (Fig. 1).
28. Proceed with adoptive transfer if adequate expression of the co-linked fluorescent reporter gene is detected.

3.2 Adoptive Transfer of Bone Marrow into Recipient Mice

1. To deplete normal bone marrow from recipient mice, irradiate recipient mice with cesium source at a lethal dose (*see* **Note 4**).
2. Take 100 μL of infected bone marrow (5×10^5 cells) into a 1 cc disposable syringe (*see* **Note 5**).
3. Dilate the tail veins of the recipient animal by placing the cage of mice under a heat lamp. Take care to ensure that the heat lamp is ~ 2 feet away from the cage top so that the animals do not over heat. Generally, 5 min under the heat lamp is sufficient to dilate the veins for injection.
4. Inject the cell suspension i.v. into each irradiated recipient animal. Maintain one irradiated animal without bone marrow transfer as positive control for efficacy of irradiation (*see* **Note 6**).
5. To prevent growth of gut bacteria, provide acidified water to irradiated animals for 14 days post-irradiation and adoptive transfer (*see* **Note 7**).

3.3 Visualization of Bone Marrow Reconstitution by Noninvasive Imaging

1. To follow bone marrow reconstitution, image mice every 5–7 days beginning at 7 days post adoptive transfer.
2. An IVIS Lumina® or equivalent noninvasive imaging machine should be used to capture luciferase signals.
3. Inject mice i.p. with 150 mg/kg of D-Luciferin (37.5 μL of a 100 mg/mL stock per 25 g mouse). [Animals may be anesthetized for injection but should be returned to the cage and allowed to awaken during uptake of the substrate.] (*see* **Note 8**).
4. Wait 15 min to allow maximum uptake of the substrate prior to imaging.
5. Anesthetize animals with 2.5%–3% isoflurane/O_2 until the animals are asleep and unmoving.
6. To increase signal sensitivity, shave the fur on the ventral surface and left side of the mouse.
7. While substrate uptake and anesthesia are ongoing, set up imaging parameters. These must be determined empirically for each experiment since the length of image acquisition will depend on the strength of the signal. A good starting point is 1 min acquisition time, with default f-stop and binning settings.
8. Position animals in the ventral position (face up) in nose cone of imaging chamber with anesthesia flowing.
9. Close chamber and acquire the image.

   Acquire additional images with shorter and longer imaging times, depending on the observed signal.
10. To detect signal in the spleen, place the animal on its right side, with the left side facing up toward the camera. Acquire several images with longer and shorter imaging times as needed to capture luminescence. Signal in the thymus will be detected by 3 weeks after adoptive transfer, and spleen signal will be detected at 5 weeks post-adoptive transfer (Fig. 2).
11. Reconstitution of B cells and T cells will be complete at 5–6 week post-adoptive transfer.

3.4 In Vitro Confirmation of Bone Marrow Reconstitution and Luciferase Expression in Lymphoid Cells

1. To confirm appropriate reconstitution of B cells and T cells, euthanize one or more animals from the group at 6 week post-transfer of labeled bone marrow.
2. As positive control, harvest one spleen from a normal syngeneic animal that has not been reconstituted with bone marrow.
3. Harvest the spleen in a complete medium.
4. Place a 70–100 μm nylon strainer on a 50 mL conical tube. Place spleen on strainer and mash with the plunger of a 3 cc syringe to dissociate the spleen cells.

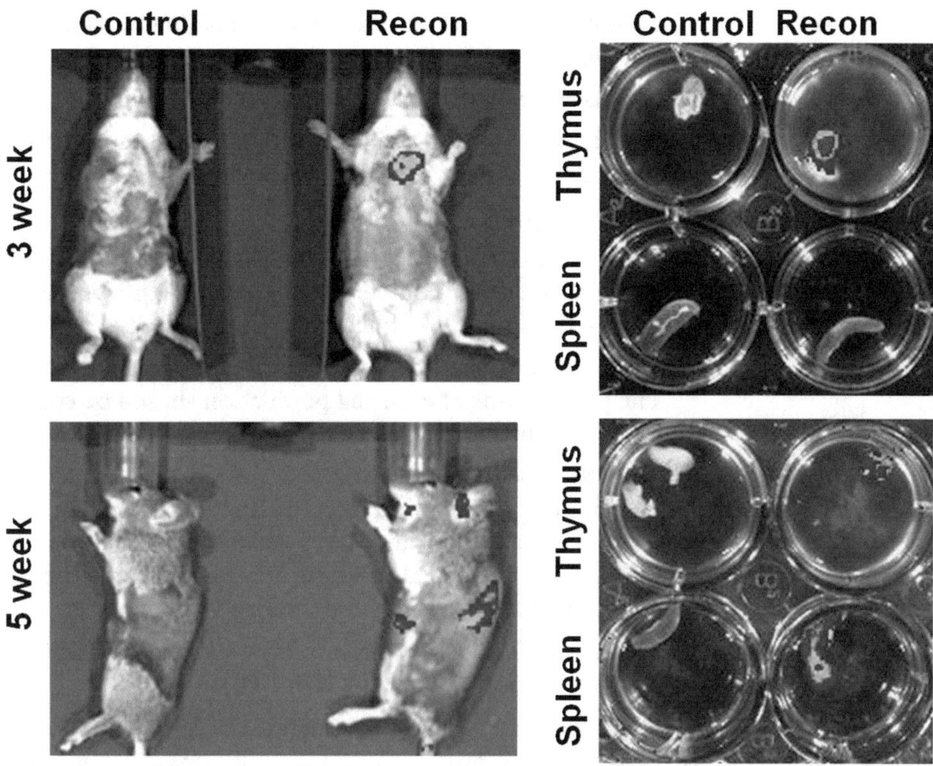

Fig. 2 Noninvasive detection of immune system reconstitution following transduction with GFPLuc labeled bone marrow. A control animal or an animal transduced with GFPLuc labeled bone marrow (Recon) is shown. Luciferase signal was detected by IVIS imaging at 3 week or 5 week after adoptive transfer. Animals were euthanized on day of imaging and organs were removed. Signal in thymus and spleen was detected using IVIS imaging. Reconstitution of the thymus is detected at 3 weeks post-reconstitution with signal observed in the spleen at 5 weeks post-reconstitution

5. When the tissue has been mashed through the strainer, pipet ~5 mL of complete medium onto the strainer to wash cells that may be stuck to the strainer.
6. Pellet the cells by centrifuging the cell suspension at $500 \times g$, 4 °C, 5 min.
7. Decant the supernatant and resuspend the cell pellet in 2.5 mL of red blood cell lysis buffer.
8. Incubate at room temperature for ~ 3 min.
9. Fill the tube with complete medium and centrifuge as in **step 5**.
10. Decant the supernatant and count cells. Aliquot 1×10^7 cells into a 15 mL conical tube. Centrifuge cells as in **step 5**, decant the supernatant, and resuspend in 1 mL of PBS/1% FBS.
11. Place 100 μL (1×10^6) spleen cells in a 5 mL FACS tube. Add fluorescently labeled antibodies specific for B220, CD4 and

CD8 in appropriate amounts per the manufacturer's guidelines (*see* **Note 9**).

12. Incubate for 15 min at 4 °C protected from light.
13. Add 1 mL of DPBS/1% FBS to each tube and centrifuge to pellet cells.
14. Repeat **step 13**.
15. Resuspend cells in 100–500 μL of PBS/1% FBS and analyze cells on a flow cytometer to determine the percentage of B220+ B cells, CD8+ T cells and CD4+ T cells.
16. Quantify the percentage of each cell type present in the spleen. The proportions of each cell population should be comparable to an untransduced control animal
17. To determine luciferase expression in a specific subset, sort the specific cell population: Place 1 mL (1×10^7) spleen cells in a 12 × 75 mm tube and stain cells with the subset specific antibody, as described in **steps 11–14**. Scale up the amount of antibody appropriately for the larger cell number.
18. Separate each cell population by flow sorting to achieve a >95% pure population of cells (*see* **Note 10**).
19. Pellet the sorted cells and resuspend in 100 μL 1× PLB.
20. Lyse an equivalent number of spleen cells from a non-transduced mouse to determine background luminescence (*See* **Note 11**).
21. Add 20 μL of LAR II substrate into a disposable luminometer test tube. Mix in 10 μL of cell lysate and immediately record luminescence in a luminometer.

4 Notes

1. Any immunocompetent strain of mouse may be used for these experiments. This chapter shows data from experiments conducted in C57BL/6 mice. Donor and recipient animals must be of the same strain and gender.
2. 5-FU (administered at 150 mg/kg) kills cycling hematopoietic cells in the marrow, thereby enriching for the quiescent stem/progenitor cells [7] (Fig. 2).
3. The marrow will be visible inside the bone, and will usually flush out as a chunk from each bone.
4. A lethal dose of irradiation from a cesium source will vary for each mouse strain [8]. For C57BL/6 mice, a lethal dose is 9 Gy (900 rad). This may be administered as one dose, or a split dose of 4.5 Gy delivered 3–4 h apart.

5. The cell number range for adequate reconstitution is $3 \times 10^5 - 1 \times 10^6$ cells per recipient. Mortality (10–50%) may be observed if less than 5×10^5 cells are injected.
6. Irradiated mice will develop anemia and will display clinical signs such as labored breathing, slow movement, inability to access food/water, ruffled fur. These symptoms are observed by day 10–14 post-irradiation. Once clinical signs are visible, the animal must be euthanized per IACUC guidelines. One irradiated animal is housed without bone marrow transfer as a positive control to ensure adequate irradiation.
7. Ciprofloxacin (0.67 mg/mL) may be added to the drinking water instead, to prevent over-growth of gut bacteria; without any treatment, animals may die before reconstitution is complete. Our experience shows that acidified water alone is sufficient to prevent gut bacterial growth during the reconstitution period.
8. Luciferin uptake is more efficient when animals are active, resulting in a stronger signal. If animals are anesthetized for injection, they should be allowed to awaken during the 15 min uptake period.
9. Antibodies specific for all markers of interest may be added to the same tube of cells, if each antibody is coupled to a different fluorochrome. Antibodies for flow cytometry are available through several different vendors. Follow the manufacturer's guidelines for amount of antibody to be added per sample. Incubate the cells in the dark to prevent photo-bleaching. A separate sample should be stained with each antibody individually, to compensate for spectral overlap of fluorochromes [9].
10. Cells stained with antigen-specific fluorescent antibodies are isolated by flow sorting using a FACS Aria® or similar machine, allowing adequate separation of individual cell populations. Alternately, cells may be isolated using magnetic beads; however, purity may be lower. Luciferase expression may vary between cell populations infected with the same construct.
11. Since bioluminescent signals are dependent on the presence of both the enzyme and substrate, background is negligible in non-transduced cells.

Acknowledgments

This work was supported by NIH 1 R21 CA124457 to P.D.

References

1. Cao YA et al (2004) Shifting foci of hematopoiesis during reconstitution from single stem cells. Proc Natl Acad Sci U S A 101:221–226. https://doi.org/10.1073/pnas.2637010100
2. Ahn SB et al (2017) Multimodality imaging of bone marrow-derived dendritic cell migration and antitumor immunity. Transl Oncol 10:262–270. https://doi.org/10.1016/j.tranon.2017.01.003
3. Edinger M et al (2003) Revealing lymphoma growth and the efficacy of immune cell therapies using in vivo bioluminescence imaging. Blood 101:640–648. https://doi.org/10.1182/blood-2002-06-1751
4. Shu CJ et al (2005) Visualization of a primary anti-tumor immune response by positron emission tomography. Proc Natl Acad Sci U S A 102:17412–17417. https://doi.org/10.1073/pnas.0508698102
5. Mitsunobu H, Teramoto J, Nishida K et al (2017) Beyond native Cas9: manipulating genomic information and function. Trends Biotechnol 35(10):983–996. https://doi.org/10.1016/j.tibtech.2017.06.004
6. Ellmeier W, Sunshine MJ, Losos K et al (1997) An enhancer that directs lineage-specific expression of CD8 in positively selected thymocytes and mature T cells. Immunity 7:537–547
7. Ogata H et al (1995) Long-term repopulation of hematolymphoid cells with only a few hemopoietic stem cells in mice. Proc Natl Acad Sci U S A 92:5945–5949
8. Grahn D, Hamilton KF (1957) Genetic variation in the acute lethal response of four inbred mouse strains to whole body X-irradiation. Genetics 42:189–198
9. Stewart CC, Stewart SJ (2004) Multiparameter data acquisition and analysis of leukocytes. Methods Mol Biol 263:45–66. https://doi.org/10.1385/1-59259-773-4:045

Chapter 11

Thymidine Kinase PET Reporter Gene Imaging of Cancer Cells In Vivo

Melissa N. McCracken

Abstract

Positron emission tomography (PET) is a three dimensional imaging modality that detects the accumulation of radiolabeled isotopes in vivo. Ectopic expression of a thymidine kinase reporter gene allows for the specific detection of reporter cells in vivo by imaging with the reporter specific probe. PET reporter imaging is sensitive, quantitative and can be scaled into larger tumors or animals with little to no tissue diffraction. Here, we describe how thymidine kinase PET reporter genes can be used to noninvasively image cancer cells in vivo.

Key words Positron emission tomography, Reporter gene, Noninvasive imaging, Thymidine kinase, [^{18}F]-FHBG, Small animal imaging, Herpes Simplex Virus Thymidine Kinase, HSV-TK, sr39TK

1 Introduction

Positron emission tomography (PET) is a nuclear imaging technology that measures the accumulation of positron emitting radiolabeled probes in vivo [1]. As the probe decays the released positrons annihilate with an electron in nearby tissue and emit two antiparallel 511 keV high-energy photons. PET detectors identify the coincident emissions from the two photons and reconstruct a quantitative 3D activity map [1]. In clinical practice the reconstruction provides a resolution of 1 cm, while small animal preclinical scanners (microPET) provide resolution at approximately 1 mm [2, 3]. In most studies a CT scan is obtained before or after the PET scan to provide anatomical information although PET scans can be obtained individually. The dual scans allow for a more precise identification of probe accumulation in target tissues. Alternatively, X-ray or MRI can be substituted for the CT scan depending on the application and availability of scanners [4].

One advantage of PET over alternative imaging modalities is the flexibility in probe design, function, and available radioisotopes. Probes can be designed to measure a vast array of

Purnima Dubey (ed.), *Reporter Gene Imaging: Methods and Protocols*, Methods in Molecular Biology, vol. 1790,
https://doi.org/10.1007/978-1-4939-7860-1_11,

biological processes including metabolism, surface epitope expression, perfusion, tracking of reporter labeled cells, or measurements of hypoxia [2, 5–7]. To date, thousands of unique PET probes have been made (The Radiosynthesis Database of PET Probes [RaDaP]). The most widely used probe [^{18}F]-FDG is a glucose analog that tracks glycolysis in vivo. [^{18}F]-FDG accounts for majority of clinical scans used for cancer diagnosis, staging, and response to therapies [1].

Complimentary to [^{18}F]-FDG for measuring total glucose metabolism is PET reporter gene imaging that tracks labeled cell populations in vivo. To date, majority of reporter genes are in preclinical development but could be directly translated into clinical practice. Reporter genes can be subdivided into three categories of transporter, extracellular, or enzymatic [6–8]. Ectopic expression of the chosen reporter gene then allows investigators to track the location of engineered cells in vivo with little to no signal from non-engineered cells when the corresponding reporter probe is utilized. Enzymatic reporters have been the most commonly used, with Herpes Simplex Virus Thymidine Kinase (HSV-TK) and variants being the majority. Other reporter gene subclasses have advantages as well as limitations. A more detailed overview of these reporter genes and alternative imaging strategies can be found in Herschman et al. and other reviews [4, 8, 9].

HSV-TK is a viral nucleoside kinase capable of phosphorylating thymidine, or non-natural nucleosides. Targeted viral-specific non-natural nucleosides are approved clinically as anti-viral pro--drugs. This class of molecules can be used for treating herpes prophylactically or to reduce total viral outbreak [10]. Approved drugs include ganciclovir, valgancyclovir, penciclovir, and acyclovir. Each drug functions through the same mechanism and is initially transported intracellularly with endogenous nucleoside transporters. Once intracellular, the drug is mono-phosphorylated by HSV-TK. Next, downstream cellular kinases then di- and tri-phosphorylate the drug. Last, the tri-phosphorylated form is incorporated into cellular DNA causing chain termination, replication halt and apoptosis [10–12]. The high efficacy in infected cells with little/low toxicity in uninfected cells provides a large therapeutic window. For these reasons, the ectopic expression of HSV-TK was first introduced as a suicide gene and allowed selective elimination of TK-expressing cells when treated with ganciclovoir [11, 12]. Follow-up studies utilized expression of TK for selective elimination of tumor cells through anti-viral therapy for HSV-TK-expressing cells [13].

The specificity of ganciclovir for HSV-TK compared to endogenous nucleoside kinases makes HSV-TK an ideal suicide gene but the same principles are needed for a robust PET reporter. The first application of HSV-TK as a reporter utilized it in SPECT imaging with a radiolabeled 5-iodo-2′-fluoro-2’deoxy-1-beta-D-

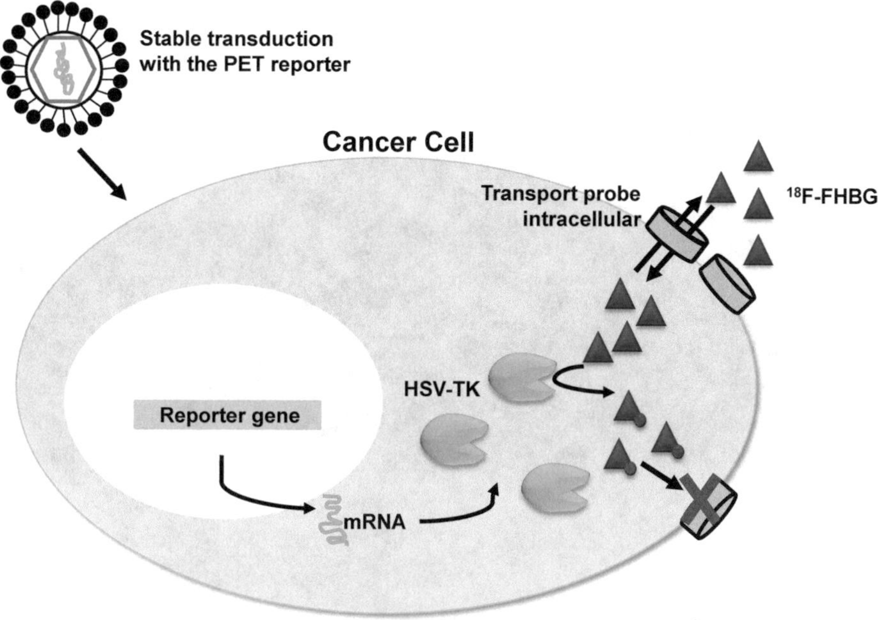

Fig. 1 PET reporter. Cancer cells are engineered to express the HSV-TK reporter through lentiviral integration. Integrated PET reporter gene will then be expressed as mRNA and protein in each cell. When animals are given [^{18}F]-FHBG host nucleoside transporters will bring the probe intracellular. Under normal conditions (no HSV-TK) the probe can freely efflux in and out of the cell. When HSV-TK is present, the reporter enzyme will phosphorylate the probe preventing efflux and allowing for intracellular accumulation

arabinofuranosyluracil (FIAU) and demonstrated the possibility of engineered reporters and probes for noninvasive imaging [14]. To increase resolution and sensitivity investigators then designed and radiolabeled PET probes for HSV-TK to be used as a PET reporter with ^{124}I and ^{18}F probes [15, 16]. Recently, preclinical studies with HSV-TK have shifted away from the longer half-life isotope ^{124}I and instead utilize an ^{18}F labeled penciclovir analog, 9-(4-[^{18}F]-fluoro-3 hydroxymethylbutyl) guanine ([^{18}F]-FHBG) [17, 18].

Cancer cells engineered to express HSV-TK allow for downstream imaging in vivo. Lentiviral transduction is the simplest method and allows for the HSV-TK reporter to be integrated into tumor cells DNA, thereby also labeling all daughter cells with the PET reporter (Fig. 1).

Cancer cells are then detected by [^{18}F]-FHBG (or other HSV-TK-specific probes) in vivo. A schematic on the setup and acquisition of HSV-TK reporter imaging in mice is displayed (Fig. 2).

In some instances, a stable cell line is not necessary or available. In these instances, alternative methods for gene delivery include non-integrating virus, electroporation, or nano-particle delivery [3, 15]. Several publications have tested the efficacy of reporter imaging in rodents using cancer cell lines with stable expression of HSV-TK. These studies identified lymphoma progression or

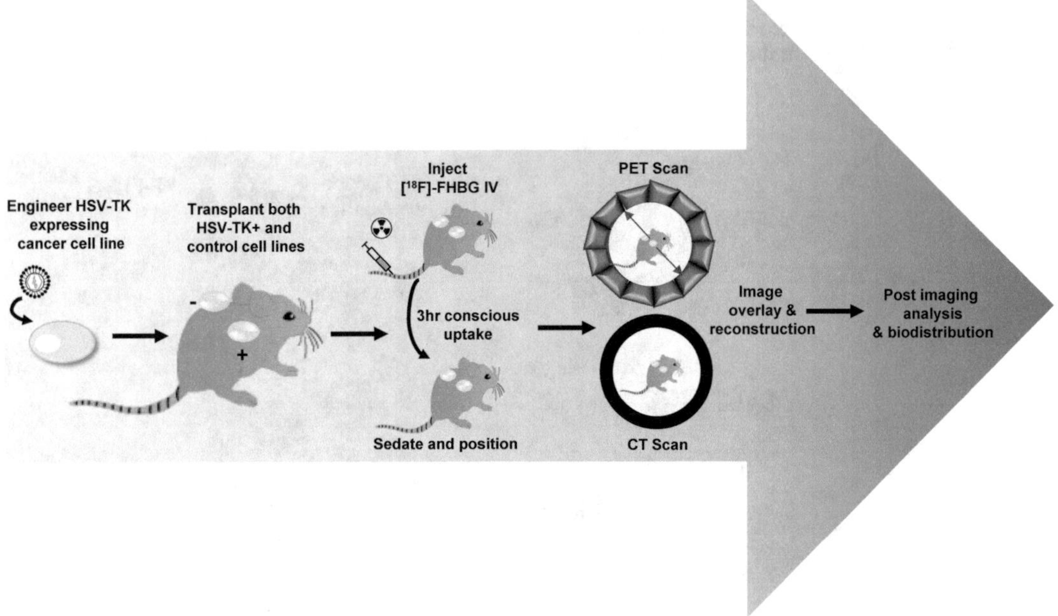

Fig. 2 Experimental flow for mouse HSV-TK reporter imaging Cancer cells are engineered to express HSV-TK by viral transduction. Stable cell lines are transplanted subcutaneous into appropriate mice. Tumors are grown to an appropriate size. Mice are injected with the reporter probe [^{18}F]-FHBG and probe accumulation/uptake for 3 h. Mice then undergo a microPET and microCT scans. Scans are overlaid and analyzed for probe distribution

regression, total cell number, quantification of transgene expression, and tumor location among other uses [16, 19–24]. In Fig. 3, investigators engineered prostate cancer cell lines to express sr39TK (a mutant form of HSV-TK) and imaged with [^{18}F]-FHBG followed by a CT scan. Figure 3b then demonstrates the sensitivity of [^{18}F]-FHBG PET imaging with increasing tumor signal as cancer cell lines are transduced with higher levels of sr39TK.

The following method provides a detailed description of how to apply HSV-TK reporter imaging to murine tumors for future studies.

2 Materials

The following materials will describe a method for TK PET reporter imaging with stably transfected cancer cells (Fig. 2). As described within the introduction, cells can be labeled through alternative methods including electroporation, adenovirus, or transient infection/transfection. Imaging methods described will cover protocols focused on ^{18}F radiolabeled acycloguanosines.

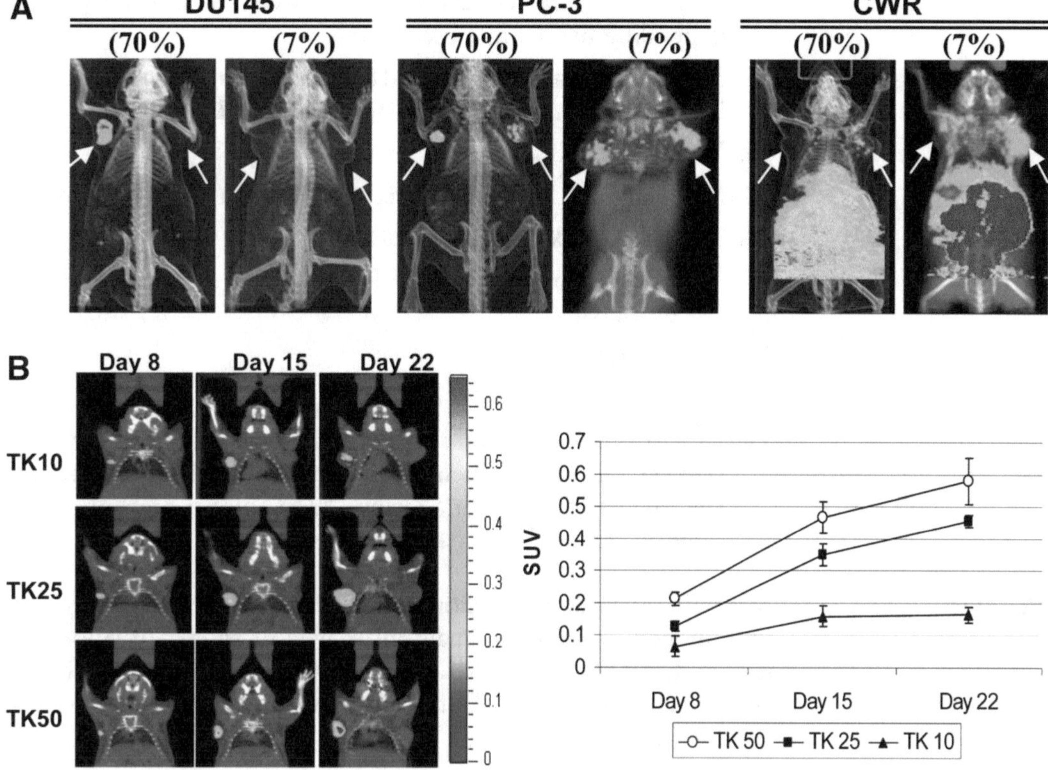

Fig. 3 PET/CT of HSV-TK expression in mice. Differential uptake of [^{18}F]-FHBG in DU-145, PC-3, and CWR22Rv.1 PCa cell lines. (**a**) Total of 7% or 70% of cells stably transduced with lentiviral vector-expressing HSV1-sr39tk-IRES-EGFP or IRES-EGFP as control were implanted on left or right shoulder, respectively. Tracer uptake seen in abdominal area of all mice is indicative of clearance route but is cropped out in DU-145 and PC-3 for clarity. Arrows indicate tumor position. (**b**) DU-145 cells transduced with increasing levels of HSV1-sr39tk have higher 18F-FHBG uptake (SUV), and intensity of signal increased over time with tumor volume ($n = 4$). This research was originally published in JNM [22]. © by the Society of Nuclear Medicine and Molecular Imaging, Inc.

2.1 Reagents

1. Cancer cell line of interest maintained as mycoplasma free.
2. Complete media for propagating and expanding the cell line in vitro.
3. Virus containing the TK reporter gene. Multiple TK reporter genes are currently developed with the most widely used one being a mutated Herpes Simplex Virus Thymidine Kinase (HSV-sr39TK). A self-inactivating virus containing HSV-sr39TK and either a fluorescent protein or selection marker is needed. The sequence of sr39TK was originally described by Black et al. and used as a PET reporter in Gambhir et al. [12, 24].

4. Polybrene (final concentration between 5 and 10 μg/mL depending on cell line used) [25].
5. Selection agent such as G418 if neomycin selection is used instead of a fluorescent reporter (*see* **Note 1**).
6. 1× PBS or HBSS.
7. Matrigel (BD Matrigel Matrix catalog #354234) (*see* **Note 2**).
8. Trypsin (0.05%), with phenol red.
9. Anesthesia that can include isoflurane or ketamine/xylazine (*see* **Note 3**).
10. Ophthalmic ointment.
11. Medical tape.
12. [^{18}F]-FHBG: The radiolabeled PET probe should be synthesized at a local radiochemistry facility within close proximity to the small animal imaging facility. Protocols for preclinical production can be found (*see* **Notes 4** and **5**).

2.2 Mice

Maintain mice at institution standards in a barrier facility. For immunocompromised animals autoclaved or irradiated laboratory rodent diet is recommended. All studies should be approved by the appropriate institutional Animal Care and Use Committees prior to conducting any imaging.

1. If using a human cell line, immunocompromised animals are necessary. These can include nude (lacking T cells), or SCID mice (lacking T/B cells and in some strains NK cells), available from commercial vendors (*see* **Note 6**).
2. If using a mouse cancer cell line, the appropriate syngeneic mouse strain from which the cell line was derived.

2.3 Equipment

1. Fluorescent activated cell sorter (FACS) machine (*see* **Note 7**).
2. Shavers.
3. Insulin syringes 23–27 gauge.
4. MicroPET scanner.
5. CT scanner—Although not entirely necessary, a co-registered CT scan allows for anatomical information. In scans where a change or diminished signal is expected, obtaining a CT scan to identify total tumor volume is useful (*see* **Note 8**).
6. Imaging chamber/bed.
7. Lead shielding.
8. Heating pad or heat lamps for warming mice after imaging.
9. Dosimeter.
10. Radiochemistry laboratory.

11. Isoflurane induction chamber if using isoflurane as the method of anesthesia.
12. Image analysis software. One free software version is Amide [26] (*see* **Note 9**).

2.4 Equipment Setup

1. MicroPET scanner.
   (a) Common scanners include: Siemens MicroPET Focus 220, Siemens Inveon microPET, or scanners from GE, PerkinElmer, Sofie Biosciences, and others.
   (b) MicroPET should be set up to acquire for 10 min and reconstruct with a filtered background projection probability algorithm.
2. CT Scanner
   (a) Common scanners include: Siemens, GE, PerkinElmer.
   (b) Scanners must be compatible with the same imaging chamber as the PET scanner to not move the mouse during PET or CT acquisition.
   (c) Set up the microCT to obtain a full body CT scan. Resolution and time can be adjusted based on imaging needs.

3 Methods

3.1 TK Reporter Gene Transduction and Selection of a Pure Reporter Gene-Expressing Cell Line

1. Produce a high titer lentivirus containing HSV-TK and a selection marker (preferred marker is GFP or similar fluorescent protein). A detailed protocol on lentiviral production is described by Tiscornia et al. [27].
2. Transduce the cancer cell of interest. A spinfection is recommended for higher infection efficiency (*see* **Note 10**).
   (a) Adherent cells—Plate cells at 30–60% confluency in 6-well dishes depending on the growth rate of the cells. The next morning aspirate approximately 50% of the media and then add either concentrated virus or viral supernatant and polybrene (typical final range of polybrene 2-10 μg/mL). Spin at 30 °C for 60 min.
   (b) Suspension cells—In a 12-well dish bring cells to 2×10^6 cells/mL. Add virus and polybrene to appropriate concentrations. Spin at 30 °C for 60 min.
   (c) Spinfection time, speed, and temperature may vary.
   (d) Place plates in the cell culture incubator at 37 °C, 5% CO_2 for 72 h.
3. If using a lentiviral construct, wait 72 h for final expression. At 72 h, cells can be sorted on fluorescent protein expression as a surrogate for HSV-TK expression. It is recommended that only the top 25% of positive cells be sorted. Verify the sort

purity and quality by performing a post sort analysis. To make an optimal reporter cell line the HSV-TK positive cells should be sorted a second time. By performing a secondary sort with more stringent parameters, cells with low expression or rare non-transduced cells will be eliminated. After FACS expand the cells in the appropriate media until needed for in vivo assays (*see* **Note 11**).

4. If using drug selection, add selection medium instead (*see* **Note 12**).

3.2 Establishing Tumor Models in Mice

1. Order the appropriate strain and number of mice. Mice should be rested for 1 week in the new barrier prior to implanting tumors.
2. Expand both the HSV-TK and control tumor cell line. On average each tumor implantation will range from 1e5 to 1e6 cells. (Some tumors establish with as little as 1e3 and some require up to 1e7.) Cells should be healthy, not overly passaged, and mycoplasma free.
3. Harvest cells into a single cell suspension and strain through a 70–100 μm cell strainer to remove clumps. Count cells and check for viability (*see* **Note 13**).
4. Wash to remove the remaining trypsin and FBS.
5. Resuspend into cold 1×HBSS at 2× the final concentration needed for injection.
6. Add 1 volume of matrigel (thawed on ice and kept cold) to bring cells to 1× concentration.
7. Place cells on ice to transport into animal barrier.
8. Example tumor implantation: Each tumor will have 1×10^6 cells in a 100 μL per tumor. Count 20×10^6 cells total. Bring cells to 20×10^6 cells/mL by adding 1 mL of 1×HBSS. Add 1 mL of matrigel to bring cells to 10×10^6 cells/mL. Anesthetize mice under 2% isoflurane.
9. Shave a clean area around where the tumor will be implanted. It is recommended to implant tumors anterior and dorsal to avoid nonspecific signal within the bladder and allow for easy visualization (Fig. 4).
10. Disinfect shaved skin with ethanol.
11. Mix cells prior to injection to create a homogenous solution.
12. Draw cells into a syringe of a 27 gauge or lower to prevent shearing. Only 1–2 injections should be drawn at a time to prevent the matrigel from solidifying in the syringe.
13. Remove all air in the syringe.
14. Create a small tent in the skin and inject cells with the bevel side up. Recommended volume for subcutaneous is 50–200 μL (usually 100 μL). After injection wait 5–10 s and then slowly

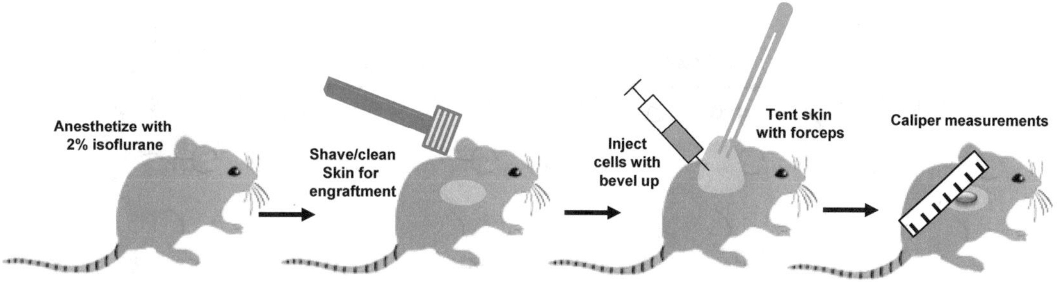

Fig. 4 Subcutaneous tumor implantation. Sedate the mouse with 2% isoflurane. Shave enough area to be able to visualize the tumor. Clean the skin with ethanol. Mix cells well and draw into a syringe. Tent the clean shaven area with forceps. Inject the tumor cells with the needle having the bevel up. Hold in place for 5–10 s prior to removing the needle. Place pressure on the injection site to prevent leaking. Monitor the tumor by size until imaging experiment

pull the needle out and place pressure at the injection site to minimize leaking.

15. Place the mouse in a recovery cage and monitor until the animal is awake and alert.
16. Monitor tumor size and growth by caliper measurements until the date of imaging.

3.3 Synthesis of PET Reporter Probe [^{18}F]-FHBG

1. Detailed synthesis instructions including weights, times, and predicted yield/purity can be found in Ponde et al. [28] (*see* **Note 14**).
2. Produce ^{18}F fluoride from ^{18}O H_2O.
3. Combine K_2CO_3, kryptofix 2.2.2, and ^{18}F.
4. Water is then evaporated from this mixture with acetonitrile under nitrogen.
5. The FHBG precursor (monomethoxytrityl-9-[4-(tosyl)-3-monomethoxytrityl-methylbutyl] guanine) is then added to the ^{18}F mixture (Fig. 5).
6. This solution is then mixed well and microwaved then cooled at room temperature. Repeat this process four times.
7. HCl is then added and the mixture is heated for 5 min at 110 °C.
8. This mixture is then allowed to cool and is then neutralized with NaOH and diluted with water to an appropriate volume for purification.
9. Solid-phase purification with an Oasis® cartridge is then performed. Begin by rinsing and priming the column with 5% methanol in water. The radioactive sample can then be loaded and rinsed to remove free unreactive ^{18}F.
10. Elute the [^{18}F]-FHBG from the column with ethanol.

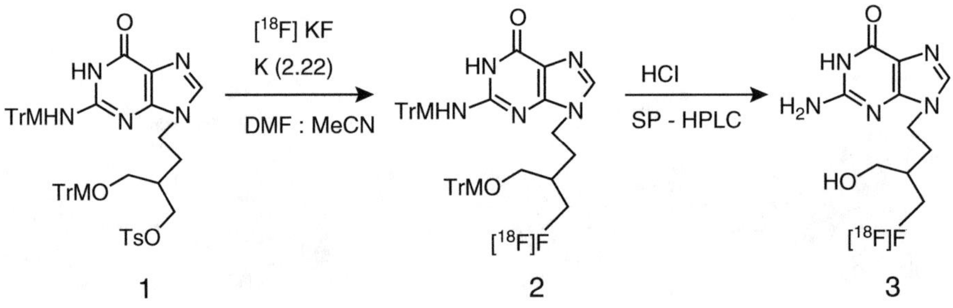

Fig. 5 [^{18}F]-FHBG synthesis. Schematic of [^{18}F]-FHBG synthesis. Reproduced with permission from Elsevier-Nuclear Medicine and Biology [28]

11. Evaporate majority of the ethanol then resuspend in water and purify on HPLC.
12. For microPET studies the HPLC product is then concentrated under vacuum and brought to a final solution of 0.9% saline to make safe for IV injection.
13. The concentrated [^{18}F]-FHBG can then be stored at room temperature in lead shielding until used. Unused [^{18}F]-FHBG should be stored in lead shielding for greater than 10 half-lives (^{18}F has a half-life of 110 min) and then disposed of as normal or chemical waste depending on the solvents used.

3.4 PET Reporter Imaging

1. Measure tumors prior to imaging. The resolution of microPET is about 1 mm; therefore tumors should be larger than this. Tumors larger than 5 mm are preferred. However, if tumors are overgrown and necrotic this will be seen on the PET scan and can interfere with analysis.
2. Synthesize [^{18}F]-FHBG (*see* Subheading 3.3).
3. Draw 200 μCi (more or less depending on microPET scanner used) into an insulin syringe, verify dose accuracy. Dilute up to a total volume of 200 μL in sterile 0.9% saline (*see* **Note 15**).
4. Inject intravenously in the tail vein. Mice can either be restrained or anesthetized for the injection.
5. Continue injections 10 min apart until all mice have been injected.
6. Allow for a 3 h conscious uptake (*see* **Note 16**).
7. Anesthetize mice 10 min prior to starting their PET/CT scans. Once animals are unconscious, perform a toe pinch to check sedation. Then apply ophthalmic ointment to the eyes.
8. Place mice in imaging chamber bed. It is recommended to tape mice with medical tape so their position remains constant in both the PET and CT scans to prevent moving.

9. Acquire the PET scan first. Standard scans are 10 min, 1 frame static acquisition (*see* **Note 17**).
10. Move the imaging chamber/bed to the CT scan. Obtain a full body CT scan.
11. As animal one is moved into the CT, place the next animal in the PET scanner. This will keep the 10 min doses and total uptake time between animals the same.
12. If this is survival imaging, place the mouse in a recovery cage on a heating pad until fully conscious (*see* **Note 18**).
13. If this is terminal imaging euthanize the mouse and perform biodistribution (*see* **Note 19**).

3.5 Image Analysis

1. Obtain reconstructed scans (*see* **Note 20**).
2. Verify that the PET and CT scans are properly overlaid.
3. Identify the bladder in the CT scan and align with the bladder in the PET scan. Adjust X, Y, and Z axes.
4. Continue adjustments of scan orientation as necessary.
5. Draw regions of interest based on CT for the subcutaneous tumors. This allows for non-biased sizing in both high and low signal tumors.
6. Apply the region of interest to the PET scans to obtain standard uptake value (SUV).

4 Notes

1. Antibiotic selection is needed if the cell line will be transplanted in syngeneic immune competent hosts to prevent rejection from the fluorescent reporter HSV-TK has not been reported to be immunogenic in mice, and it should be tolerated in vivo.
2. Matrigel is sold in normal, high concentration, and growth factor reduced. Some tumor cell lines survive better in vivo when injected together with matrigel, thereby ensuring consistent tumor take. Other cell lines do not require matrigel and can be implanted without it.
3. Anesthesia needs to be administered during the entire PET and CT scan since animals must be anesthetized to remain immobile for PET and CT scans. The recommended dose is 2% isoflurane to keep mice sedated during the entire process. Check with EH&S to determine how to properly use and install isoflurane induction systems. Ketamine is a controlled substance, check with your animal oversight committee on the proper way to obtain and use in mice.

4. Synthesis of [^{18}F]-FHBG should only be done by a well-trained radiochemist in a dedicated radiosynthesis laboratory.
5. [^{18}F]-FHBG can by synthesized in a number of ways. The initial synthesis was described by Alauddin et al. [29]. Later studies changed the synthesis to be faster, higher yield, one pot, or carrier free [17, 24, 28, 30].
6. Mice can be bred in house or ordered from commercial vendors. All mice should be rested for at least 1 week in the new facility prior to beginning an experiment or tumor implantation. Shipping and transport can cause high stress levels in rodents and may cause irregular or abnormal tumor growth.
7. Fluorescent activated cell sorter (FACS) instrument is only necessary if sorting the cancer cell line on fluorescent protein expression. Cells should be sorted in sterile conditions and should be cultured with antibiotics after primary and secondary sort.
8. A CT scan is not required for PET imaging but improves the ability to determine exact tissue locations. Other alternatives are MRI or X-ray. If a secondary anatomical scan is required, the imaging chamber should be adapted to fit both machines to prevent any movement between scans. Some companies sell dual PET/CT instruments that allow both images to be acquired on the same machine without changing the animal's position.
9. There are several softwares available for data analysis. It is important to know the file format needed for each to ensure that image acquisition and reconstruction are performed in the correct format.
10. A separate non-transduced cell line should be maintained as a negative control for background [^{18}F]-FHBG accumulation. Spinfection protocols vary based on cell type, virus, and lab. It is best to find a method that provides reproducible high infection rates.
11. Lentivirus will have peak and stable expression after 72 h while retrovirus has stable expression after 48 h. In both the cases it is best to wait until stable expression occurs prior to sorting. Sorting the top 25% of positive cells will ensure a high and uniform expression of HSV-TK. Cells can then be expanded and resorted to ensure a pure population. For cancer cells that are large or sensitive to sorting, a slow sort with a large nozzle will help increase viability post-sort.
12. If drug selection is used, selection can begin 48–72 h after lentiviral infection. Selection should be maintained through

several passages, but is recommended until cells are transplanted in vivo.

13. Cell viability prior to tumor implantation is crucial. Cells should not be confluent, overgrown, or in poor condition. Viability greater than 90% is preferred. Cell counts should be based on live cells only.
14. Based on the available equipment or preferred synthesis methods within the radiochemistry laboratory, an alternative probe production protocol can be used. The method described is for preclinical studies.
15. The total dose needed per mouse is dependent on the scanner minimum and maximum ranges. Prior to imaging, the appropriate range of activity (dose corrected for the 3 h uptake) needs to be calculated.
16. Uptake time can be shortened in some instances. The uptake time of 3 h helps to reduce nonspecific signal in the GI, kidneys, and bladder.
17. Scan times can be adjusted for increased signal, or to obtain a dynamic image. For most subcutaneous studies, a 10 min scan is sufficient.
18. After scanning, place the animals and cages in a designated area that is either protected by lead shielding or is isolated to prevent unintentional radiation exposure. After ten half-lives, animals can be returned to the normal animal barrier.
19. All animal tissue and material used in the biodistribution should be kept in an isolated freezer with a radiation warning until the tissue is fully decayed (10 half-lives). After the material can be disposed of as biohazardous waste.
20. Filtered background projection is recommended for acquisition and reconstruction. A detailed description on image analysis and quantification is available in an alternative chapter.

Acknowledgment

M.N.M. is supported by the Stanford Dean's Fellowship and the A.P. Giannini Foundation.

References

1. Phelps ME (2000) Positron emission tomography provides molecular imaging of biological processes. Proc Natl Acad Sci U S A 97:9226–9233
2. Cherry SR, Gambhir SS (2001) Use of positron emission tomography in animal research. ILAR Journal/National Research Council, Institute of Laboratory Animal Resources 42:219–232

3. Gambhir SS (2002) Molecular imaging of cancer with positron emission tomography. Nat Rev Cancer 2:683–693
4. Kircher MF, Gambhir SS, Grimm J (2011) Noninvasive cell-tracking methods. Nat Rev Clin Oncol 8:677–688
5. Serdons K, Verbruggen A, Bormans GM (2009) Developing new molecular imaging probes for PET. Methods 48:104–111
6. Acton PD, Zhou R (2005) Imaging reporter genes for cell tracking with PET and SPECT. The Quarterly Journal of Nuclear Medicine and Molecular Imaging: Official Publication of the Italian Association of Nuclear Medicine 49:349–360
7. Gelovani Tjuvajev J, Blasberg RG (2003) In vivo imaging of molecular-genetic targets for cancer therapy. Cancer Cell 3:327–332
8. Herschman HR (2004) PET reporter genes for noninvasive imaging of gene therapy, cell tracking and transgenic analysis. Crit Rev Oncol Hematol 51:191–204
9. McCracken MN, Tavare R, Witte ON, Wu AM (2016) Advances in PET detection of the antitumor T cell response. Adv Immunol 131:187–231
10. Saral R, Burns WH, Laskin OL, Santos GW, Lietman PS (1981) Acyclovir prophylaxis of herpes-simplex-virus infections. N Engl J Med 305:63–67
11. Tiberghien P, Reynolds CW, Keller J et al (1994) Ganciclovir treatment of herpes simplex thymidine kinase-transduced primary T lymphocytes: an approach for specific in vivo donor T-cell depletion after bone marrow transplantation? Blood 84:1333–1341
12. Black ME, Newcomb TG, Wilson HM, Loeb LA (1996) Creation of drug-specific herpes simplex virus type 1 thymidine kinase mutants for gene therapy. Proc Natl Acad Sci U S A 93:3525–3529
13. Blumenthal M, Skelton D, Pepper KA, Jahn T, Methangkool E, Kohn DB (2007) Effective suicide gene therapy for leukemia in a model of insertional oncogenesis in mice. Molecular therapy: The Journal of the American Society of Gene Therapy 15:183–192
14. Tjuvajev JG, Stockhammer G, Desai R et al (1995) Imaging the expression of transfected genes in vivo. Cancer Res 55:6126–6132
15. Gambhir SS, Barrio JR, Wu L et al (1998) Imaging of adenoviral-directed herpes simplex virus type 1 thymidine kinase reporter gene expression in mice with radiolabeled ganciclovir. Journal of nuclear medicine: official publication, Society of Nuclear Medicine 39:2003–2011
16. Tjuvajev JG, Avril N, Oku T et al (1998) Imaging herpes virus thymidine kinase gene transfer and expression by positron emission tomography. Cancer Res 58:4333–4341
17. Penuelas I, Boan JF, Marti-Climent JM et al (2002) A fully automated one pot synthesis of 9-(4-[18F]fluoro-3-hydroxymethylbutyl) guanine for gene therapy studies. Molecular imaging and biology: MIB: The Official Publication of the Academy of Molecular Imaging 4:415–424
18. Yaghoubi S, Barrio JR, Dahlbom M et al (2001) Human pharmacokinetic and dosimetry studies of [(18)F]FHBG: a reporter probe for imaging herpes simplex virus type-1 thymidine kinase reporter gene expression. Journal of Nuclear Medicine : Official Publication, Society of Nuclear Medicine 42:1225–1234
19. Le LQ, Kabarowski JH, Wong S, Nguyen K, Gambhir SS, Witte ON (2002) Positron emission tomography imaging analysis of G2A as a negative modifier of lymphoid leukemogenesis initiated by the BCR-ABL oncogene. Cancer Cell 1:381–391
20. Hustinx R, Shiue CY, Alavi A et al (2001) Imaging in vivo herpes simplex virus thymidine kinase gene transfer to tumour-bearing rodents using positron emission tomography and. Eur J Nucl Med 28:5–12
21. Su H, Forbes A, Gambhir SS, Braun J (2004) Quantitation of cell number by a positron emission tomography reporter gene strategy. Molecular imaging and biology: MIB: the Official Publication of the Academy of Molecular Imaging 6:139–148
22. Johnson M, Karanikolas BD, Priceman SJ et al (2009) Titration of variant HSV1-tk gene expression to determine the sensitivity of 18F-FHBG PET imaging in a prostate tumor. Journal of nuclear medicine: Official Publication, Society of Nuclear Medicine 50:757–764
23. Moolten FL, Wells JM, Heyman RA, Evans RM (1990) Lymphoma regression induced by ganciclovir in mice bearing a herpes thymidine kinase transgene. Hum Gene Ther 1:125–134
24. Gambhir SS, Bauer E, Black ME et al (2000) A mutant herpes simplex virus type 1 thymidine kinase reporter gene shows improved sensitivity for imaging reporter gene expression with positron emission tomography. Proc Natl Acad Sci U S A 97:2785–2790
25. Davis HE, Morgan JR, Yarmush ML (2002) Polybrene increases retrovirus gene transfer efficiency by enhancing receptor-independent

virus adsorption on target cell membranes. Biophys Chem 97:159–172

26. Loening AM, Gambhir SS (2003) AMIDE: a free software tool for multimodality medical image analysis. Mol Imaging 2:131–137
27. Tiscornia G, Singer O, Verma IM (2006) Production and purification of lentiviral vectors. Nat Protoc 1:241–245
28. Ponde DE, Dence CS, Schuster DP, Welch MJ (2004) Rapid and reproducible radiosynthesis of [18F] FHBG. Nucl Med Biol 31:133–138
29. Alauddin MM, Conti PS (1998) Synthesis and preliminary evaluation of 9-(4-[18F]-fluoro-3-hydroxymethylbutyl)guanine ([18F]FHBG): a new potential imaging agent for viral infection and gene therapy using PET. Nucl Med Biol 25:175–180
30. Shiue GG, Shiue CY, Lee RL et al (2001) A simplified one-pot synthesis of 9-[(3-[18F] fluoro-1-hydroxy-2-propoxy)methyl]guanine ([18F]FHPG) and 9-(4-[18F]fluoro-3-hydroxymethylbutyl)guanine ([18F]FHBG) for gene therapy. Nucl Med Biol 28:875–883

Chapter 12

Ex Vivo Radiolabeling and In Vivo PET Imaging of T Cells Expressing Nuclear Reporter Genes

Maxim A. Moroz, Pat Zanzonico, Jason T. Lee, and Vladimir Ponomarev

Abstract

Recent advances in T cell-based immunotherapies from bench to bedside have highlighted the need for improved diagnostic imaging of T cell trafficking in vivo and the means to noninvasively investigate failures in treatment response. T cells expressing tumor-associated T cell receptors (TCRs) or engineered with chimeric antigen receptors (CARs) face multiple challenges, including possible influence of genetic engineering on T cell efficacy, inhibitory effects of the tumor microenvironment, tumor checkpoint proteins and on-target, off-tissue toxicities (Kershaw et al., Nat Rev Cancer 13:525–541, 2013; Corrigan-Curay et al., Mol Ther 22:1564–1574, 2014; June et al., Sci Trans Med 7:280–287, 2015; Whiteside et al., Clin Cancer Res 22:1845–1855, 2016; Rosenberg and Restifo, Science 348:62–68, 2015). Positron emission tomography (PET) imaging with nuclear reporter genes is potentially one of the most sensitive and noninvasive methods to quantitatively track and monitor function of adoptively transferred cells in vivo. However, in vivo PET detection of T cells after administration into patients is limited by the degree of tracer accumulation per cell in situ and cell density in target tissues. We describe here a method for ex vivo radiolabeling of T cells, a reliable and robust technique for PET imaging of the kinetics of T cell biodistribution from the time of administration to subsequent localization in targeted tumors and other tissues of the body. This noninvasive technique can provide valuable information to monitor and identify the potential efficacy of adoptive cell therapies.

Key words T cell, Immunotherapy, Adoptive cell therapy, PET, Human nuclear reporter gene, Reporter probe, Ex vivo radiolabeling, Tumor microenvironment

1 Introduction

Technologies to assess the migration, survival, and function of antigen-specific T cells in vivo hold promise to improve cellular immunotherapies. Several imaging modalities have been investigated for this purpose including positron emission tomography (PET), magnetic resonance imaging (MRI), and two-photon microscopy. While two-photon microscopy is an invasive technique for ex vivo imaging of immune cell trafficking using fluorescent reporter genes [1, 2], PET and MRI are noninvasive in vivo imaging techniques that permit real-time, longitudinal monitoring of adoptively transferred T cells. For MRI, phagocytic macrophages

Purnima Dubey (ed.), *Reporter Gene Imaging: Methods and Protocols*, Methods in Molecular Biology, vol. 1790,
https://doi.org/10.1007/978-1-4939-7860-1_12,

and monocytes are co-incubated with superparamagnetic iron oxide (SPIO) nanoparticles or perfluorocarbon (PFC) emulsion prior to adoptive transfer and subsequent imaging [3]. These agents are complexed with a cationic transfection agent to permit imaging of non-phagocytic cells.

PET imaging of ex vivo radiolabeled T cells with or without stably expressing reporter genes has been demonstrated successfully for noninvasive cell tracking in vivo [4–7]. The technique involves three general steps: (1) stable expression of a reporter gene (optional depending on labeling technique), (2) ex vivo radiolabeling by co-incubating target cells with radiotracer, and (3) adoptive transfer of cells and in vivo PET imaging. Some systems require expression of a reporter gene, which functions to trap the radiotracer intracellularly during ex vivo radiolabeling. These genes include herpes simplex virus thymidine kinase (HSV-TK, Fig. 1) and humanized reporter genes such as deoxycytidine kinase (dCKDM), norepinephrine transporter (hNET), and sodium-iodide symporter (hNIS) [8].

Koehne et al. demonstrated PET and gamma camera imaging of ex vivo and in vivo radiolabeled adoptively transferred T cells and their selective accumulation in HLA-matched and Epstein-Barr virus-positive (EBV+) tumors, but not in EBV^- or HLA-mismatched tumors (Fig. 2) [4]. The percentage of infiltrating T cells in tumor and spleen closely correlated with the doses of radioactivity accumulated at each site. Additionally, radiolabeled T cells retained their capacity to eliminate target-specific tumors [4].

While PET reporter gene imaging techniques vary in detection sensitivity, T cells can be imaged in mice with microPET scanners and are within clinically relevant range of clinical PET scanners. The ability to identify populations as low as 1×10^5 T cells has been shown (Fig. 3). In vivo PET imaging of ex vivo radiolabeled antigen-specific T cells is directly translatable to current adoptive cellular therapy protocols in the clinic and can provide critical information about therapeutic efficacy.

The following describes the methodology for ex vivo radiolabeling of reporter gene-expressing T cells with PET radiotracers and subsequent in vivo PET imaging to assess T cell biodistribution. Other adoptively transferred cell protocols should, in theory, be amenable to this imaging technique and could prove valuable for in vivo assessment of cellular therapy.

2 Materials

2.1 Reporter Gene Constructs and Virus Production

1. Viral construct bearing transcriptional promoter (constitutive or inducible), reporter gene, targeting receptor (e.g., CAR), and selection marker (e.g., green fluorescent protein, GFP).
2. Virus-producing cells: PG13 or Phoenix Ampho-Ecotropic are generally efficient for most retroviral productions and are available through the American Type Culture Collection (ATCC).

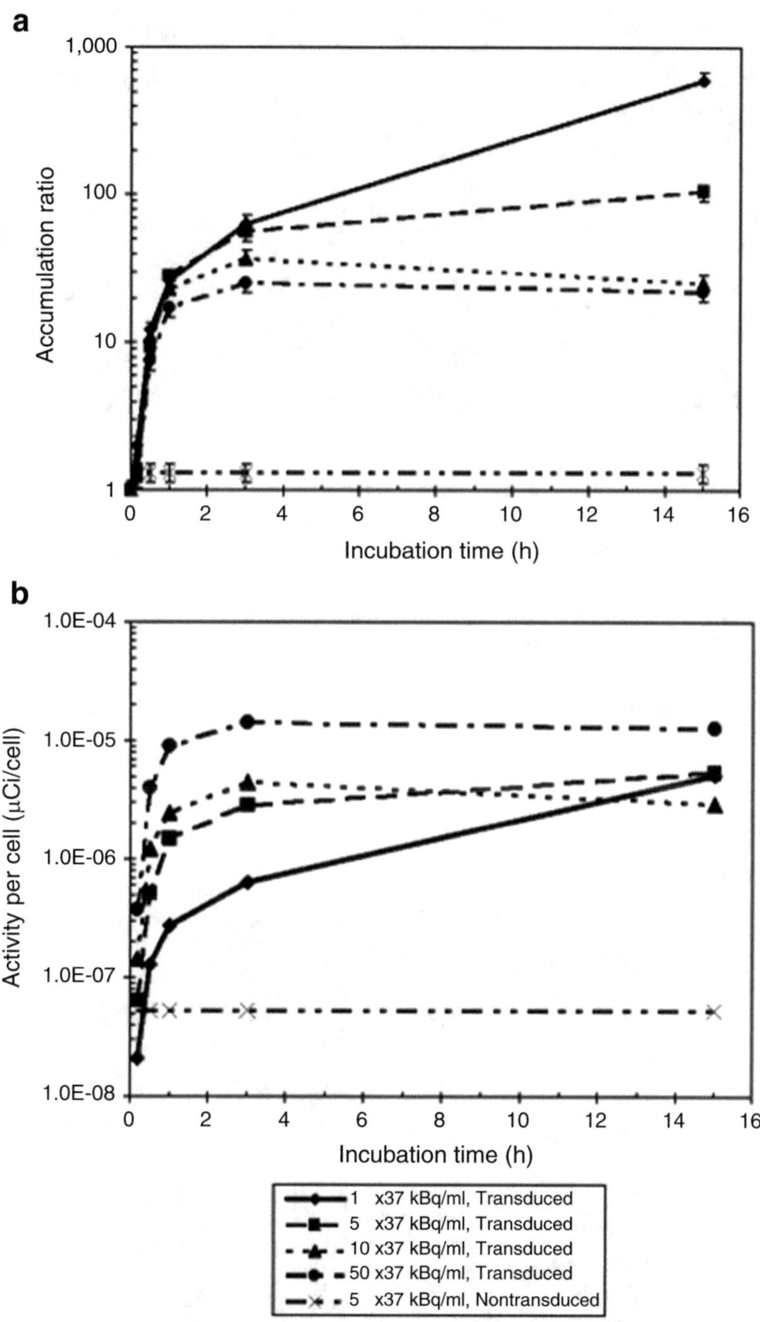

Fig. 1 Dynamics of ex vivo radiolabeling of HSV-TK+ lymphocytes, expressed as (**a**) the accumulation ratio and (**b**) the activity per cell (µCi/cell) of 131I-FIAU as a function of incubation time in 131I-FIAU-containing medium for radioactivity concentrations ranging from 1 to 50 µCi/mL. Adapted from Koehne et al. [4] with permission from the publisher

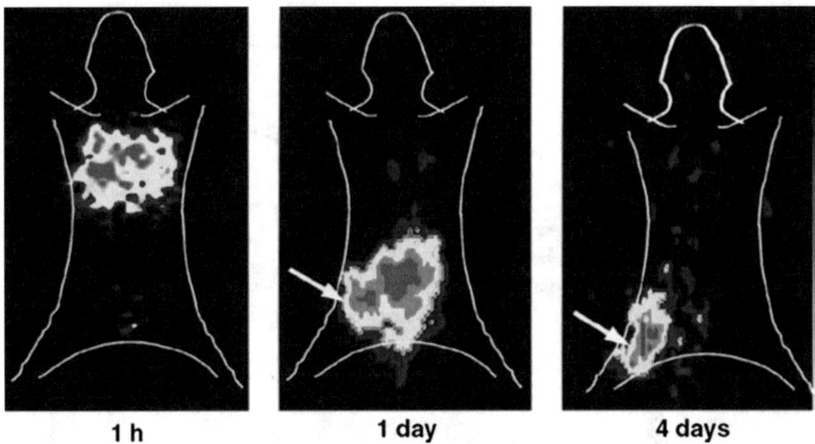

Fig. 2 Representative serial planar gamma camera images of SCID mice bearing a human EBV lymphoma xenograft at 1 h, 1 day, and 4 days following tail vein injection of 3×10^7 autologous EBV-specific T cells transduced with NIT+ and radiolabeled in vitro with 131I-FIAU. For anatomic orientation, manually drawn body contours of the mouse are shown. The arrows in the 1- and 4-day images identify the tumor. The NIT+ EBV-specific T cells were radiolabeled with 131I-FIAU to the MTD, that is, the 827-cGy nuclear absorbed dose indicated in Fig. 3. The images were obtained with an Adac Vertex+ digital gamma camera (Adac, Milpitas, CA, USA) fitted with a high-energy high-resolution (HEHR) collimator and using a 364-keV ± 10% photopeak energy window for ^{131}I. Adapted from Koehne et al. [4] with permission from the publisher

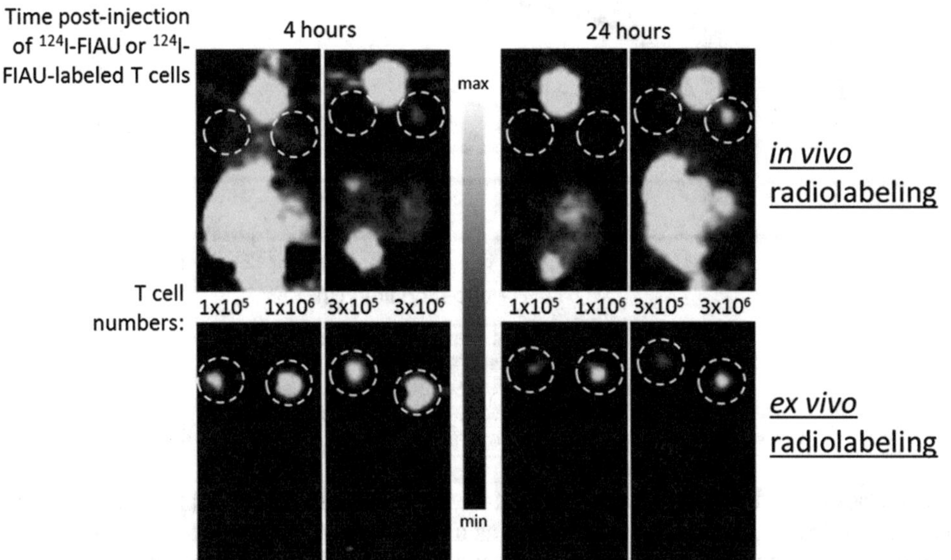

Fig. 3 A 30-fold improvement in in vivo microPET detection sensitivity of T cells injected subcutaneously when radiolabeled ex vivo with ^{124}I-FIAU prior to implantation in mice compared to in vivo radiolabeling through systemic intravenous injection of ^{124}I-FIAU. Unpublished data from Vladimir Ponomarev et al.

3. X-tremeGENE 9 (Roche, 06365787001) or similar reagents for transfection of virus-producing cells with reporter gene-bearing vectors.

2.2 T Cell Isolation and Expansion from Whole Blood or Buffy Coat

1. Whole blood or buffy coat (available from regional blood banks or blood donations).
2. 1× Phosphate-buffered saline (PBS).
3. Lymphocyte separation medium (LSM; Corning, 25-072-CI or similar agent), a polysucrose and diatrizoate solution designed for isolating lymphocytes from blood by centrifugation. Store at 25 °C.
4. Red blood cell lysis buffer. Store at 25 °C, away from light.
5. Phytohemagglutinin (PHA). Stock solution prepared in sterile PBS at 1 mg/mL. Store at −20 °C. Anti-CD3/CD28 Dynabeads can be used as an alternative for PHA for stimulation purposes at a ratio of three Dynabeads per one T cell (Fisher Scientific, 111.32D).
6. T cell media: RPMI 1640 media (containing nonessential amino acids, 10 mM HEPES, 1 mM sodium pyruvate, 2 mM L-glutamine, 1.5 g/L sodium bicarbonate, 4.5 g/L glucose) supplemented with 1% penicillin/streptomycin, 10% fetal calf serum, and 50 μM β-mercaptoethanol.
7. IL-2, available in many stock formulations (final concentration 20 IU per mL of media).

2.3 Reporter Gene Transduction and T Cell Maintenance

1. RetroNectin (Fisher, T100B) or similar reagent. Stock is 2.5 mg and stored at −20 °C.
2. IL-15 (1000× stock is 10 mg/mL).
3. For CAR T cells: antigen-presenting cells (e.g., PSMA) growing in exponential phase will be required, it is beneficial to modify antigen-presenting cells (APCs) to also express co-stimulatory molecules (e.g., B7).
4. For constructs that include antibiotic resistance genes: an antibiotic, e.g., gentamicin (G418), will be required.
5. For constructs that include a fluorescent reporter gene or that can be detected with an antibody labeled with fluorophores: fluorescence activated cell sorting (FACS) will be required.
6. For long-term storage, T cells can be cryopreserved using DMSO-containing cell-freezing media.
7. Untreated and cell-culture-treated plastic T-175 flasks and six-well plates.

2.4 Ex Vivo Radiolabeling

Ensure all equipment is and the radiolabeling workspace is approved for work with radioactive materials.

1. Incubator with shaking platform, set at 37° C, 5% CO_2.
2. Cell viability counter, e.g., ViCell.
3. FACS sorting tubes.
4. Cell-culture-treated plastic T-175 flasks and six-well plates.
5. ^{51}Cr chromate for ^{51}Cr release assay of T cell cytotoxicity.
6. Automated gamma counter.

2.5 PET Imaging

1. MicroPET scanner for animal imaging. Many commercial scanners are available designed for whole-body imaging of mice with relatively high sensitivity and spatial resolution.
2. CT or MRI scanner. PET data benefit greatly from anatomical co-registration, so it is highly recommended to combine PET with CT or MRI imaging.
3. Image analysis software (*see* Subheading 4).

2.6 Other Materials and Equipment

1. 1× phosphate-buffered saline (PBS).
2. 0.05% or 0.25% trypsin.
3. Isoflurane in oxygen and vaporizer.
4. Untreated and cell culture-treated plastic T-175 flasks and six-well plates.
5. 50 mL conical tubes.
6. 10 or 20 mL serological pipettes.
7. Benchtop centrifuge with temperature control and plate holders.

3 Methods

3.1 T Cell Transduction, Expansion, and Preparation

Please *see* Chapter 13, steps 3.1–4 in Lee et al., *Imaging T Cell Dynamics and Function Using PET and Human Nuclear Reporter Genes.* Figure 4 below shows a schematic representation of the transduction and imaging workflow.

3.2 Ex Vivo Radiolabeling of T Cells

1. Before radiolabeling, assess T cell viability (trypan blue exclusion assay), proliferation (cell growth), expression of TCR/CAR (e.g., flow cytometry), functional status (activation upon antigen presentation), cytotoxic potential (^{51}Cr release assay).
2. Animal formulation: T cells can be prepared in T cell culture media at desired concentrations (e.g., 1–10 × 10^6 T cells per mL of media).
3. Add radioactivity to T cells: for animal formulation, resuspend pelleted T cells in radioactive media and transfer to untreated

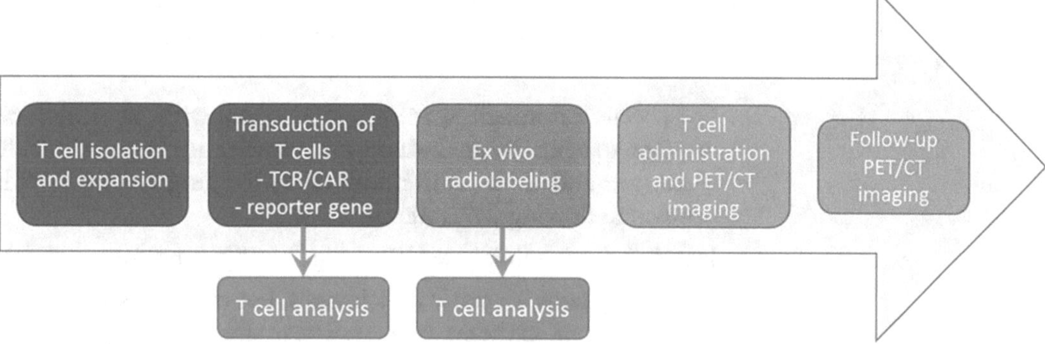

Fig. 4 Summary workflow for ex vivo radiolabeling and in vivo PET/CT imaging of T cells

tissue culture flasks/plates. Media radioactivity concentration up to 30 μCi/mL and incubation for 2 h does not adversely affect T cells [9].

4. Place resuspended cells in an incubator for a minimum of 2 h at 37 °C and 5% CO_2 on a cell culture rocker/shaker.
5. Prepare ex vivo radiolabeled T cells for injection. For animal imaging, collect and centrifuge T cells at 400 × *g* for 5 min. Safely remove and discard radioactive media. Resuspend T cells in 100–250 μL saline or non-radioactive, serum-free media for injections. Obtain an aliquot of cells for further analysis (*see* **step** 7). Maintain cells on ice until administration.
6. Measure amount of radioactivity per T cell. To optimize the activity per cell, alter the radioactivity concentration in media, concentration of T cells, and/or duration of ex vivo labeling. These parameters should be determined empirically for each type of radiopharmaceutical.
7. After radiolabeling, assess T cell viability (trypan blue exclusion assay), proliferation (cell growth), expression of TCR/CAR (e.g., flow cytometry), functional status (activation upon antigen presentation), cytotoxic potential (^{51}Cr release assay). Compare results with **step 1** to determine whether radiolabeling is detrimental to T cells (*see* Subheading 4, **Notes 1–5**).
8. For further investigation of the influence of the radiolabeling procedure on T cell health, repeat **step 6** and monitor overall cell proliferation for the next 48–72 h.

3.3 PET Imaging of T Cell Biodistribution

To observe immediate trafficking of T cells after injection, "dynamic" PET imaging should be conducted, e.g., acquire list-mode PET data starting at the time of T cell injection and continuing through 1–2 h post-injections. Otherwise, "static" (single time frame) PET imaging is performed to obtain T cell bio distributions at various time points (*see* Subheading 4, **Note 6**).

Follow all institutional, local, state and federal ethical and safety regulations. Anesthetics should be used according to approved techniques.

1. For preclinical imaging, anesthetize animal with 2% isoflurane in pure oxygen in an induction chamber for approximately 5–10 min and then transfer animal to imaging chamber with nose cone flowing 2% isoflurane.
2. Inject/infuse radiolabeled T cells, generally intravenously (i.v.).
3. Acquire dynamic or static PET images. For dynamic scans, inject T cells i.v. via catheter (e.g., tail vein for rodents) or direct injection immediately prior to starting PET acquisition. A slow, 10–20 s i.v. injection is recommended for rodents.
4. It would be beneficial to start with dynamic imaging for first 2 h to observe initial migration and homing. This can be followed with static imaging at later time points. The timing will depend partly on half-life of the isotope and partly on T cell biodistribution and targeting.
5. After each PET imaging, acquire CT image for anatomical co-registration and PET attenuation correction.
6. Reconstruct raw images and perform image analysis. Quantitation and image data is generally presented in units of "percent injected dose per gram of tissue" (%ID/g) or normalized to background (e.g., nonspecific tissue).

4 Notes

1. For proper use of ^{51}Cr release assay it is important to select a suitably narrow photopeak energy window for measuring ^{51}Cr (151 kEV) and use a substantial concentration for target cell uptake (up to 100 μCi per 1×10^6 target cells).
2. The ^{51}Cr release assay should be performed using T cells with same experimental radiopharmaceutical, but untreated with ^{51}Cr to calculated background.
3. Ex vivo radiolabeled T cells will be the most beneficial when used with long half-life radionuclides such as ^{124}I, ^{89}Zr, and ^{64}Cu; however it is important to note that the diagnostic value of PET biodistribution studies will decline as T cells die and/or proliferate in vivo, the latter causing a dilution of the activity per cell.
4. It is important to assess total amount of intracellular radioactivity in experimental cells to optimize for T cell dosage and optimal parameters of imaging such as scanner sensitivity and resolution.

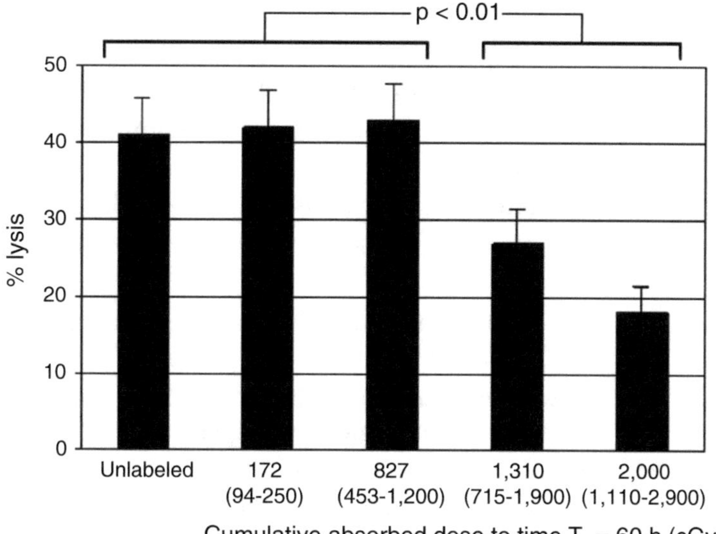

Fig. 5 Dose-dependent in vitro immune cytotoxicity of ^{131}I-FIAU-radiolabeled NIT+ cells against BCLCs determined by a ^{51}Cr-release cytotoxicity assay at a target:effector ratio of 20:1. Values indicated represent the calculated median cumulative absorbed doses to the effector-cell nuclei projected to the reference time $T_\beta = 60$ h after a 2-h incubation in ^{131}I-FIAU-containing medium, that is, the absorbed doses assuming 0.5 of the intracellular activity and cumulated activity is in the cytoplasm and 0.5 is in the nucleus. The values in parentheses represent the respective ranges of the calculated nuclear absorbed doses, with the lower limit corresponding to all of the intracellular activity being in the cytoplasm and the upper limit corresponding to all of the intracellular activity being in the nucleus. These data represent the results of triplicate determinations. The error bars represent the standard error of the mean (SEM). Adapted from Zanzonico et al. [9] with permission from the publisher

5. Cell-level dosimetry and radioactivity dose-dependent toxicity for ex vivo radiolabeled T cells and radioactivity dose-dependent T cell immune cytotoxicity should be evaluated (Fig. 5) [9].
6. Imaging ex vivo radiolabeled cells is informative and can assess therapy efficacy, but in vivo cell division will dilute intracellular tracer concentrations (particularly when imaging longer-lived isotopes) and significant cell death may increase tissue background due to the presence of free tracer. These situations may limit the comparison of PET images with true T cell numbers in vivo and are more pronounced in extended studies (e.g., on the order of days) [9].

Assay of T Cell Accumulation Ratio (AR)

1. Weigh one micro-centrifuge tube labeled "Cells (C)" and two gamma counting tubes, one labeled "Medium (M)" and the other labeled "Wash (W)."

2. Transfer the 1 mL of radiolabeled T cells (from **step 3** above) into the micro-centrifuge tube (labeled "cells (C)").
3. Centrifuge the T cells at 400 × *g* for 5 min to pellet the cells.
4. Decant the medium into the counting tube labeled "Medium (M)."
5. Wash the cells by resuspending the pellet in fresh media.
6. Centrifuge the cell suspension at 400 × *g* for 5 min to pellet the cells.
7. Decant the wash medium into the tared counting tube labeled "Wash (W)."
8. Re-weigh the micro-centrifuge tube and the two counting tubes to determine their respective gross weights.
9. Subtract the tare weights of each tube from the gross weights of each tube to determine the net weight of the cells (plus any wash adherent to the cells), the media, and the wash media.
10. For 1 × 10^6 cells, the net weight of the "Cells (C)" tube will be due almost entirely to the adherent wash in that tube. Therefore, determine the count rate specifically for the labeled cells as follows:

$$\begin{matrix}\text{Count Rate (cpm)}\\ \text{in Labeled Cells}\end{matrix} = \begin{matrix}\text{Net Count Rate (cpm)}\\ \text{in "Cells (C)" Tube}\end{matrix} - \frac{\begin{matrix}\text{Net Count Rate (cpm)}\\ \text{in "Wash (W)" Tube}\end{matrix}}{\begin{matrix}\text{Net Weight (gm)}\\ \text{of Wash Medium}\\ \text{in "Wash (W)" Tube}\end{matrix}} \times \begin{matrix}\text{Net Weight (gm)}\\ \text{of "Cells (C)" Tube}\end{matrix}$$

11. Calculate the cpm/gm of cells:

$$\text{cpm/gm of cells} = \frac{\text{Count Rate (cpm) in Labeled Cells}}{\text{Net Weight (gm) of "Cells (C)" Tube}}$$

12. Calculate the cpm/gm of medium:

$$\text{cpm/gm of medium} = \frac{\begin{matrix}\text{Net Count Rate (cpm)}\\ \text{in "Medium (M)" Tube}\end{matrix} + \begin{matrix}\text{Net Count Rate (cpm)}\\ \text{in "Wash (W)" Tube}\end{matrix}}{\text{Net Weight (gm) of "Medium (M)" Tube}}$$

13. Finally, calculate the accumulation ratio (AR):

$$\text{AR} = \frac{\text{cpm/gm of cells}}{\text{cpm/gm of medium}}$$

AR values between **50** and **100** are expected.

Acknowledgments

This work was supported by NIH P50 CA86438, R01 CA163980 and R01 CA161138 grants, Mr. William H. Goodwin and Mrs. Alice Goodwin and the Commonwealth Foundation for Cancer Research and The Experimental Therapeutics Center of Memorial Sloan Kettering Cancer Center, NIH Small-Animal Imaging Research Program (SAIRP), NIH Shared Instrumentation Grant No 1 S10 RR020892-01, NIH Shared Instrumentation Grant No 1 S10 RR028889-01, and NIH Center Grants P30 CA08748 and P30 CA08748.

References

1. Asperti-Boursin F, Real E, Bismuth G, Trautmann A, Donnadieu E (2007) CCR7 ligands control basal T cell motility within lymph node slices in a phosphoinositide 3-kinase-independent manner. J Exp Med 204:1167–1179
2. Salmon H, Rivas-Caicedo A, Asperti-Boursin F, Lebugle C, Bourdoncle P, Donnadieu E (2011) Ex vivo imaging of T cells in murine lymph node slices with widefield and confocal microscopes. J Vis Exp: JoVE (53):e3054
3. Ahrens ET, Bulte JW (2013) Tracking immune cells in vivo using magnetic resonance imaging. Nat Rev Immunol 13:755–763
4. Koehne G, Doubrovin M, Doubrovina E et al (2003) Serial in vivo imaging of the targeted migration of human HSV-TK-transduced antigen-specific lymphocytes. Nat Biotechnol 21:405–413
5. Adonai N, Nguyen KN, Walsh J et al (2002) Ex vivo cell labeling with 64Cu-pyruvaldehyde-bis (N4-methylthiosemicarbazone) for imaging cell trafficking in mice with positron-emission tomography. Proc Natl Acad Sci U S A 99:3030–3035
6. Bansal A, Pandey MK, Demirhan YE et al (2015) Novel (89)Zr cell labeling approach for PET-based cell trafficking studies. EJNMMI Res 5:19
7. Liu Z, Li Z (2014) Molecular imaging in tracking tumor-specific cytotoxic T lymphocytes (CTLs). Theranostics 4:990–1001
8. Yaghoubi SS, Campbell DO, Radu CG, Czernin J (2012) Positron emission tomography reporter genes and reporter probes: gene and cell therapy applications. Theranostics 2:374–391
9. Zanzonico P, Koehne G, Gallardo HF et al (2006) [131I]FIAU labeling of genetically transduced, tumor-reactive lymphocytes: cell-level dosimetry and dose-dependent toxicity. Eur J Nucl Med Mol Imaging 33:988–997

Chapter 13

Imaging T Cell Dynamics and Function Using PET and Human Nuclear Reporter Genes

Jason T. Lee, Maxim A. Moroz, and Vladimir Ponomarev

Abstract

Adoptive cell transfer immunotherapy has demonstrated significant promise in the treatment of cancer, with long-term, durable responses. T cells expressing T cell receptors (TCRs) that recognize tumor antigens, or engineered with chimeric antigen receptors (CARs) can recognize and eliminate tumor cells even in advanced disease. Positron emission tomography (PET) imaging with nuclear reporter genes, a noninvasive method to track and monitor function of engineered cells in vivo, allows quantitative, longitudinal monitoring of these cells, including their expansion/contraction, migration, retention at target and off-target sites, and biological state. As an additional advantage, some reporter genes also exhibit "suicide potential" permitting the safe elimination of adoptively transferred T cells in instances of adverse reaction to therapy. Here, we describe the production of human nuclear reporter gene-expressing T cells and noninvasive PET imaging to monitor their cell fate in vivo.

Key words T cell, Immunotherapy, PET, Human nuclear reporter gene, Reporter probe, Chimeric antigen receptors, Nucleoside kinases

1 Introduction

Immunotherapy with tumor-reactive T cells is a rapidly growing and exceptionally promising personalized cancer therapy, achieving durable disease remission across many cancers [1, 2]. These T cells include isolated tumor-infiltrating lymphocytes (TILs), circulating T cells, or T cells engineered to express either T cell receptors (TCRs) or chimeric antigen receptors (CARs) [3]. CARs are synthetic receptors that allow for antigen recognition, T cell activation, and co-stimulation to augment T cell functionality and viability [4, 5]. Recent success achieved with adoptive transfer of CAR+ T cells that recognize the CD19 antigen in patients with hematologic malignancies [6] and the prospect of implementing similar strategies for solid tumors [7] has established T cell immunotherapy as a promising treatment for various types of cancer. There has been

Purnima Dubey (ed.), *Reporter Gene Imaging: Methods and Protocols*, Methods in Molecular Biology, vol. 1790, https://doi.org/10.1007/978-1-4939-7860-1_13,

rapid growth in the number of clinical trials and commercialization to further develop the technology.

Nevertheless, acquired tumor resistance and activation of immunosuppressive pathways may limit responses to immunotherapy [8, 9]. Longitudinal assessment of adoptively transferred therapeutic T cells would be beneficial to optimize therapy [10, 11]. Currently, the ability to monitor these cell populations once infused into patients is limited and highlights the need for noninvasive imaging technologies such as positron emission tomography (PET) using reporter gene-reporter probe systems [12]. Such imaging paradigms provide information on the spatial distribution and functional status of T cells through the use of viral constructs that carry different reporter genes under control of constitutive (Fig. 1) and/or inducible promoters (Fig. 2). Generally, the systems leverage the same gene transfer technology already optimized to instruct T cells to recognize tumor-associated antigens [13, 14].

Clinical proof-of-concept studies have demonstrated the feasibility of imaging T cells in patients [16]. Potential immunogenicity of current viral transgenes warrants the use of human-based

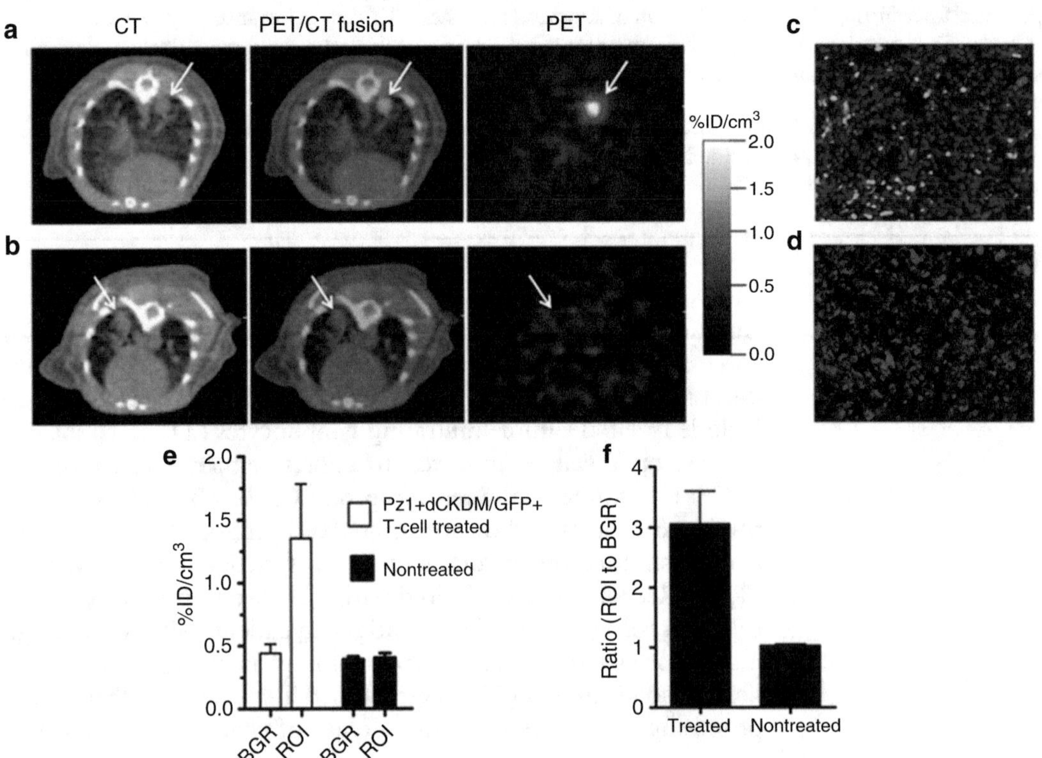

Fig. 1 PET/CT imaging of T cells expressing a constitutive PET reporter gene (dCKDM) and CAR targeting PSMA tumor antigen (Pz1). ^{18}F-FEAU accumulation by PET co-localized with tumor regions identified by CT, indicated by the arrow [15]

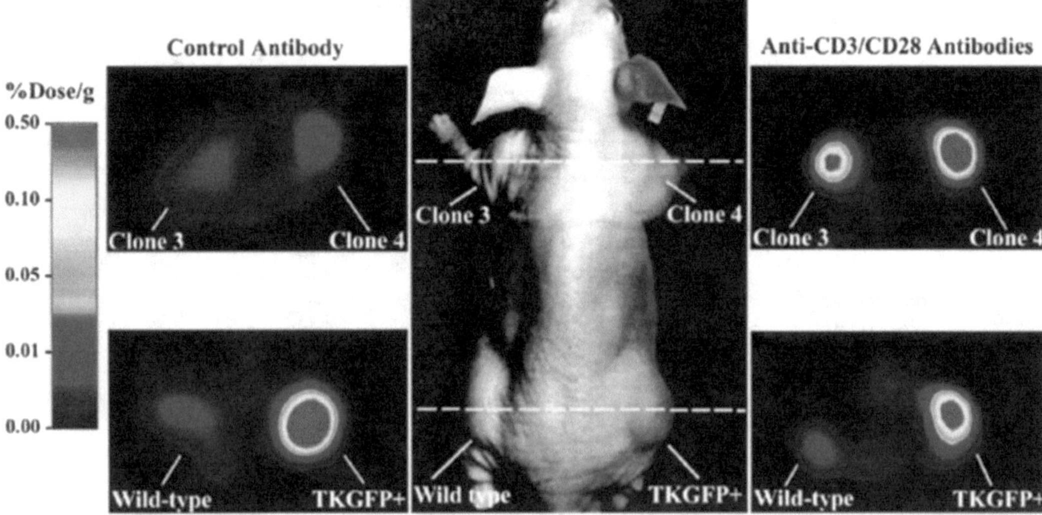

Fig. 2 ^{124}I-FIAU PET imaging of Jurkat T cells expressing an inducible (clone 3 and 4) or constitutive PET reporter gene (TKGFP), treated with control or anti-CD3/CD28 antibodies [17]

reporter systems. Reporter genes such as variants of human deoxycytidine kinase (dCK), thymidine kinase (TK), norepinephrine transporter (NET), sodium iodide symporter (NIS), dopamine 2 receptor (D2R), and carcinoembryonic antigen (CEA) are of human origin and, therefore, likely non-immunogenic [12]. They are designed to trap the radiolabeled reporter probe inside the cell (dCK, TK2), facilitate probe transport inside the cell (NET, NIS), or act as receptors for the probe (D2R, SSTR2, CEA) (Fig. 3). PET probes are radiolabeled with short (e.g., ^{18}F, ^{68}Ga) or long (e.g., ^{124}I, ^{89}Zr) half-life isotopes, and are small molecule compounds (e.g., FEAU, FESP, MFBG), antibodies/antibody variants, or peptides. Reporter gene-reporter probe pairings exhibit different biodistributions and sensitivities (Fig. 4, *see* Subheading 4, **Note 1**).

Molecular reporter systems are designed to monitor constitutive or inducible reporter gene expression [18]. The former permits the monitoring of cell trafficking and population dynamics [16, 19–22]. The latter, when placed under particular transcriptional control, links reporter gene expression to a desired biological phenomenon such as T cell activation [17, 23]. Together, the two complementary systems provide a more comprehensive understanding of the in vivo fate of adoptively transferred T cells, than either method alone (*see* Subheading 4, **Note 2**).

The following provides the methods for the production of reporter gene-expressing CAR+ T cells and PET imaging of their fate in vivo. Methods described here may also be adapted for other cell-based therapies such as dendritic cell vaccines and adoptive transfer of natural killer cells.

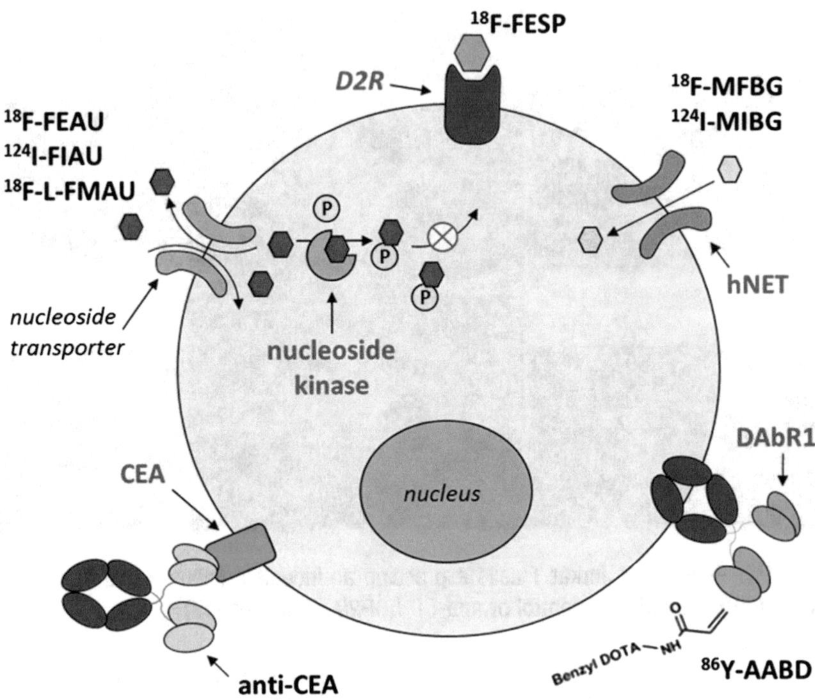

Fig. 3 Types of available human reporter gene imaging systems. Reporter genes and reporter probes are labeled in red and black bolded text, respectively

2 Materials

2.1 Reporter Gene Constructs and Virus Production

1. Viral construct bearing transcriptional promoter (constitutive or inducible), reporter gene, targeting receptor (e.g., CAR) and selection marker (e.g., green fluorescent protein, GFP). *For an inducible reporter system, the selection marker must be placed under a separate constitutive promoter to avoid, T cell activation during transduction and selection for a T cell activation-dependent promoter.*
2. Virus-producing cells: PG13, H29, or Phoenix Amphotropic are generally efficient for most retroviral productions and are available through the American Type Culture Collection (ATCC) (*see* Subheading 4, **Note 3**).
3. X-tremeGENE 9 (Roche, 06365787001) or similar reagents for transfection of virus-producing cells with reporter gene-bearing vectors.

2.2 T Cell Isolation and Expansion from Whole Blood or Buffy Coat

1. Whole blood or buffy coat (available from regional blood banks or blood donations).
2. 1× Phosphate-buffered saline (PBS).

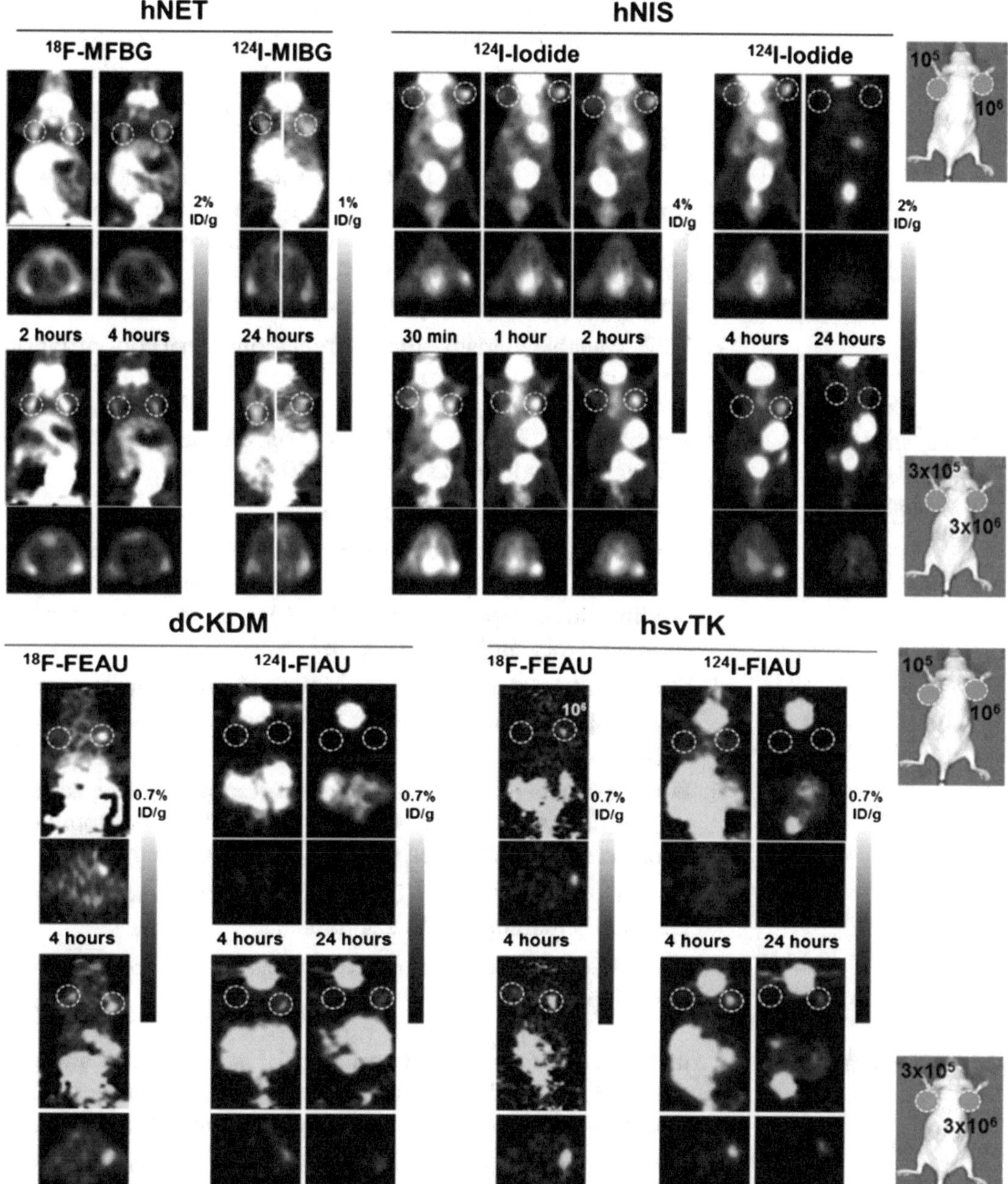

Fig. 4 In vivo PET imaging of human T cells transduced with various reporter genes in combination with their respective reporter probes [24]

3. Lymphocyte separation medium (LSM; Corning, 25–072-CI), a polysucrose and diatrizoate solution designed for isolating lymphocytes from blood by centrifugation. Store at 25 °C.
4. Red blood cell lysis buffer. Store at 25 °C, away from light.

5. Phytohemagglutinin (PHA). Stock solution prepared in sterile PBS at 1 mg/mL. Store at −20 °C. Antio-*CD3/CD28 Dynabeads can be used as an alternative for PHA for stimulation purposes at a ratio of three dynabeads per one cell (Fisher Scientific, 111.32D).*
6. T cell media: RPMI 1640 media (containing nonessential amino acids, 10 mM HEPES, 1 mM sodium pyruvate, 2 mM L-glutamine, 1.5 g/L sodium bicarbonate, 4.5 g/L glucose) supplemented with 1% penicillin/streptomycin, 10% fetal calf serum, and 50 μM β-mercaptoethanol.
7. IL-2, available in many stock formulations (final concentration 20 IU per mL of media).

2.3 Reporter Gene Transduction and T Cell Maintanence

1. RetroNectin (Fisher, T100B) or similar product. Stock is 2.5 mg of powder and stored at −20 °C.
2. IL-15 (1000× stock is 10 mg/mL).
3. For CAR T cells: antigen-presenting cells (e.g., PSMA) growing in exponential phase will be required, it is beneficial to modify antigen-presenting cells (APCs) to also express co-stimulatory molecules (e.g., B7).
4. For constructs that include antibiotic resistance genes: an antibiotic, e.g., gentamicin (G418, Invitrogen, 10131035), will be required.
5. For constructs that include either fluorescent reporter gene or can be detected with an antibody labeled with fluorophores: fluorescence activated cell sorting (FACS) will be required.
6. For long-term storage, T cells can be cryopreserved using DMSO-containing cell-freezing media.
7. Untreated and cell-culture-treated plastic T-175 flasks and six-well plates.

2.4 PET Imaging

1. microPET scanner. Many commercial scanners are available designed for whole body imaging of mice with relatively high sensitivity and spatial resolution (*see* Subheading 4, **Notes 14–17**).
2. microCT or microMRI scanner. PET data can benefit greatly from anatomical co-registration, so it is highly recommended to combine PET with CT or MRI imaging.
3. Image analysis software (*see* Subheading 4, **Notes 14–17**).

2.5 Other Materials and Equipment

1. 1× PBS.
2. 0.05% or 0.25% trypsin.
3. Isoflurane in oxygen.
4. 50 mL conical tubes.
5. 10 or 20 mL serological pipettes.
6. Benchtop centrifuge with temperature control and plate holders.

3 Methods

3.1 Production of Reporter Gene-Containing Virus

Viruses for transducing reporter genes can be produced by transient transfection of the viral construct into producer cells (H29 or Phoenix Ampho) or by viral transduction of stable producer cells (e.g., ATCC® CRL-10686™ (PG13)) clonally selected for high titer.

1. Transient transfection using H29 or Phoenix Ampho producer cells: Thaw and culture cells (generally in a 6-well or 10 cm plate) to achieve 50–70% confluency for transfection. *Cells growing in exponential phase are best for transfection and produce higher viral titer.*
2. Measure concentration of viral construct using spectrophotometer.
3. Transfect producer cells using X-tremeGENE (or similar) transfection agent: Add 2–10 μg of DNA in 1 mL of media with no serum and 30 μL of transfection reagent. Incubate for 20 min at room temperature. Apply transfection agent to cells drop-wise and gently mix by swirling plate to avoid disturbing cells.
4. Incubate for24 h at 37 °C, 5% CO_2, then replace media with fresh media supplemented with serum.
5. After 24–48 h, collect viral supernatant and filter through 0.45 μm filters.
6. For developing a stable retroviral producer cell line, PG13 producer cells have to be plated on the 10 cm dish and reach 40–50% confluence to be treated with H29 supernatant in the presence of polybrene (8 μg, Sigma, AL-118) for 24 h.
7. After 48 h post transduction, PG13 cells have to be assessed, using flow cytometry, either by measuring expressing of fluorescent reporter gene (if present) or by direct measurement of gene of interest using fluorescent immunostaining.
8. Collect viral supernatant from stably transduced PG13 cells every 24 h and filter through 0.45 μm filters. Supplement PG13 cells with fresh media.

3.2 T Cell Isolation and Expansion (Day 1)

1. Dilute blood (or buffy coat) in PBS at a ratio of 1:2.
2. Add 15 mL LSM in conical tubes (number of tubes depends on volume of diluted blood).
3. To each conical tube, slowly and with tube at an angle add 15–20 mL diluted blood to LSM. Avoid mixing or disturbing LSM layer.
4. Centrifuge tubes at 400 × *g*, 20 min at 25 °C. *Lymphocytes will become visible as a thin white layer below the plasma, second layer from the top.*

5. Collect lymphocytes into new 50 mL conical tubes using a serological pipette.
6. Wash 1: top off with PBS and centrifuge at 500 × *g*, 10 min at 25 °C.
7. Aspirate supernatant leaving behind pellet (lymphocytes).
8. Wash 2: resuspend pellet with 25 mL PBS and centrifuge at 500 × *g*, 10 min at 25 °C.
9. Aspirate the supernatant.
10. RBC lysis: resuspend pellet with 5 mL RBC lysis buffer.
11. Incubate suspension for 5 min at 25 °C.
12. Wash 3: resuspend pellet with 25 mL PBS and centrifuge at 500 × *g*, 10 min at 25 °C.
13. Aspirate the supernatant.
14. Stimulation of T cells: resuspend lymphocytes in T cell media containing PHA (2 μg/mL) or anti-CD3/CD28 beads at a concentration of 1 × 10^6 cells/mL and plate in T-25 flasks.
15. Incubate T cells for 48 h at 37 °C, 5% CO_2.

3.3 T Cell Transduction (Days 2–4)

1. On day 2, dilute RetroNectin in PBS to working concentration of 15 μg/mL.
2. Coat untreated 6-well plates with 1 mL RetroNectin working solution per well (will need one well per 1 × 10^6 T cells plated).
3. Seal plates with parafilm to maintain sterility and prevent evaporation. Store overnight at 4 °C or in room temperature for 2 h.
4. On day 3, collect and count T cells from culture. *T cells should be in suspension, but some may have adhered to the plates and should be harvested by gentle pipetting using a serological pipet.*
   (a) Collect cells in a 50 mL conical tube. To remove adhered T cells, add 5 mL 0.25% trypsin to the T-25 flask(s) and incubate at 37 °C for 5 min. Stop trypsinization by adding 10 mL T cell media and combine with collected cells.
   (b) Centrifuge at 500 × *g*, 5 min at 4 °C.
   (c) Resuspend pellet in 50 mL T cell media and count. Place cells on ice.
5. Pellet desired number of T cells for transduction at 500 × *g*, 5 min at 4 °C.
6. From virus producer plates, collect supernatant containing virus and filter through 0.45 μm syringe filters. *Replace media in virus producer plates for subsequent transductions.*

7. Supplement virus media with IL-2 at a final concentration of 20 IU/mL. *IL-2 is used in the initial T cell expansion, and replaced by IL-15 thereafter.*
8. Resuspend pellet in filtered virus media at 1×10^6 T cells/3 mL virus media and place on ice.
9. Remove RetroNectin from 6-well plates.
10. Add 1 mL PBS + 10% FCS to each well and incubate plates in an incubator at 37 °C for 30 min.
11. Remove PBS/FCS solution and wash RetroNectin-coated plates once with regular PBS.
12. Plate T cells on RetreoNectin-coated plates in 3 mL of supernatant/well (equal to 1×10^6 cells/well). It is possible to use two sets of supernatants for simultaneous transduction of T cells with two vectors. Up to 6 mL of the final mix can be used per well.
13. Spinonculate.
    (a) Wrap each plate in parafilm.
    (b) Spin plates at $100 \times g$ at 4 °C for 1 h.
    (c) Incubate plates at 37 °C, 5% CO_2.
    (d) Repeat transductions after 4–6 h, and similarly the next day for a total of four transductions.
    - Perform Subheading 3.2, **steps 6** and 7.
    - Spin T cell plates at $500 \times g$ for 5 min.
    - Aspirate ~2 mL old virus and refresh with 3 mL fresh virus.
    - Perform Subheading 3.3, **step 13a–c** as these steps are required to improve the transduction efficacy.
14. At 24 h after the last transduction, spin T cell plates at $500 \times g$ for 5 min.
15. Aspirate media and resuspend in fresh T cell media supplemented with IL-15 (10 ng/mL) and maintain in an incubator until use. Replace this media every 7 days or as needed depending on confluency.

3.4 Transduced T Cell Selection (Day 5+)

1. Depending on the viral construct used, transduced T cells can be selected for based on one or a combination of several methods:
    (a) Fluorescence-activated cell sorting of T cells by companion fluorescent reporter gene or fluorescence staining of transgene. For example, a nuclear reporter gene co-expressed with GFP permits FACS selection based on GFP expression.
    (b) Antibiotic selection. For example, nuclear reporter gene constructs containing the neomycin-resistance gene will

render T cells resistant to G418 exposure (e.g., 0.5 μg/mL for 10–14 days will kill off non-transduced T cells).

(c) Coculturing of T cells on antigen-presenting cells will lead to lysis of APCs and rapid expansion of CAR+ T cells relative to CAR-T cells. *Monitor T cells frequently during the co-incubation with APCs. If you observe rapid growth of antigen presenting cells, despite T cell presence, removal of T cells and re-application with a larger T cell to APC ratio is recommended.*

3.5 T Cell Administration and PET Imaging

Prepare and handle animals according to institutionally approved ethical and safety regulations. Anesthetics should be used according to approved techniques.

Dedicated microPET or microPET+CT/MRI scanners can be used for maximum PET sensitivity and resolution as well as anatomical correlation.

1. Prepare T cells at the desired concentration for injection. For example, a concentration of 1–10 × 10^6 cells/100 μL saline for a total dose of 2–20 × 10^6 reporter gene-positive T cells can be used. Keep cells on ice prior to injection.
2. Inject T cells intravenously (i.v.) via tail vein catheter or direct injection into conscious mice. Slow i.v. injection via tail vein is recommended in a volume of 100–250 μL.
3. Inject PET probe intravenously and allow 1 h time for probe biodistribution prior to PET imaging. The PET probe should be administered within 15 min of T cell injection to observe early stages of T cell migration if using a constitutive reporter system. PET probes can also be administered at specific time points of interest for repetitive imaging of constitutive and/or inducible systems, allowing for the probe to decay to background between imaging sessions.
4. For PET imaging, anesthetize animal in an induction chamber with 2% isoflurane mixed in air or pure oxygen for approximately 5–10 min.
5. Transfer animal to a nose cone, ideally placed on a heating pad to maintain physiological temperature.
6. Place animal on PET scanner bed in nose cone and acquire PET image (e.g., 10 min acquisition).
7. Acquire CT image for anatomical co-registration and PET attenuation correction.
8. Reconstruct raw images and perform image analysis. *Quantitation and image data is generally presented in units of "percent injected dose per gram of tissue" (%ID/g) or normalized to background* (e.g., *nonspecific tissue*). At the end of Subheading 3, add the following sentence: Fig. 5 shows a diagram of the work flow for virus production, transduction, and imaging.

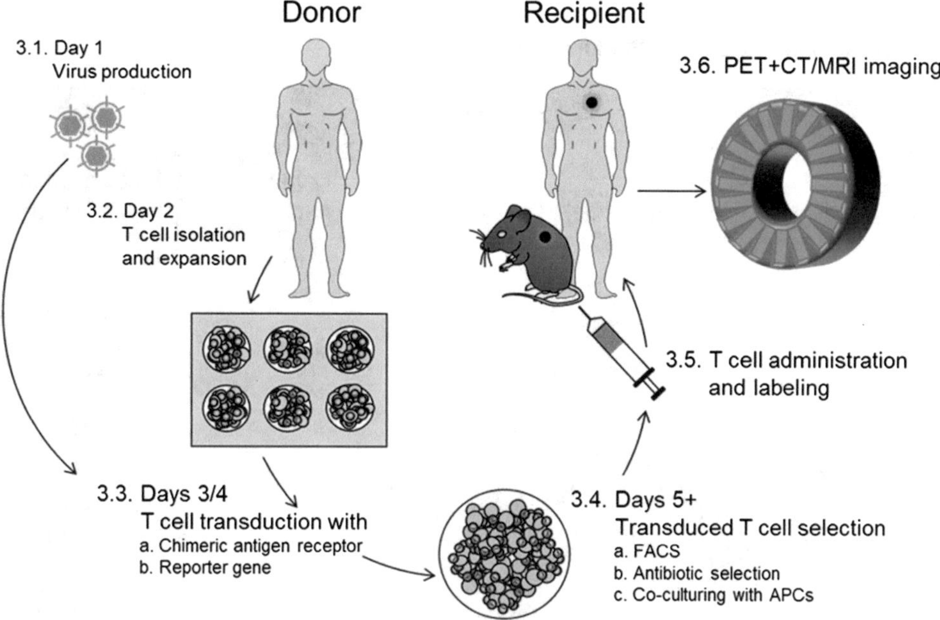

Fig. 5 Summary of T cell preparation and in vivo PET imaging workflow

4 Notes

1. Reporter gene-reporter probe systems. A large family of human reporter gene-reporter probe systems is available with different properties (Table 1). In general, selection of the best system is dependent on the location of the target tissue, timing of imaging needed, high reporter transgene expression in target cells and ideal dosimetry for clinical translation. Reporter probes differ in isotope used for labeling, ease of synthesis, radiochemical yield and, together with the reporter gene, sensitivity. In our hands, we determined the in vivo lower limit of T cell detection for several reporter systems in the range of 1×10^5 cells per 50 μL volume (Fig. 3).
2. Constitutive versus inducible reporters. Reporter gene systems can be engineered to report on the spatial distribution of target cells (e.g., T cell tumor targeting) or their functional state (e.g., T cell activation). The former is achieved by placing reporter transgenes under constitutive promoters ("always on") [15], and the latter, under inducible promoters such as one regulated by an NFAT transcriptional response element [17]. Reporter genes and CAR constructs [25] are generally available in the form of retroviral or lentiviral constructs and can be generated or acquired via collaborations or plasmid repositories like Addgene (https://www.addgene.org).

Table 1
Human reporter gene-reporter probe imaging systems

Human reporter gene	Probe (half-life)	Optimal approximate probe biodistribution time (h)	Primary probe excretion route	Probe overlap with normal tissue(s)
Deoxycytidine kinase mutants (hdCK)	^{18}F-FEAU (109 mins)	1	Renal	Intestines, gallbladder, kidneys, bladder
	^{124}I-FIAU (4.18 days)	1	Renal	Intestines, gallbladder, thyroid, stomach, kidneys, bladder
Thymidine kinase mutants (hTK2)	^{18}F-L-FMAU (109 mins)	1	Renal	Intestines, gallbladder, kidneys, bladder
Sodium-iodide symporter (hNIS)	^{124}I-iodide (4.18 days)	2	Renal	Salivary gland, thyroid, stomach, kidneys, bladder
Norepinephrine transporter (hNET)	^{18}F-MFBG (109 mins)	4	Renal and hepatobiliary	Salivary gland, intestines, kidneys, bladder
	^{124}I-MIBG (4.18 days)	24	Renal and hepatobiliary	Salivary gland, intestines, thyroid, kidneys, bladder
Human estrogen receptor α ligand binding domain (hERL)	^{18}F-FES (109 mins)	1	Renal and hepatobiliary	Intestines, liver, kidneys, bladder
Human somatostatin receptor subtype 2 (hSSTr2)	^{68}Ga-DOTATOC	1	Renal	Kidneys, bladder
Dopamine 2 receptor (D2R)	^{18}F-FESP (109 mins)	3	Renal and hepatobiliary	Intestines, liver, kidneys, bladder
Membrane-anchored anti-polyethylene glycol antibody (anti-PEG)	^{124}I-PEG-SHPP (4.18 days)	24	Renal and hepatobiliary	Liver, thyroid
Anti-DOTA antibody fragment (DAbR1)	^{86}Y-AABD	24	Renal and hepatobiliary	Liver, intestine
Carcino-embryonic antigen (CEA)	^{124}I anti-CEA antibody fragment (4.18 days)	24	Renal	Thyroid, kidneys

3. Stable viral producers. To avoid variations of viral titer, the highest-titer PG13 clones are selected as viral producers for T cell transduction. Perform single-cell sorting (e.g., for the highest-expressing fluorescent gene selection marker) followed by determining viral titer of several selected clones using robust target cells (e.g., HEK 293 fibroblasts). The clone with the highest expression and titer is expanded and several stocks are frozen. Subsequently, supernatant is prepared from a culture that is 80–90% confluent, and up to 6 mL of supernatant per 1×10^6 T cells is used for transduction.
4. Transduction selection. Companion selection markers are available to permit selection of reporter gene-positive cells and enumerate their reporter transgene expression. Generally, fluorescence reporter genes are engineered downstream of PET reporter genes and ex vivo selection is performed by FACS.
5. T cell expansion in vitro. During initial isolation and expansion of T cells, when using PHA for stimulation expect T cell numbers to drop by 50% in 48 h and fast expansion after 72 h (depending on the donor, this can range from 10- to 50-fold). When using anti-CD3/CD28 beads, only a marginal decrease (5–10%) of cells can be observed 24 h after stimulation, which will be followed by moderate (2–5 fold) expansion in the next 72–96 h. For best viability and rate of expansion, maintain T cells at a concentration of approximately $1\text{–}2 \times 10^6$ per mL In general, it is best to minimize T cell doublings between isolation and adoptive transfer to ensure greater survival and expansion in vivo.
6. T cell stimulation in vitro. Freshly transduced T cells can be incubated in media supplemented with IL-15 for up to 7 weeks from transduction. At 4–5 weeks after transduction, cells need to be re-stimulated on specific APCs or nonspecifically such as with anti-CD3/CD28 beads at a ratio of 1 bead to 10 cells. To reduce the influence of increased cytokine production, it is preferable to wait 3–5 days after stimulation before in vivo administration.
7. T cell dynamics in vivo. Optimal PET imaging times for observing T cell dynamics in vivo is specific to the system being studied. Depending on the health of T cells injected, the injected population contracts within the first days of engraftment in animals followed by their concentration, proliferation and possible activation at target sites and lymphoid organs such as draining lymph nodes and spleen. Initial therapeutic response is generally rapid leading to significant reduction in T cell numbers that parallels reduction in tumor burden.
8. Suicide gene potential. Some reporter genes also exhibit "suicide potential," which allows for the elimination of adoptively

transferred T cells using drugs such as ganciclovir, gemcitabine, or bromovinyldeoxyuridine. This ensures safety of the adoptive cell therapy if T cells are causing adverse effects, e.g., graft-versus-host disease.

9. T cell radiation sensitivity. Proliferating T cells are sensitive to radiation exposure. For example, T cells exposed to median nuclear absorbed doses up to 830 cGy showed no reduction in immune cytotoxicity of APCs [26].
10. Optimal probe uptake time in vivo depends on probe biodistribution but is generally 1–3 h and up to 48 h after injection of the probe. Doses generally range between 3–16 MBq (~80–400 μCi) depending on PET scanner sensitivity and probe properties (e.g., the injected dose of I-124 is increased due to lower emission of positrons by this isotope).
11. Working with radioactive iodine. Radioactive iodine can be absorbed by the thyroid gland leading to adverse effects such as hypothyroidism. Researchers working with radioactive iodine should take additional precautions such as by conducting thyroid scans before and after handling the probe to monitor iodine exposure, and radiochemists should handle potentially airborne radioactive iodine in certified radioiodine fume hoods.
12. PET imaging. Depending on the amount of probe used and its percentage of positron emissions, recommended PET acquisition times are generally between 5–20 min for single, static images. After administration of T cells, image as early as possible to determine T cell migration and distribution. Dynamic scans can be helpful. Ex vivo-labeled T cells can be monitored sequentially within a period of 8–10 half-lives of the radioisotope used.
13. Animal handling. Position the animal on the scanner bed to permit easy discrimination of the area of interest, e.g., spread out arms and legs. PET produces 3-dimensional tomographic images, but overlap of target and normal tissues may prevent delineation of target areas due to signal spillover and limitations of scanner resolution.
14. PET scanners. Several preclinical combined PET/CT systems exist. The G8 PET/CT (Sofie Biosciences, Inc) is a BGO-based scanner with a PET sensitivity of 14% at center field of view and spatial resolution of 1.5 mm full-width-half-maximum using maximum-likelihood expectation maximization (MLEM) reconstruction. It includes a heated platform for maintaining animal physiological temperatures. The combined Inveon PET/CT (Siemens) is an LSO-based scanner with a PET sensitivity of 10% at the center field of view and spatial resolution of 1.5 mm full-width-half-maximum using three-

dimensional ordered-subset expectation maximization plus maximum a posteriori (3DOSEM + MAP) reconstruction.

15. Image reconstruction and corrections. Many image reconstruction algorithms exist. Generally, iterative (e.g., ML-EM, OSEM), compared to analytical (filtered back-projection), image reconstruction methods produce more accurate quantitation and superior contrast recovery coefficients at the expense of increased computation time. It may provide better detection of small sites of interest, although this is limited to inherent scanner properties. Since image reconstruction is performed after data acquisition, comparing reconstruction methods on the same dataset is possible. Additionally, correction factors such as for dead-time, random coincidences, scatter, normalization, and attenuation should be applied.
16. Quantification of imaging data. General quantitation of PET image data is adopted from traditional pharmacology and is presented as standardized uptake value (SUV), units of "percent injected dose per gram of tissue" (%ID/g) or normalized to a background tissue within the subject (e.g., target tissue divided by nonspecific tissue) [27]. Keeping accurate records of radioactive doses injected, and times of injection and scans are important for accurate quantitation.
17. Image analysis software. A variety of PET image analysis software are available, many of which are free for non-commercial use. Programs that are routinely maintained include AMIDE [28], ImageJ [29], OsiriX [30], and others. A list of free imaging software can be found at http://www.idoimaging.com. In general, these software are also able to co-register PET with CT or MRI data for anatomical localization of PET signal.

Acknowledgments

This work was supported by the NIH P50 CA86438, R01 CA163980, and R01 CA161138 grants, Mr. William H. Goodwin and Mrs. Alice Goodwin and the Commonwealth Foundation for Cancer Research and The Experimental Therapeutics Center of Memorial Sloan-Kettering Cancer Center, NIH Small-Animal Imaging Research Program (SAIRP), NIH Shared Instrumentation Grant No. 1 S10 RR020892-01, NIH Shared Instrumentation Grant No. 1 S10 RR028889-01, and NIH Center Grant P30 CA08748.

References

1. Rosenberg SA, Restifo NP (2015) Adoptive cell transfer as personalized immunotherapy for human cancer. Science 348(6230):62–68
2. Couzin-Frankel J (2013) Breakthrough of the year 2013. Cancer immunotherapy. Science 342(6165):1432–1433
3. Fesnak AD, June CH, Levine BL (2016) Engineered T cells: the promise and challenges of cancer immunotherapy. Nat Rev Cancer 16 (9):566–581
4. Sadelain M, Brentjens R, Riviere I (2013) The basic principles of chimeric antigen receptor design. Cancer Discov 3(4):388–398
5. Cartellieri M et al (2010) Chimeric antigen receptor-engineered T cells for immunotherapy of cancer. J Biomed Biotechnol 2010:956304
6. Sadelain M (2015) CAR therapy: the CD19 paradigm. J Clin Invest 125(9):3392–3400
7. Morello A, Sadelain M, Adusumilli PS (2016) Mesothelin-targeted CARs: driving T cells to solid tumors. Cancer Discov 6(2):133–146
8. Restifo NP, Smyth MJ, Snyder A (2016) Acquired resistance to immunotherapy and future challenges. Nat Rev Cancer 16 (2):121–126
9. Moynihan KD et al (2006) Eradication of large established tumors in mice by combination immunotherapy that engages innate and adaptive immune responses. Nat Med 22 (12):1402–1410
10. Lucignani G et al (2006) Molecular imaging of cell-mediated cancer immunotherapy. Trends Biotechnol 24(9):410–418
11. Akins EJ, Dubey P (2008) Noninvasive imaging of cell-mediated therapy for treatment of cancer. J Nucl Med 49(Suppl 2):180S–195S
12. Yaghoubi SS et al (2012) Positron emission tomography reporter genes and reporter probes: gene and cell therapy applications. Theranostics 2(4):374–391
13. Sadelain M (2009) T-cell engineering for cancer immunotherapy. Cancer J 15(6):451–455
14. Wang X, Riviere I (2016) Clinical manufacturing of CAR T cells: foundation of a promising therapy. Mol Ther Oncolytics 3:16015
15. Likar Y et al (2010) A new pyrimidine-specific reporter gene: a mutated human deoxycytidine kinase suitable for PET during treatment with acycloguanosine-based cytotoxic drugs. J Nucl Med 51(9):1395–1403
16. Yaghoubi SS et al (2009) Noninvasive detection of therapeutic cytolytic T cells with 18F-FHBG PET in a patient with glioma. Nat Clin Pract Oncol 6(1):53–58
17. Ponomarev V et al (2001) Imaging TCR-dependent NFAT-mediated T-cell activation with positron emission tomography in vivo. Neoplasia 3(6):480–488
18. Minn I et al (2014) Molecular-genetic imaging of cancer. Adv Cancer Res 124:131–169
19. Shu CJ et al (2009) Quantitative PET reporter gene imaging of CD8+ T cells specific for a melanoma-expressed self-antigen. Int Immunol 21(2):155–165
20. McCracken MN et al (2015) Noninvasive detection of tumor-infiltrating T cells by PET reporter imaging. J Clin Invest 125 (5):1815–1826
21. Dobrenkov K et al (2008) Monitoring the efficacy of adoptively transferred prostate cancer-targeted human T lymphocytes with PET and bioluminescence imaging. J Nucl Med 49 (7):1162–1170
22. Dubey P et al (2003) Quantitative imaging of the T cell antitumor response by positron-emission tomography. Proc Natl Acad Sci U S A 100(3):1232–1237
23. Hoekstra ME et al (2015) Assessing T lymphocyte function and differentiation by genetically encoded reporter systems. Trends Immunol 36 (7):392–400
24. Moroz MA et al (2015) Comparative analysis of T cell imaging with human nuclear reporter genes. J Nucl Med 56(7):1055–1060
25. Sadelain M, Frassoni F, Riviere I (2000) Issues in the manufacture and transplantation of genetically modified hematopoietic stem cells. Curr Opin Hematol 7(6):364–377
26. Zanzonico P et al (2006) [131I]FIAU labeling of genetically transduced, tumor-reactive lymphocytes: cell-level dosimetry and dose-dependent toxicity. Eur J Nucl Med Mol Imaging 33(9):988–997
27. Thie JA (2004) Understanding the standardized uptake value, its methods, and implications for usage. J Nucl Med 45(9):1431–1434
28. Loening AM, Gambhir SS (2003) AMIDE: a free software tool for multimodality medical image analysis. Mol Imaging 2(3):131–137
29. Schneider CA, Rasband WS, Eliceiri KW (2012) NIH image to ImageJ: 25 years of image analysis. Nat Methods 9(7):671–675
30. Rosset A, Spadola L, Ratib O (2004) OsiriX: an open-source software for navigating in multidimensional DICOM images. J Digit Imaging 17 (3):205–216

Chapter 14

Positron Emission Tomography Imaging of Tumor Apoptosis with a Caspase-Sensitive Nano-Aggregation Tracer [^{18}F]C-SNAT

Zixin Chen and Jianghong Rao

Abstract

Cellular apoptosis is an important criterion for evaluating the efficacy of cancer therapies. We have developed a new small molecule probe ([^{18}F]C-SNAT) for positron emission tomography (PET) imaging of apoptosis. [^{18}F]C-SNAT, when activated by caspase-3 and glutathione reduction, undergoes intramolecular cyclization followed by self-assembly to form nano-aggregates in apoptotic cells. This unique mechanism creates preferential retention of gamma radiation signals in targeted cells and thus enables the detection of apoptosis using PET, a sensitive and clinically practical technique. This protocol describes the chemical synthesis, radiolabeling and PET imaging of apoptosis using this probe.

Key words Positron emission tomography (PET), Imaging, Apoptosis, Caspase-3, Nano-aggregation, Radiolabeling, "Click" reaction

1 Introduction

Early therapeutic responses serve as important prognostic indicators of outcome in cancer therapies and can be used as guidance for subsequent therapies. As we gain deeper understandings of the heterogeneity of tumors, techniques that measure early therapeutic responses are gaining more attention in the coming age of precision medicine. With these techniques, patients who respond poorly to prescribed therapies can be identified earlier, so their physicians can intervene early on and switch to a more appropriate course of treatment to increase the patients' chance of survival. Current clinical methods to assess treatment response are based on size measurements of tumors using computerized tomography (CT) or magnetic resonance imaging (MRI) under the guidelines of the Response Evaluation Criteria In Solid Tumors (RECIST) [1]. However, RECIST-based size measurements do not have the sensitivity for early assessment because measurable changes in

Purnima Dubey (ed.), *Reporter Gene Imaging: Methods and Protocols*, Methods in Molecular Biology, vol. 1790,
https://doi.org/10.1007/978-1-4939-7860-1_14,

tumor sizes may take weeks or months to become apparent after treatment initiation. Furthermore, tumor shrinkage may not occur in the case of cytostatic and molecularly targeted therapy even when the treatment is effective. Positron emission tomography (PET) imaging of fluorine-18 labeled deoxyglucose ([^{18}F]FDG) metabolism in tumors can provide a functional measurement, as described by the PET Response Criteria in Solid Tumors (PERSIST) [1]. PERSIST considers a decrease in the [^{18}F]FDG metabolism as positive treatment response assuming fewer living tumor cells; however, since [^{18}F]FDG uptake is not limited to tumor cells, higher metabolism in nearby inflammatory or hypoxic tissues, which are often associated with cancer treatments, for example, in radiotherapy, may offset the decrease in the tumor metabolism even when the treatment is effective, resulting in false negative results. Thus, new imaging methods that can better monitor the changes in underlying biochemistry even preceding morphological changes of the tumors are still much needed.

Apoptosis is an important cell death pathway that proceeds through a cascade of events and eventually leads to morphological changes and disassembly of cells [2]. Increasing tumor cell apoptosis has been shown to have a positive correlation with the efficacy of anticancer therapies [3], which supports the use of cell death as the surrogate biomarker to monitor treatment responses in tumor. Extensive efforts have been put into developing imaging probes based on the molecular markers associated with apoptosis such as redistribution of phosphatidylserine and activation of caspases [3–6]. For example, annexin V is a 36-kDa endogenous protein that binds with high affinity to the head group of phosphatidylserine and the binding is minimally affected when annexin V is conjugated to a reporting group such as radioactive or fluorescent labels. Various annexin V imaging probes have been reported including ^{99m}Tc-Annexin V that has been evaluated clinically for imaging chemotherapy-induced apoptosis in human cancer [7] and other diseases [8] but has failed to progress beyond phase II/III clinical trials due to its poor biodistribution profile [9].

Compared with large proteins like annexin V, small molecule probes have a number of advantages including: (1) small molecules can be easily functionalized or chemically optimized to improve their activity; (2) they are typically cleared faster from circulation after infusion to provide a generally lower background; and (3) they are less prone to elicit immunologic responses [9]. Caspases are a class of enzymes that are involved in the apoptosis pathway. Caspases can be divided into upstream initiators (caspases-1, -2, -4, -5, -8, -10) and downstream executors (caspases-3, -6, -7, -9) [10]. The downstream caspases are responsible for operating at the end of the apoptosis cascade to cleave substrates. For example, caspase-3 plays a major role in the proteolysis of a large number of substrates including poly(ADP-ribose) polymerase (PARP) [10] and has become an important molecular target for imaging apoptosis.

Both peptide-based and small molecule-based probes have been reported for imaging caspase-3/7, such as competitive inhibitors derived from isatin sulfonamide [11, 12] and activity based probes that can form covalent bond with the enzymes. Activity-based probes such as [^{125}I] M808 [13], FLICA [14], and Apomab [15] exploit the inherent cysteine protease reactivity of caspases to form irreversible covalent bonds between the enzyme and the probe. This approach does not take advantage of catalytic activity of enzymes and the imaging signal is potentially limited by binding site saturation. Another approach is to detect the enzymatic activity with substrate-based probes, such as caged-luminescent [16], -fluorescent [17–20], and -radiolabeled [21] probes. These substrate-based probes do not form covalent bonds with the enzyme after caspase cleavage and thus promise higher signal and potentially better imaging contrast. The luminescent and fluorescent probes however are limited to preclinical research settings due to the requirement of protein engineering and poor light penetration in biological tissues. Furthermore, the activation mechanisms for designing these optical probes cannot be applied to designing PET imaging probes since PET imaging contrast can only be generated through preferential uptake and retention of radioactivity.

Our group has recently developed a new strategy for designing caspase-imaging probes [22–26] based on a bioorthorgonal cyclization reaction between cyanoquinoline and cysteine. The probe is constituted with a cyanoquinoline on one end and a cysteine residue on the other end, which is caged with the peptide sequence Asp-Glu-Val-Asp (DEVD) that is specific for caspases-3 and -7 and disulfide. Upon cleavage of the peptide by caspases and reduction of the disulfide by intracellular glutathione, the cyanoquinoline and the un-caged terminal cysteine undergo rapid condensation reaction to form macrocycles, which subsequently self-assemble through hydrophobic interactions to form nano-aggregates in vivo. Because the formation of nanoparticles enhances their cellular retention, this mechanism may serve as a general approach to designing activatable probes for imaging the activity of enzymes. Using peptide substrate DEVD for caspase-3 and -7, we have designed a series of molecular probes for imaging caspase-3/7 with different imaging modalities including fluorescence [22], MRI [24], and PET imaging [23, 25, 26].

For PET imaging, the prosthetic group with an ^{18}F label was introduced onto the precursor through copper (I)-catalyzed "click" reaction to generate [^{18}F]C-SNAT. As control, **1-ctrl** was synthesized with unnatural D-peptide sequence and nonreducible methylthiol that cannot be activated by caspase-3 and glutathione (Fig. 1). This probe was first used for in vivo PET imaging of

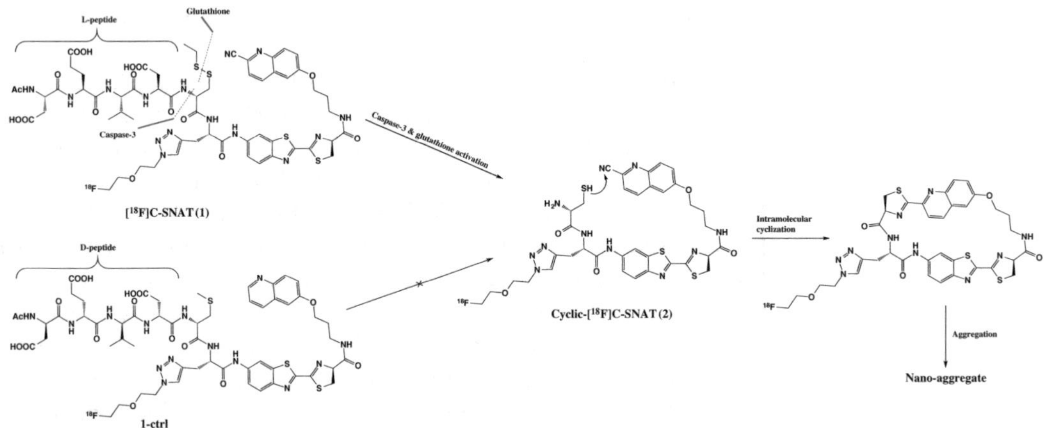

Fig. 1 Mechanisms of activation, cyclization and aggregation of [^{18}F]C-SNAT for PET imaging of caspase-3/7 activity

chemotherapy-induced apoptosis in tumor xenografts in nude mice. A mouse implanted subcutaneously with HeLa tumor cells received intratumoral injection of 0.2 mg of doxorubicin. PET imaging with [^{18}F]C-SNAT 4 days posttreatment detected a 1.9-fold signal increase in treated tumors compared with untreated tumor and a maximum of seven-fold increase in the uptake ratio between tumor and muscle at 182 min post-injection [23]. In another study [25], mice bearing HeLa tumor xenografts received three intravenous injections of doxorubicin (8 mg/kg) in saline suspension on days 0, 4, and 8, followed by PET scanning on day 10. There was a significantly higher tumor-to-muscle ratio of 3.9 ± 0.9 (2.5 ± 0.6%ID/g in tumor and 0.6 ± 0.4%ID/g in muscle) in treated mice than in untreated mice (2.2 ± 1.9: 1.6 ± 0.2%ID/g in tumor and 0.7 ± 0.1%ID/g in muscle). A - two-tissue compartment model was used to calculate pharmacokinetic rate constants [25], which showed a significant increase in delivery and accumulation of the tracer after the systemic chemotherapeutic treatment. Delivery of [^{18}F]C-SNAT to the tumor tissue, quantified as K_1, increased from 0.31 g/mL/min in untreated mice to 1.03 g/mL/min in treated mice, a measurement closely related to changes in blood flow. Accumulation of [^{18}F]C-SNAT, quantified as k_3, increased from 0.03 to 0.12 min^{-1}, proving a higher retention of [^{18}F]C-SNAT in treated tumors that is independent of changes in blood flow.

[^{18}F]C-SNAT has been compared to other reported apoptosis tracers such as ^{18}F–FDG, ^{99m}Tc-Annexin V, and ^{18}F–ML-10 in the same cell lines and tumor models [26]. In drug-treated EF-4 lymphoma cells, ^{18}F–FDG, ^{99m}Tc- Annexin V, and [^{18}F]C-SNAT cell-associated radioactivity correlated well to levels of cell death ($R^2 > 0.8$; $P < 0.001$), but no correlation was observed for ^{18}F–ML-10. PET imaging with [^{18}F]C-SNAT of EL-4 tumor treated with etoposide showed 2.1-fold higher ^{18}F activity than control mice without drug treatment. While ^{99m}Tc-Annexin V uptake in treated tumor increased by 1.4-fold, its binding did not correlate to ex vivo TUNEL staining of tissue sections. PET imaging with ^{18}F–FDG or ^{18}F–ML-10 did not detect statistically significant differential responses between treated and untreated mice [26]. In addition, [^{18}F]C-SNAT demonstrated a trend of increasing uptake over time, which is consistent with the proposed aggregation mechanism. These results have demonstrated that this novel apoptosis PET tracer will not only be useful for studying cancer biology in the research setting but also potentially useful for monitoring drug responses in the clinical setting.

Here, we describe the protocol for the preparation of [^{18}F]C-SNAT and PET imaging of drug-induced apoptosis in mice bearing tumor xenografts.

2 Materials

2.1 Synthesis of Precursors of Probe 3a And Control Probe 3b

All chemicals can be purchased from commercial sources unless otherwise specified.

1. N-Boc-propargylglycine.
2. 4-methylmorpholine.
3. Isobutyl chloroformate.
4. 6-amino-2-cyanobenzothiazole.
5. Trifluoroacetic Acid (TFA).
6. N-Boc-S-Trt-D-cysteine.
7. *N,N,N′,N′*-Tetramethyl-*O*-(1*H*-benzotriazol-1-yl)uronium hexafluorophosphate (HBTU).
8. Diisopropylethylamine (DIPEA).
9. Tris(2-carboxyethyl)phosphine hydrochloride (TCEP•HCl).
10. Triisopropylsilane (TIPS).
11. 2-(Ethyldisulfanyl)pyridine.
12. Methyl iodide.
13. Tetraethyleneglycol di(p-toluenesulfonate).
14. Sodium azide.
15. 1 M HCl.
16. Brine.
17. Sodium bicarbonate ($NaHCO_3$).
18. Magnesium sulfate ($MgSO_4$).
19. Tetrahydrofuran (THF).
20. Ethyl acetate (EtOAc).

21. Hexane.
22. Dichloromethane (DCM).
23. Dimethylformamide (DMF).
24. Methanol (MeOH).
25. Silica gel.

Instrument

26. Analytical, semi-preparative or preparative HPLC system.
27. Rotary evaporator.
28. Hot/stir plate.
29. Oil bath.
30. Lyophilizer.

2.2 Radiosynthesis

All chemicals can be purchased from commercial sources unless otherwise specified.

1. Anion-exchange resin cartridge (Macherey-Nagel Chromafix 30-PS-HCO_3).
2. 4,7,13,16,21,24-Hexaoxa-1,10-diazabicyclo[8.8.8]hexacosane (Kryptofix 222).
3. Potassium carbonate.
4. Acetonitrile (CH_3CN).
5. Dimethylsulfoxide (DMSO).
6. C18 Sep-Pak cartridge.
7. Diethyl ether.
8. Sodium sulfate (Na_2SO_4).
9. Helium gas.
10. 1 M HEPES buffer.
11. Copper sulfate ($CuSO_4$).
12. Sodium ascorbate.
13. Ethanol.

Instrument

14. Analytical and semi-prep HPLC systems with gamma radiation detectors.
15. Tracerlab FX-FN module (GE Healthcare, USA).
16. PETtrace cyclotron (GE Healthcare, USA).

2.3 PET Imaging

1. Nude mice.
2. HeLa cells or other cell lines of choice.
3. Catheters.
4. Doxorubincin.

5. Saline.
6. Syringes.
7. Infrared warming pad.

Instrument

8. R4 microPET scanner (Siemens Medical Solutions, USA).
9. PET imaging processing software (Siemens Inveon Research Workplace software v.4.0 or other appropriate software).

3 Methods

3.1 Synthesis of Precursors (3a & 3b) for Radioisotope Labeling (Fig. 2)

1. Synthesis of **4**:

   Prepare a solution of N-Boc-propargylglycine (384 mg, 1.8 mmol), 4-methylmorpholine (330 mL, 3.0 mmol) and isobutyl chloroformate (195 mL, 1.5 mmol) in THF (3 mL) and stir at 0 °C for 2 h. Add 6-Amino-2-cyanobenzothiazole (175 mg, 1.0 mmol) in THF (5 mL) to the solution at 0 °C and keep it stirred for 12 h at room temperature. Quench the reaction with aqueous 1 M HCl (3 mL) and extract the

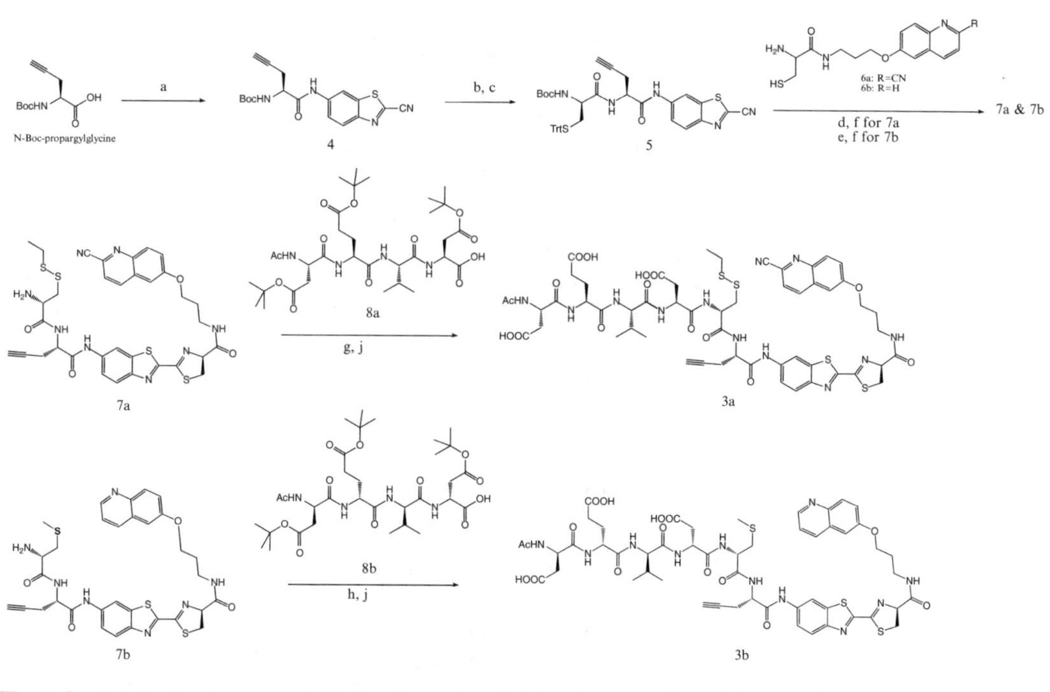

Fig. 2 Synthesis of precursors **3a** & **3b**. (**a**) iso-Butyl chloroformate, 4-methylmorpholine, THF, 0 °C, 2 h and then 6-amino-2-cyanobenzothiazole, THF, 0 °C to r.t., 12 h; (**b**) 50% TFA in DCM, r.t., 1 h; (**c**) N-Boc-S-Trt-D-Cysteine, HBTU, DIPEA, DMF, r.t.; 2 h. (**d**) **6a**, DIPEA, DMF, r.t., 30 min; (**e**) **6b**, DIPEA, DMF, 30 min; (**f**) 50% TFA in DCM, r.t., 1 h and then 2-(ethyldisulfanyl) pyridine, MeOH, r.t., 2 h; (**g**) Ac-DEVD-OH (**8a**), HBTU, DIPEA, THF, r.t., 1 h; (**h**) Ac-devd-OH (**8b**), HBTU, DIPEA, THF, r.t., 1 h; (**i**) CH_3I, TCEP·HCl, DIPEA, DMF, 1 h; (**j**) 50% TFA in DCM, r.t., 2 h

resulting mixture with EtOAc (40 mL) and H_2O (40 mL). Wash the organic phase with saturated $NaHCO_3$ (40 mL) and dry with $MgSO_4$. Filter the organic layer and evaporate under reduced pressure to afford the crude product. Purify the crude product with silica gel chromatography (Hexane: EtOAc = 1:1) to afford the product **4** (296 mg, 85%).

2. Synthesis of **5**:

   Add compound **4** (300 mg, 0.81 mmol) to a solution of 1:1 DCM/TFA (6 mL) at room temperature and keep the solution stirred for 1 h. Evaporate the solvent and remaining TFA under reduced pressure. Dissolve the crude residue, N-Boc-S-Trt-D-cysteine (394 mg, 0.85 mmol), HBTU (323 mg, 0.85 mmol), and DIPEA (442 μL, 2.5 mmol) in DMF (5 mL) and keep the solution under stirring for 1 h at room temperature. Extract the resulting solution with EtOAc (30 mL) and water (30 mL). Wash the organic layer with brine (40 mL × 2) and dry with $MgSO_4$. Filter the organic layer to remove $MgSO_4$ and evaporate the solvent under reduced pressure to afford the crude product. Purify the crude product with silica gel chromatography (Hexane: EtOAc = 1:1) to afford the dipeptide **5** (464 mg, 80%).

3. Synthesis of 7**a**:

   Prepare a solution of compound **5** (143 mg, 0.2 mmol), quinolone **6a** (89 mg, 0.2 mmol), TCEP•HCl (115 mg, 0.4 mmol), and DIPEA (418 μL, 2.4 mmol) in DMF (5 mL) and keep it stirred for 30 min at room temperature. Evaporate the solvent under reduced pressure. Dissolve the resulting residue in a solution of DCM:TFA:TIPS (1: 1: 0.05) and stir at room temperature for 1 h to remove both N-Boc and S-Trt groups. Evaporate the solvent under reduced pressure and remove the residual TFA under high vacuum. Re-dissolve the crude product in MeOH (5 mL), followed by addition of 2-(ethyldisulfanyl)pyridine (68 mg, 0.4 mmol). Stir the resulting solution for 2 h at room temperature. Purify the crude product by HPLC to afford the desired product 7**a** (88 mg, 51% from **5**).

4. Synthesis of 7**b**:

   Dissolve compound **5** (72 mg, 0.1 mmol), quinolone **6b** (42 mg, 0.1 mmol), TCEP•HCl (58 mg, 0.2 mmol), and DIPEA (209 μL, 1.2 mmol) in DMF (3 mL) and keep the solution stirred for 30 min at room temperature, followed by evaporation under reduced pressure. Dissolve the resulting residue in a solution of DCM:TFA:TIPS (1:1:0.05) and keep it under stirring at room temperature for 1 h to remove both N-Boc and S-Trt groups, followed by evaporation under reduced pressure to remove the solvent. After another evaporation under high vacuum to further remove the residual TFA, re-dissolve the crude residue in MeOH (3 mL) together with 2-(ethyldisulfanyl)-pyridine (34 mg, 0.2 mmol) and keep the solution stirred for 1 h at room temperature. Purify the crude product by preparative HPLC to afford the desired product **7b** (33 mg, 40% from **5**).

5. Synthesis of **8a** and **8b**:

   Prepare the protected peptide Ac-Asp(tBu)-Glu(tBu)-Val-Asp (tBu)-OH (Ac-DEVD-OH) and control protected D-peptide through standard solid phase peptide synthesis.

6. Synthesis of **3a**(Fig. 3):

   Prepare a solution of **7a** (15 mg, 17.4 μmol), **8a** (18 mg, 26.1 μmol), HBTU (10 mg, 26.4 μmol) and DIPEA (16 μL, 87 μmol) in THF (2 mL) and keep it stirred for 1 h at room temperature. Dilute the solution with EtOAc (30 mL) and wash with brine (30 mL × 2). After drying the organic phase with $MgSO_4$, filter the solution, and evaporate the solvent under reduced pressure. Then treat the resulting crude residue by DCM:TFA:TIPS (1.0:1.0:0.05) for 1 h to remove the protecting groups. After the evaporation under reduced pressure, purify the crude product by preparative HPLC to afford the probe **3a** (15 mg, 2.0 μmol, 69% from **7a**).

7. Synthesis of **3b**:

   Prepare a solution of **7b** (13 mg, 15.6 μmol), **8b** (22 mg, 31.2 μmol), HBTU (12 mg, 31.2 μmol) and DIPEA (13.5 mL, 78 μmol) in THF (2 mL) and keep it stirred for 1 h at room temperature. Evaporate the solvent under reduced pressure and purify the crude product with preparative HPLC to afford 11 mg (7.9 μmol) of protected peptide. Dissolve the purified peptide (11 mg, 7.9 μmol) in DMF (1 mL) and add TCEP.HCl (4.5 mg, 16 μmol), DIPEA (20 μL, 0.1 mmol) and methyl iodide (1.9 μL, 30 μmol) to the solution at room temperature. Keep the resulting solution stirred for 40 min before evaporation under reduced pressure. Then dissolve the resulting residue in DCM:TFA:TIPS (1.0:1.0:0.05) solution to remove the tert-butyl group. After 1 h, evaporate the solvent under reduced pressure and purify the crude product by preparative HPLC to afford the control probe **3b** (7 mg, 6.0 μmol, 38% from **7b**).

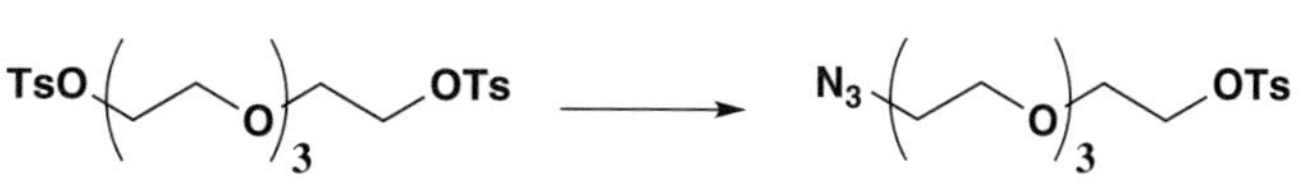

Fig. 3 Synthesis of radiolabeling precursor **9**; conditions: sodium azide, DMF, 100 °C, overnight

8. Synthesis of **9**:

   Dissolve tetraethyleneglycol di(p-toluenesulfonate) (5 g, 10 mmol) and sodium azide (0.65 g, 10 mmol) in DMF (30 mL) and heat it at 100 °C under stirring overnight. After the reaction is cooled down, dilute the reaction solution with ethyl acetate (200 mL) and wash with water (3 ×200 mL) and brine (100 mL). Then dry the organic layer over $MgSO_4$ and concentrate the solution under reduced pressure. Purify the crude residue with silica gel chromatography (Hexane: EtOAc = 4:1) to afford the product **9** (700 mg, 19%) as colorless oil.

3.2 Radiosynthesis (Fig. 4)

1. Synthesis of **10**:

   A fully automated synthesis procedure in a Tracerlab FX-FN module is used for the radiosynthesis. First, produce no-carrier added [^{18}F]fluoride via the ^{18}O(p,n)^{18}F nuclear reaction by irradiation of enriched [^{18}O]H_2O in a PETtrace cyclotron. Trap [^{18}F]Fluoride on an anion-exchange resin cartridge (pre-conditioned with 1 mL of EtOH, 1 mL of H_2O and then 1 mL of air) and elute with a solution of Kryptofix 222 (K2.2.2) (15 mg) and potassium carbonate (3 mg) in H_2O (0.1 mL) and CH_3CN (0.9 mL). Following azeotropic drying, add compound **9** (3.0 mg in 1.0 mL of dry DMSO) to the K[^{18}F]F/K2.2.2 complex, and heat the mixture for 20 min at 110 °C to yield **10**. After cooling down to room temperature, purify the reaction mixture on a semi-preparative HPLC (Eluent A: H_2O + 0.1% TFA, B: CH_3CN + 0.1% TFA; Gradient: 0–2 min 5% B, 2–30 min 5–65% B, 30–40 min 60–95% B; Flow rate: 5.0 mL/min). Collect the fraction corresponding to the peak of the desired product in a round bottom flask containing sterile water (20 mL), and then transfer to an adjacent customized module for solid phase extraction (SPE) using a C18 Sep-Pak cartridge (pre-conditioned with 10 mL of EtOH, 10 mL of H_2O). Elute **10** trapped on C-18 cartridge with diethyl ether (2 mL) through a Na_2SO_4 cartridge into a 5 mL V-vial with a stirring bar in the customized module. Remove the diethyl ether under helium stream for 60 to 90 s at ambient temperature and reconstitute the dried labeling agent with THF (50 μL) for next step click chemistry.

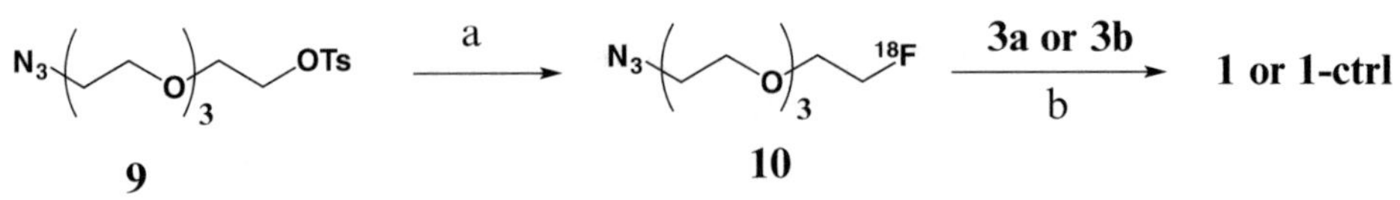

Fig. 4 Radiosynthesis of ^{18}F–labeled tracer and control tracer. (**a**) K[^{18}F]F/K2.2.2, 110 °C, 20 min; (**b**) $CuSO_4$, sodium ascorbate, HEPES, DMSO, 40 °C, 20 min

2. Synthesis of **1**:

   Prepare a solution of **10** in THF (50 μL) and add **3a** (1.2 mg, 1 mmol) in 1 M HEPES solution (100 μL), $CuSO_4$ (300 mM, 10 μL) and sodium ascorbate (300 mM, 10 μL). Keep the reaction mixture at 40 °C for 20 min. Dilute the crude product with 2 mL of water and purify on a semi-preparative HPLC (Eluent A: H_2O + 0.1% TFA, B: CH_3CN + 0.1% TFA; Gradient: 0–2 min 10% B, 2–40 min 10–60% B, 40–50 min 95% B, 50–60 min 10% B; Flow rate: 5.0 mL/min). Formulate the final product **1** in saline with 10% ethanol by solid phase extraction.

3. Synthesis of **1-ctrl**:

   To a THF solution of **10** (50 μL), add 1 M HEPES/DMSO (1:1) solution (50 μL) of **3b** (0.5 mg, 0.4 mmol), $CuSO_4$ (300 mM, 14 μL) and sodium ascorbate (300 mM, 14 μL), and keep the reaction mixture at 40 °C for 20 min. Dilute the crude product with 2 mL water and purify on a semi-prep HPLC (Eluent A: H_2O + 0.1% TFA, B: CH_3CN + 0.1% TFA; Gradient: 0–2 min 10% B, 2–40 min 10–40% B, 40–50 min 95% B, 50–60 min 10% B; Flow rate: 5.0 mL/min). Formulate the final product **1-ctrl** in saline with 10% ethanol by solid phase extraction (Fig. 5).

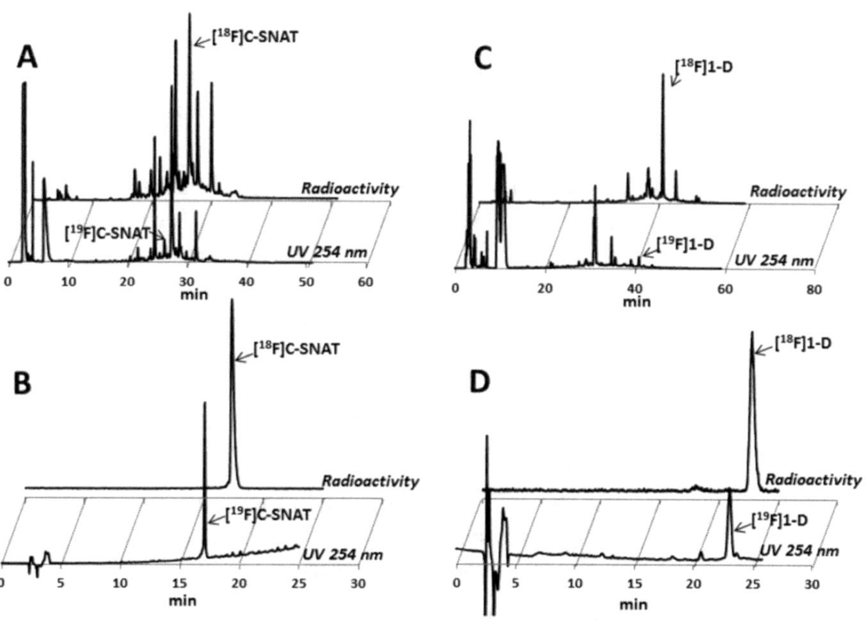

Fig. 5 (**a**) Semi-Prep HPLC chromatogram of crude [^{18}F/^{19}F]**1**; (**b**) Analytical HPLC chromatogram of purified [^{18}F/^{19}F]**1**; (**c**) Semi-Prep HPLC chromatogram of crude [^{18}F/^{19}F]**1-ctrl**; (**d**) Analytical HPLC chromatogram of purified [^{18}F/^{19}F]**1-ctrl**. (Reproduced from ref. [23] with permission from *John Wiley and Sons*)

3.3 PET Imaging

1. Inject three groups of mice (4–6 mice in each group, 6–7 week-old nude mice) with 1-2 × 10^6 HeLa cells on the right shoulders. Monitor tumor xenograft growth by caliper measurement for 10–14 days until the tumors reach 5–10 mm in size.
2. Inject two groups of animals with 0.2 mg of doxorubicin formulated in 0.2 mL of saline intravenously on days 0, 4, and 8 before the imaging experiment. One control group will receive no treatment.
3. On the day of scanning, move the animals from their housing area to the PET scanner around 1 h prior to the imaging. Anesthetize the mice with 2% isoflurane at a flow rate of 2 L/min and insert a catheter into the tail vein.
4. Inject 100 μL of heparinized saline (100 IU/mL heparin) i.v. to maintain patency of the catheter and vein, followed by regular small injections to keep patency and to hydrate the mice during the procedure.
5. Place one group of treated mice and one group of untreated mice into a custom-made 4×4 bed in an R4 microPET scanner, 4 mice at a time with isoflurane anesthesia throughout the whole image acquisition.
6. Perform a 15 min CT scan before the tracer injection.
7. Inject about 200 μCi (7.4 MBq in 100 μL formulation) of probe **1** intravenously to each mouse through the catheter.
8. Acquire a 120-min dynamic PET scan.
9. Apply eye lubricant to maintain moisture in the eyes and use a heating pad to maintain body temperature during the imaging period.
10. As an additional control, perform a similar scan using the control tracer **1-ctrl** (about 200 μCi in 100 μL formulation) in a third group of treated animals. This can be done the same day or a different day depending on the availability of the tracer.
11. Euthanize the mice following IACUC guidelines immediately after imaging acquisition to collect tumor tissues for further histological studies. For longitude imaging, mice may be returned to a holding area for 10 h to allow the radioactivity to decay.
12. Bin the PET data into 21 frames, and reconstruct each frame using 2-dimensional ordered-subset expectation maximization with arc and scatter correction.
13. Reconstruct one frame (15 min from 45 to 60 min) using 3-dimensional ordered-subset expectation maximization with arc and scatter correction. Representative coregistered PET/CT images are shown in Fig. 6.

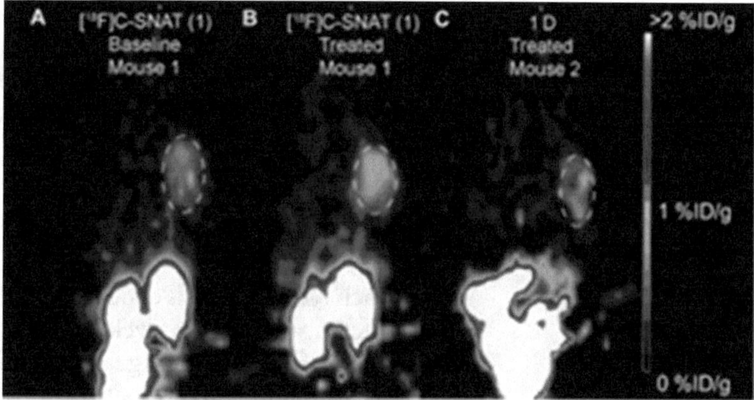

Fig. 6 Representative coregistered [^{18}F]C-SNAT PET/CT images from 2 mice with xenographed HeLa tumors. (**a**) Untreated mouse. (**b**) Treated mouse. Summed images from 45 to 60 min and reconstructed using 3-dimensional ordered-subset expectation maximization. White circles mark tumors. (Reproduced from ref. [25] with permission from Society of Nuclear Medicine and Molecular Imaging, Inc.)

14. Measure tracer activity over time in the PET image using CT as an anatomical guidance.
15. Analyze the reconstructed images by making volumes of interest (VOI), one on the tumor and one located on the left shoulder containing the muscle/bone.
16. The percent of injected dose per gram tissue (%ID/g) can be calculated in each VOI. Calculate and normalize the tumor uptake using the percentage of the injected dose per gram (%ID/g) and a normalization factor (NFX) calculated as: $ID*NFX = ID*AUCx/AUC_{mean}$, where AUCx is individual mouse's muscle activity (area under the curve in the selected areas of muscle of mouse X) and AUCmean is the average activity in the selected areas of muscle of all mice.
17. Calculate the effect of treatment as the difference in uptake of probe **1** in mice without and with treatment.

4 Notes

1. The cyanobenzothiazole moiety is susceptible to hydrolysis under basic aqueous condition. During the synthesis of **4**, **5**, and 7, if an organic base is used, immediate quenching with acid in an ice bath after reaction completion is necessary to minimize the hydrolysis and obtain high yields.
2. Radiosynthesis of **10** using the automatic module is extremely moisture sensitive. In order to ensure a high production yield

at this step, the precursor **9** should be dried under high vacuum overnight before the experiment or stored at −20 °C in sealed vials. Anhydrous solvent should be used for the reaction.

3. In order to insure high reproducibility of the radiosynthesis protocol, a "cold" trial experiment using the non-radioactive ^{19}F analog should be run before the actual "hot" experiment to establish the formula, time for the reactions and also the HPLC purification methods.
4. For each radiosynthesis experiment, the minimally required ^{18}F radioactivity from the cyclotron production can be roughly calculated from the dosage needed for each mouse, the yield for each step from trial experiments, and radioactivity decay for the time needed for the experiment.
5. For tumor implantation, different tumor types may have different time span to grow to the appropriate sizes.

References

1. Wahl RL, Jacene H, Kasamon Y et al (2009) From RECIST to PERCIST: evolving considerations for PET response criteria in solid tumors. J Nucl Med 50(Suppl 1):122S–150S. https://doi.org/10.2967/jnumed.108.057307
2. Okada H, Mak TW (2004) Pathways of apoptotic and non-apoptotic death in tumour cells. Nat Rev Cancer 4(8):592–603. https://doi.org/10.1038/nrc1412
3. Brindle K (2008) New approaches for imaging tumour responses to treatment. Nat Rev Cancer 8(2):94–107. https://doi.org/10.1038/nrc2289
4. De Saint-Hubert M, Prinsen K, Mortelmans L et al (2009) Molecular imaging of cell death. Methods 48(2):178–187. https://doi.org/10.1016/j.ymeth.2009.03.022
5. Blankenberg FG (2008) In vivo detection of apoptosis. J Nucl Med 49(Suppl 2):81S–95S. https://doi.org/10.2967/jnumed.107.045898
6. Zeng W, Wang X, Xu P et al (2015) Molecular imaging of apoptosis: from micro to macro. Theranostics 5(6):559–582. https://doi.org/10.7150/thno.11548
7. Belhocine T, Steinmetz N, Hustinx R et al (2002) Increased uptake of the apoptosis-imaging agent (99m)Tc recombinant human Annexin V in human tumors after one course of chemotherapy as a predictor of tumor response and patient prognosis. Clin Cancer Res 8(9):2766–2774
8. Kietselaer BL, Reutelingsperger CP, Heidendal GA et al (2004) Noninvasive detection of plaque instability with use of radiolabeled annexin A5 in patients with carotid-artery atherosclerosis. N Engl J Med 350(14):1472–1473. https://doi.org/10.1056/NEJM200404013501425
9. Reshef A, Shirvan A, Akselrod-Ballin A et al (2010) Small-molecule biomarkers for clinical PET imaging of apoptosis. J Nucl Med 51(6):837–840. https://doi.org/10.2967/jnumed.109.063917
10. Villa P, Kaufmann SH, Earnshaw WC (1997) Caspases and caspase inhibitors. Trends Biochem Sci 22(10):388–393
11. Nguyen QD, Smith G, Glaser M et al (2009) Positron emission tomography imaging of drug-induced tumor apoptosis with a caspase-3/7 specific [18F]-labeled isatin sulfonamide. Proc Natl Acad Sci USA 106(38):16375–16380. https://doi.org/10.1073/pnas.0901310106
12. Zhou D, Chu W, Rothfuss J et al (2006) Synthesis, radiolabeling, and in vivo evaluation of an 18F-labeled isatin analog for imaging caspase-3 activation in apoptosis. Bioorg Med Chem Lett 16(19):5041–5046. https://doi.org/10.1016/j.bmcl.2006.07.045
13. Methot N, Vaillancourt JP, Huang J et al (2004) A caspase active site probe reveals high fractional inhibition needed to block DNA fragmentation. J Biol Chem 279(27):27905–27914. https://doi.org/10.1074/jbc.M400247200

14. Bedner E, Smolewski P, Amstad P et al (2000) Activation of caspases measured in situ by binding of fluorochrome-labeled inhibitors of caspases (FLICA): correlation with DNA fragmentation. Exp Cell Res 259(1):308–313. https://doi.org/10.1006/excr.2000.4955
15. Edgington LE, Berger AB, Blum G et al (2009) Noninvasive optical imaging of apoptosis by caspase-targeted activity-based probes. Nat Med 15(8):967–973. https://doi.org/10.1038/nm.1938
16. Laxman B, Hall DE, Bhojani MS et al (2002) Noninvasive real-time imaging of apoptosis. Proc Natl Acad Sci USA 99 (26):16551–16555. https://doi.org/10.1073/pnas.252644499
17. Bullok K, Piwnica-Worms D (2005) Synthesis and characterization of a small, membrane-permeant, caspase-activatable far-red fluorescent peptide for imaging apoptosis. J Med Chem 48(17):5404–5407. https://doi.org/10.1021/jm050008p
18. Ai HW, Hazelwood KL, Davidson MW et al (2008) Fluorescent protein FRET pairs for ratiometric imaging of dual biosensors. Nat Methods 5(5):401–403. https://doi.org/10.1038/nmeth.1207
19. Bardet PL, Kolahgar G, Mynett A et al (2008) A fluorescent reporter of caspase activity for live imaging. Proc Natl Acad Sci USA 105 (37):13901–13905. https://doi.org/10.1073/pnas.0806983105
20. Johnson JR, Kocher B, Barnett EM et al (2012) Caspase-activated cell-penetrating peptides reveal temporal coupling between endosomal release and apoptosis in an RGC-5 cell model. Bioconjug Chem 23(9):1783–1793. https://doi.org/10.1021/bc300036z
21. Bauer C, Bauder-Wuest U, Mier W et al (2005) 131I-labeled peptides as caspase substrates for apoptosis imaging. J Nucl Med 46 (6):1066–1074
22. Ye DJ, Shuhendler AJ, Cui LN et al (2014) Bioorthogonal cyclization-mediated in situ self-assembly of small-molecule probes for imaging caspase activity in vivo. Nat Chem 6 (6):519–526. https://doi.org/10.1038/Nchem.1920
23. Shen B, Jeon J, Palner M et al (2013) Positron emission tomography imaging of drug-induced tumor apoptosis with a Caspase-triggered Nanoaggregation probe. Angew Chem Int Ed 52(40):10511–10514. https://doi.org/10.1002/Anie.201303422
24. Ye D, Shuhendler AJ, Pandit P et al (2014) Caspase-responsive smart gadolinium-based contrast agent for magnetic resonance imaging of drug-induced apoptosis. Chem Sci 4 (10):3845–3852. https://doi.org/10.1039/C4SC01392A
25. Palner M, Shen B, Jeon J et al (2015) Preclinical kinetic analysis of the Caspase-3/7 PET tracer 18F-C-SNAT: quantifying the changes in blood flow and tumor retention after chemotherapy. J Nucl Med 56(9):1415–1421. https://doi.org/10.2967/jnumed.115.155259
26. Witney TH, Hoehne A, Reeves RE et al (2015) A systematic comparison of 18F-C-SNAT to established radiotracer imaging agents for the detection of tumor response to treatment. Clin Cancer Res 21(17):3896–3905. https://doi.org/10.1158/1078-0432.CCR-14-3176

Chapter 15

Practical Guidelines for Cerenkov Luminescence Imaging with Clinically Relevant Isotopes

Nikunj B. Bhatt, Darpan N. Pandya, William A. Dezarn, Frank C. Marini, Dawen Zhao, William H. Gmeiner, Pierre L. Triozzi, and Thaddeus J. Wadas

Abstract

Cerenkov luminescence imaging (CLI) is a relatively new imaging modality that utilizes conventional optical imaging instrumentation to detect Cerenkov radiation derived from standard and often clinically approved radiotracers. Its research versatility, low cost, and ease of use have increased its popularity within the molecular imaging community and at institutions that are interested in conducting radiotracer-based molecular imaging research, but that lack the necessary resources and infrastructure. Here, we provide a description of the materials and procedures necessary to conduct a Cerenkov luminescence imaging experiment using a variety of imaging instrumentation, radionuclides, and animal models.

Key words Cerenkov luminescence imaging, Isotope, Radiation, Radiotherapy, Antibody, Nanoparticle, Peptide, Reporter gene expression, Optical imaging

1 Introduction

Molecular imaging is defined as the noninvasive, visualization, characterization, and measurement of biological processes at the molecular and cellular levels in living organisms using 2-or 3-dimensional imaging techniques such as positron emission tomography, single photon computed tomography, magnetic resonance imaging, optical imaging, and ultrasound [1]. This dynamic scientific discipline has had a significant impact on health care since it enhances precision medicine strategies through improving patient diagnosis, risk stratification, and monitoring therapy response [2]. Preclinically, molecular imaging has enabled scientists to expand their knowledge of cellular function in health and disease; rapidly identify novel biomarkers for diagnosis and prognosis, and accelerate drug discovery and therapeutic development while reducing research costs in academia and industry [3].

Purnima Dubey (ed.), *Reporter Gene Imaging: Methods and Protocols*, Methods in Molecular Biology, vol. 1790, https://doi.org/10.1007/978-1-4939-7860-1_15,

Cerenkov luminescence imaging (CLI) is a new imaging modality that continues to gain popularity within the molecular imaging community since it utilizes conventional optical imaging instrumentation to detect Cerenkov radiation [4–9]. Cerenkov radiation, first described in the early twentieth century [10, 11], is electromagnetic radiation in the ultra-violet and blue portion of the visible spectrum that is emitted when charged particles, such as positrons (β^+) or beta minus (β^-) particles, travel beyond the speed of light in a dielectric medium [7, 12]. For example, as a β^- particle travels with superluminal velocity through water, it creates a non-homogeneous electromagnetic field among the water molecules within the medium. As homogeneity to the electromagnetic field is restored, Cerenkov radiation is emitted and can be detected with charge-coupled devices designed to detect bioluminescent and fluorescent light. Figure 1 illustrates this principle and its application to CLI. Since the discovery of Cerenkov radiation, additional publications have described the physics behind this phenomenon and its potential applications to molecular imaging research [12–16]. Moreover, since CLI was first reported by Robertson and coworkers [17], scientists have expanded its applications to include clinical CLI [18–24]; CLI-monitored gene expression [25–28]; and the CLI-based, high-throughput screening of imaging agents [29–33], nanoparticles [34–40] and radiotherapeutics [41–44].

The adaptability of CLI to a variety of research questions will only serve to increase its popularity among molecular imaging scientists. However, considering this imaging modality's relatively low cost and ease of use, it has the potential to dramatically impact the investigations of those who are not molecular imaging scientists, but wish to utilize molecular imaging techniques to answer fundamental questions related to their scientific research. This document has been prepared with these scientists as the primary audience, and provides a description of the materials and procedures necessary to conduct a Cerenkov luminescence imaging experiment.

2 Materials

Prepare all solutions using ultrapure water (18 MΩ-cm resistivity (25 °C)) and analytical grade reagents. Prepare and store all reagents at room temperature (unless indicated otherwise).

1. An appropriate radiotracer to probe the biological phenomenon of interest (*see* **Note 1**). Use appropriate shielding for storage.
2. An appropriate mouse model (*see* **Note 2**).

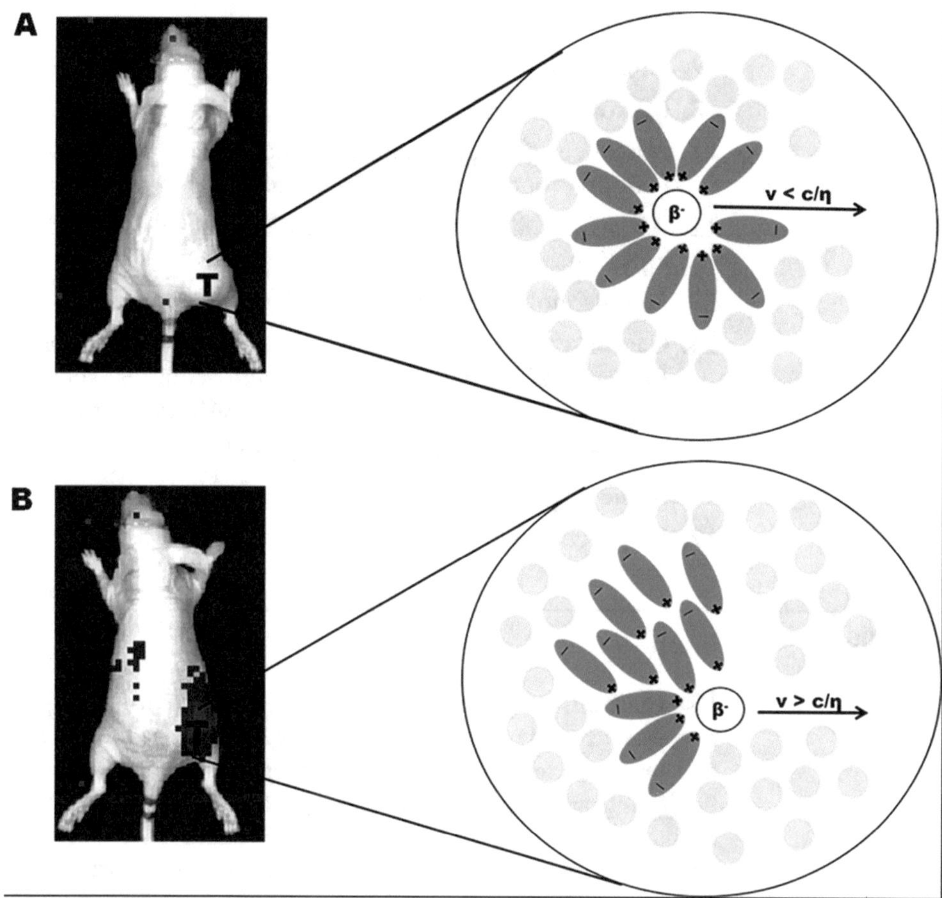

Fig. 1 Illustration depicting the generation of Cerenkov radiation. (**A**) A tumor (**T**) bearing mouse injected with a radiotracer that emits charged (β^-) particles, which travel with subluminal velocities ($v < c/\eta$). These particles are unable to distort the electromagnetic field among the surrounding water molecules and Cerenkov radiation is not generated at the site of radiotracer localization. (**B**) A tumor (**T**) bearing mouse injected with a radiotracer that emits charged (β^-) particles, which travel with superluminal velocities ($v > c/\eta$). These particles distort the electromagnetic field among the surrounding water molecules. As this distortion in the electromagnetic field is removed, Cerenkov radiation is produced and is detected by the optical imaging instrumentation. The red color in B is a software-generated pseudo-color, which denotes radiotracer accumulation and detection of Cerenkov radiation. Light gray circles represent bulk water molecules. Dark gray ellipsoids represent water molecules interacting with the charged particles. Arrows represent the paths of the particles

3. An optical imaging system with applicable software and computer interface (*see* **Note 3**).
4. A rodent anesthesia system (*see* **Note 4**).
5. Isofluorane (USP) or equivalent inhalant anesthetic and non-reflective black paper (Edmunds Optics; 54–571).
6. Non-reflective black tape (ThorLabs; T743–2.0).
7. Geiger Counter (Ludlum Measurements, Inc.; Model 3 with 44–9 GM pancake detector).

8. Dissection tools and pipettes.
9. Pipette tips.
10. Microfuge tubes.
11. Absorbent blue pads and spare mouse cage(s) with adsorbent bedding, food and water (*see* **Note 5**).
12. 0.5 mL insulin syringe with fixed 29-guage needle for animal injection.
13. 70% alcohol in a spray bottle and alcohol wipes.
14. Gamma counter such as the Wizard® gamma counter (Perkin Elmer; 2470–0020) or scintillation counter such as the TRI-CARB 4810TR (Perkin Elmer; A481000) (*see* **Note 6**).
15. Radioactive dose calibrator (*see* **Note 7**).
16. Saline or phosphate buffered saline (PBS).
17. Radioactive decontaminant.

3 Methods

Use Caution! Radioactive materials (RAM) emit ionizing radiation and are extremely dangerous. They are colorless, odorless, tasteless, and are detected only with an appropriate survey meter. Before beginning any experiments, seek approval from your institution's Radiation Safety committee, Environmental Health and Safety committee, Animal Resources Program and Institutional Animal Care and Use committee. Observe safe work practices and ALARA (**A**s **L**ow **A**s **R**easonably **A**chievable) rules associated with RAM. Use appropriate personal protective equipment such as lab coats; gloves; safety goggles; Teflon® sleeve and shoe covers; dosimetry badges and environmental controls such as lead and Plexiglas® materials to minimize radiation exposure. It is advisable to never work alone with RAM, and to regularly use a survey meter to determine hand, foot, or body contamination. Always use the survey meter to assess work areas before and after experiments. Follow your institution's guidelines for handling RAM contamination. Dispose of RAM and contaminated materials using protocols established by your institution's Radiation Safety committee.

3.1 Evaluating a CLI Phantom

1. Pipette 200 (7400), 100 (3700), 50 (1850), 25 (925), 12 (444), 6 (222) and 0 (0) μCi (kBq) of radioactivity into seven separate clear Eppendorf tubes. Adjust the volume in each tube to 200 μL with saline and seal.
2. Confirm the total radioactivity in each microfuge tube using a dose calibrator that has been configured to detect the radionuclide of interest.

3. Place the tubes on non-reflective black paper in the optical imaging system chamber. They may be fixed to the paper with non-reflective black tape if necessary (*see* **Note 8**).
4. Image the tubes (Initial settings: f-stop: 2; binning: 1, FOV: B; background correction applied; 1 min acquisition time; bioluminescent mode). These settings are listed as a reference.
5. Using the optical imaging system software, draw regions-of-interest (ROI) around the areas of detected luminescence and calculate the radiance within the ROI.
6. Using productivity software, plot the average radiance on the ordinate (Y) axis and the activity in each tube on the abscissa (X) axis. Perform linear regression analysis to determine the correlation coefficient between the observed radiance and dispensed activity (*see* **Note 9**).

3.2 Cerenkov Luminescence Imaging In Vivo

1. Prepare the radiotracer in a suitable injection buffer such as medical saline or PBS (*see* **Note 10**).
2. Anesthetize the animal to be imaged. Supply heat to the animal during the injection process. This can be accomplished using a heating pad underneath an absorbent blue pad.
3. Inject each animal with the formulated radiotracer (*see* **Note 11**).
4. After injection, return the animal to its cage and allow the animal to recover from anesthesia. The animal should be able to ambulate efficiently and not be in distress.
5. After the prescribed biodistribution period, anesthetize the animal as in Subheading 3.2, **step 2** (*see* **Note 12**).
6. Place the anesthetized animal on non-reflective black paper in the imaging chamber and the animal's nose in the anesthesia nose cone of the imaging system.
7. Take a photograph of the animal in the imaging chamber to verify the animal is positioned within the instrument's field of view (FOV).
8. Image the animal in bioluminescence or fluorescence mode to detect the Cerenkov radiation emanating from the animal (*see* **Notes 13**, **14**, and **15**). If using fluorescent mode, the excitation lamp must be off and short wavelength filter sets removed.
9. After in vivo imaging is completed, the animal may be returned to its cage for further imaging in the future (*see* **Note 16**).
10. Using the optical imaging system software, draw ROIs around the areas of detected luminescence and calculate the radiance associated with the ROIs (*see* **Notes 17** and **18**).

4 Notes

1. Consult your Radiology and Nuclear Medicine Departments for the availability of CLI-applicable radiotracers. Vendors such as PETNET Solutions (https://usa.healthcare.siemens.com/molecular-imaging/petnet-solution), Cardinal Health (http://www.cardinalhealth.com/en/product-solutions/pharmaceutical-products/nuclear-medicine/radiopharmaceuticals.html), Perkin Elmer (http://www.perkinelmer.com/category/radiochemicals), or Nordion (http://www.nordion.com/) sell radiotracers that can be used in CLI experiments.
2. In general, due to the absorbance of Cerenkov radiation by deep tissue, subcutaneous tumors are visualized more easily than orthotopic tumors within the body cavity. Also, the presence of fur will cause optical scattering and reduce the observed Cerenkov luminescence signal detected by the instrument. If necessary, depilate the animal before radiotracer injection. Use clippers to remove bulk fur followed by a depilatory cream to remove any fine fur from the animal. Consult your institution's veterinary staff for an appropriate protocol.
3. Consult the optical imaging instrument manufacturer to determine if your particular instrument is configured to detect Cerenkov radiation.
4. An inhalant anesthesia system is preferred for anesthetizing the rodent during radiotracer injection. Typically, the optical imaging system will be configured with an anesthesia machine that delivers inhalant anesthesia in a stream of medical oxygen to the rodent while in the imaging chamber. Inhalant anesthesia is preferred over the use of injected anesthetics since delivery of the former is more consistent. It reduces the possibility of animal movement during the imaging session.
5. These should be available from the institution's animal resources program. Transferring the animals to new cages at any point after radiotracer injection reduces the animal's exposure to radioactive materials in the bedding. This also minimizes body surface contamination of the animal, which may increase the background luminescence signal during the imaging session.
6. Gamma counters and liquid scintillation counters detect radiation in different ways. Gamma counters measure the gamma ray photons emitted by a decaying radionuclide. This is a "dry" technique. If using a gamma counter, ensure that the energy window is configured to detect the gamma photon(s) of interest. Liquid scintillation counting is a "wet" technique used primarily to detect alpha or beta particles emitted from a decaying radionuclide. Liquid scintillation counters measure the

radioactivity in a sample by detecting luminescence, which is generated when charged particles interact with a liquid scintillant that has been mixed with the radioactive material. If using a liquid scintillation counter, scintillation fluid, and scintillation vials with cap will be required.

7. Be sure your instrument is configured to detect the radionuclide of interest.
8. The tubes should be arranged in the center of the instrument's FOV. This can be accomplished by laying the sealed tubes on their sides in a circular pattern on non-reflective black paper, and taking a photograph of the tubes in the imaging chamber to verify their position.
9. The better the agreement between the calculated value and the theoretical value of 1.00, the more meaningful the correlation between the dispensed activity and the Cerenkov radiation detected by the instrument.
10. The injection volume should not exceed 250 μL, or as defined by your institution's IACUC.
11. Tail vein injection is preferred since it delivers the radiotracer directly into the circulatory system.
12. The imaging of animals injected with small molecule radiotracers can begin immediately. The imaging of animals injected with large molecular weight radiotracers (i.e., a radiolabeled antibody or nanoparticle) should be delayed for 12–24 h to allow for the accumulation of the radiotracer at the tissue of interest and systemic clearance.
13. For radiotracers that emit prompt Cerenkov radiation, imaging can occur immediately. When Cerenkov radiation is produced by the daughter decay products of alpha particle emitting radionuclides, secular equilibrium must be achieved before imaging. For ^{225}Ac this period is 10 h, and reference 13 lists equilibrium periods for additional alpha particle emitting radionuclides.
14. During imaging, keep the animal under anesthesia. While the number of animals imaged at any one time will be dependent upon the injected radiotracer and instrument settings, it is recommended that not more than three animals be imaged at the same time.
15. Table 1 lists several CLI applications. While the instrumentation settings are provided, they should be utilized as an initial reference only. Final imaging parameters should be determined empirically and optimized beforehand by imaging one mouse that has been injected with the radiotracer. Once the imaging parameters have been optimized, all other mice can be injected with the radiotracer and imaged using the finalized imaging

Table 1
Summarized imaging parameters of selected applications involving Cerenkov luminescence imaging

Entry	Radiotracer	Activity injected (MBq/μCi)	Application	Data collection parameters and notes	Biological model	Reference
1	[^{18}F]F-FDG	7.3/270	In vivo tumor visualization	IVIS 100/200 bioluminescence mode, 1 min data acquisition, 1 h post-injection (p.i.)	CWR22-RV-1 human prostate xenograft	[17]
2	[^{18}F]F-FHBG	8.1/300	Reporter gene expression/ tumor visualization	IVIS 200 bioluminescence mode, 1 h and 2 h p.i. data acquisition	C6 rat glioma xenograft transfected with HSV1-tk reporter gene system	[26]
3	[^{124}I]NaI	11/297	Reporter gene expression in human mesenchymal stem cells (MSCs)	IVIS 100 bioluminescence mode, 1 min data acquisition, 0–8 days p.i.	Athymic nude mice injected with Fluc-hNIS transfected MSCs	[27]
4	[^{90}Y]Y-DOTA-30F11	11/300	In vivo visualization of systemic radiotherapy delivery	IVIS Spectrum fluorescence mode (lamp off), 1.5 min acquisition time (0–3 d p.i.), f-stop: 1; binning: 4; FOV: B; cosmic ray normalization, flat field correction and background correction applied	Athymic nude mice bearing murine myeloid SJL leukemia cells, SJLB6F1/J mice, SJL/J mice	[41]
5	[^{177}Lu]Lu-DOTA-30F11	11/300	In vivo visualization of systemic radiotherapy delivery	IVIS Spectrum fluorescence mode (lamp off), 1.5 min acquisition time (0–3 d p.i.), f-stop: 1; binning: 4; FOV: B; cosmic ray normalization, flat field correction and background correction applied	Athymic nude mice bearing murine myeloid SJL leukemia cells, SJLB6F1/J mice, SJL/J mice	[41]
6	[^{225}Ac]Ac-DOTA-c (RGDyK)	1.9/50	In vivo visualization of systemic radiotherapy delivery	IVIS 100, fluorescence mode (lamp off), 5 min acquisition time (24 h p. i.), f-stop: 2; binning: 1; FOV: B; background correction applied	Athymic nude mice bearing human U87 mg xenografts	[43]

7	[^{89}Zr]Zr-DFO-J591 mAb	11/300	In vivo tumor visualization	IVIS 200 bioluminescence mode, 1 min acquisition time (24–96 h p.i.), f-stop: 1; binning: Medium; FOV: B; background correction applied	Athymic nude mice bearing human LNCAP xenografts	[9]
8	[^{64}Cu]Cu-DOTA-anti-GD2 mAb	11/300	In vivo tumor visualization	IVIS Spectrum 1 min acquisition (0–48 h p.i.), f-stop: 1; binning 16; FOV: 12.5 cm; cosmic ray, flat field and background corrections applied.	SHO mice bearing $GD2^+$ neuroblastoma xenografts	[45]
9	[^{18}F]F-FDG	15/400	Nanoparticle mediated biomarker imaging	IVIS 200 0.5 min acquisition	Athymic nude mice bearing SCC7 or BT20 xenografts	[16]

parameters. This practice reduces radiotracer waste, and utilizes time more efficiently when short-lived radiotracers are being used in CLI applications.

16. After the final imaging time point, additional data can be obtained through ex vivo imaging of the animal's organs and tissues. This is accomplished by euthanizing the animal, removing organs and tissues of interest, and imaging them on non-reflective black paper in the imaging chamber with the parameters established for the in vivo imaging experiments.
17. Background correction can be performed through (a) use of dark images acquired at the equivalent instrument settings immediately before experimental image collection, or (b) ROI analysis of a region in the same experimental image but remote from the area of interest.
18. Radiotracer in vivo specificity, retention, and clearance can be determined from comparing the average radiance observed in each tissue or by generating target tissue-to-non-target tissue ratios (T/NT = average radiance of target tissue/average radiance of non-target tissue).

Acknowledgments

This work was supported by NIH grant NIH P30 CA012197, DoD grant W81XWH-13-1-0125, and The United States Department of Energy Office of Science-Isotope Program in the Office of Nuclear Physics.

References

1. Mankoff DA (2007) A definition of molecular imaging. J Nucl Med 48(6):18N–21N
2. James ML, Gambhir SS (2012) A molecular imaging primer: modalities, imaging agents, and applications. Physiol Rev 92(2):897–965
3. Chen ZY, Wang YX, Lin Y et al (2014) Advance of molecular imaging technology and targeted imaging agent in imaging and therapy. Biomed Res Int 2014:819324–819334
4. Boschi F, Spinelli AE (2014) Cerenkov luminescence imaging at a glance. Curr Mol Imaging 3(2):106–117
5. Chin PTK, Welling MM, Meskers SCJ (2013) Optical imaging as an expansion of nuclear medicine: Cerenkov-based luminescence vs fluorescence-based luminescence. Eur J Nucl Med Mol Imaging 40(8):1283–1291
6. Das S, Thorek Daniel LJ, Grimm J (2014) Cerenkov imaging. Adv Cancer Res 124:213–234
7. Mitchell GS, Gill RK, Boucher DL et al (2011) In vivo Cerenkov luminescence imaging: a new tool for molecular imaging. Philos Trans A Math Phys Eng Sci 369(1955):4605–4619
8. Thorek DL, Robertson R, Bacchus WA et al (2012) Cerenkov imaging - a new modality for molecular imaging. Am J Nucl Med Mol Imaging 2(2):163–173
9. Ruggiero A, Holland JP, Lewis JS et al (2010) Cerenkov luminescence imaging of medical isotopes. J Nucl Med 51(7):1123–1130
10. Cerenkov P (1937) Visible radiation produced by electrons moving in a medium with velocities exceeding that of light. Phys Rev 52:378–379
11. Cerenkov P (1934) Visible emission of clean liquids by action of gamma irradiation. Dokl Akad Nauk SSSR 2(2):451–454
12. Xu Y, Liu H, Cheng Z (2011) Harnessing the power of radionuclides for optical imaging:

Cerenkov luminescence imaging. J Nucl Med 52(12):2009–2018

13. Ackerman NL, Graves EE (2012) The potential for Cerenkov luminescence imaging of alpha-emitting radionuclides. Phy Med Biol 57(3):771–783
14. Gill RK, Mitchell GS, Cherry SR (2015) Computed Cerenkov luminescence yields for radionuclides used in biology and medicine. Phys Med Biol 60(11):1–18
15. Lewis MA, Kodibagkar VD, Oz OK et al (2010) On the potential for molecular imaging with Cerenkov luminescence. Opt Lett 35 (23):3889–3891
16. Thorek DL, Ogirala A, Beattie BJ et al (2013) Quantitative imaging of disease signatures through radioactive decay signal conversion. Nat Med 19(10):1345–1350
17. Robertson R, Germanos MS, Li C et al (2009) Optical imaging of Cerenkov light generation from positron-emitting radiotracers. Phys Med Biol 54(16):N355–N365
18. Grootendorst MR, Cariati M, Pinder SE et al (2017) Intraoperative assessment of tumor resection margins in breast-conserving surgery using 18F-FDG Cerenkov luminescence imaging - a first-in-human feasibility study. J Nucl Med 58(6):891–898. https://doi.org/10.2967/jnumed.116.181032
19. Grootendorst MR, Cariati M, Purushotham A et al (2016) Cerenkov luminescence imaging (CLI) for image-guided cancer surgery. Clin Transl Imaging 4(5):353–366
20. Holland JP, Normand G, Ruggiero A et al (2011) Intraoperative imaging of positron emission tomographic radiotracers using Cerenkov luminescence emissions. Mol Imaging 10(3):177–186
21. Hu H, Cao X, Kang F et al (2015) Feasibility study of novel endoscopic Cerenkov luminescence imaging system in detecting and quantifying gastrointestinal disease: first human results. Eur Radiol 25(6):1814–1822
22. Hu Z, Ma X, Qu X et al (2012) Three-dimensional noninvasive monitoring Iodine-131 uptake in the thyroid using a modified Cerenkov luminescence tomography approach. PLoS One 7(5):e37623
23. Kothapalli S-R, Liu H, Liao JC et al (2012) Endoscopic imaging of Cerenkov luminescence. Biomed Optics Express 3 (6):1215–1225
24. Spinelli AE, Ferdeghini M, Cavedon C et al (2013) First human Cerenkography. J Biomed Optics 18(2):20502
25. Jeong SY, Hwang M-H, Kim JE et al (2011) Combined Cerenkov luminescence and nuclear imaging of radioiodine in the thyroid gland and thyroid cancer cells expressing sodium iodide symporter: initial feasibility study. Endocr J 58 (7):575–583
26. Liu H, Ren G, Liu S et al (2010) Optical imaging of reporter gene expression using a positron-emission-tomography probe. J Biomed Opt 15(6):060505
27. Wolfs E, Holvoet B, Gijsbers R et al (2014) Optimization of multimodal imaging of mesenchymal stem cells using the human sodium iodide symporter for PET and Cerenkov luminescence imaging. PLoS One 9(4):e94833
28. Yang W, Qin W, Hu Z et al (2012) Comparison of Cerenkov luminescence imaging (CLI) and gamma camera imaging for visualization of let-7 expression in lung adenocarcinoma A549 cells. Nucl Med Biol 39(7):948–953
29. Fan D, Zhang X, Zhong L et al (2015) 68Ga-Labeled 3PRGD2 for dual PET and Cerenkov luminescence imaging of Orthotopic human Glioblastoma. Bioconjug Chem 26 (6):1054–1060
30. Kim D-H, Choe Y-S, Choi J-Y et al (2011) Binding of 2-[18F]fluoro-CP-118,954 to mouse acetylcholinesterase: microPET and ex vivo Cerenkov luminescence imaging studies. Nucl Med Biol 38(4):541–547
31. Natarajan A, Habte F, Liu H et al (2013) Evaluation of 89Zr-rituximab tracer by Cerenkov luminescence imaging and correlation with PET in a humanized transgenic mouse model to image NHL. Mol Imaging Biol 15 (4):468–475
32. Robertson R, Germanos MS, Manfredi MG et al (2011) Multimodal imaging with (18)F-FDG PET and Cerenkov luminescence imaging after MLN4924 treatment in a human lymphoma xenograft model. J Nucl Med 52 (11):1764–1769
33. Zhang X, Kuo C, Moore A et al (2013) In vivo optical imaging of interscapular brown adipose tissue with 18F-FDG via Cerenkov luminescence imaging. PLoS One 8(4):e62007
34. Black KCL, Zhegalova N, Sultan DH et al (2016) In vivo fate tracking of degradable nanoparticles for lung gene transfer using PET and ^Cerenkov imaging. Biomaterials 98:53–63
35. Guo W, Sun X, Jacobson O et al (2015) Intrinsically radioactive [64Cu]CuInS/ZnS quantum dots for PET and optical imaging: improved radiochemical stability and controllable Cerenkov luminescence. ACS Nano 9 (1):488–495
36. Lee SB, Ahn SB, Lee S-W et al (2016) Radionuclide-embedded gold nanoparticles

for enhanced dendritic cell-based cancer immunotherapy, sensitive and quantitative tracking of dendritic cells with PET and Cerenkov luminescence. NPG Asia Mat 8(6): e281–e288

37. Lee SB, Yoon GS, Lee S-W et al (2016) Combined positron emission tomography and Cerenkov luminescence imaging of sentinel lymph nodes using PEGylated radionuclide-embedded gold nanoparticles. Small 12 (35):4894–4901
38. Ma X, Kang F, Xu F et al (2013) Enhancement of Cerenkov luminescence imaging by dual excitation of Er3+, Yb3+–doped rare-earth microparticles. PLoS One 8(10):e77926
39. Thorek DLJ, Das S, Grimm J (2014) Molecular imaging using nanoparticle quenchers of cerenkov luminescence. Small 10 (18):3729–3734
40. Wang Y, Liu Y, Luehmann H et al (2013) Radioluminescent gold nanocages with controlled radioactivity for real-time in vivo imaging. Nano Lett 13(2):581–585
41. Balkin ER, Kenoyer A, Orozco JJ et al (2014) In vivo localization of 90Y and 177Lu Radioimmunoconjugates using Cerenkov luminescence imaging in a disseminated murine Leukemia model. Cancer Res 74 (20):5846–5854
42. Chakravarty R, Chakraborty S, Sarma HD et al (2016) 90Y/177Lu-labelled Cetuximab immunoconjugates: radiochemistry optimization to clinical dose formulation. J Label Compd Radiopharm 59(9):354–363. https://doi.org/10.1002/jlcr.3413
43. Pandya DN, Hantgan R, Budzevich MM et al (2016) Preliminary therapy evaluation of 225Ac-DOTA-c(RGDyK) demonstrates that cerenkov radiation derived from 225Ac daughter decay can be detected by optical imaging for in vivo tumor visualization. Theranostics 6 (5):698–709
44. Wright CL, Zhang J, Tweedle MF (2015) Theranostic imaging of Yttrium-90. BioMed Res Inter 2015:481279
45. Maier FC, Schmitt J, Maurer A et al (2016) Correlation between positron emission tomography and Cerenkov luminescence imaging in vivo and ex vivo using 64Cu-labeled antibodies in a neuroblastoma mouse model. Oncotarget 7(41):67403–67411. https://doi.org/10.18632/oncotarget.11795

Chapter 16

Synthesis, Purification, Characterization, and Imaging of Cy3-Functionalized Fluorescent Silver Nanoparticles in 2D and 3D Tumor Models

Jessica Swanner and Ravi Singh

Abstract

Silver nanoparticles (AgNPs) have a high affinity for sulfhydryl (thiol) groups, which can be exploited for functionalization with various tracking and targeting moieties. Here, we describe how to reliably and reproducibly functionalize AgNPs with the fluorescent moiety cyanine3-polyethelyne glycol (5000 molecular weight)-thiol (Cy3-PEG_{5000}-SH). We also demonstrate how to purify and characterize Cy3-functionalized AgNPs (Cy3-AgNPs). Additionally, we describe how these Cy3-AgNPs can be imaged in 2D and 3D tumor models, providing insight into cellular localization and diffusion through a tumor spheroid, respectively.

Key words Silver, Nanomaterials, Fluorescence, Imaging, 3D tumor models

1 Introduction

Silver nanoparticles (AgNPs) are the most widely applied nanomaterial for both commercial and clinical biomedical applications. Due to their anti-bacterial properties, AgNPs have been adapted for use in disinfectants for aseptic environments, as surface coatings for neurosurgical shunts and venous catheters, and in bone cement. They have also been shown to enhance wound healing and improve skin regeneration [1]. Preclinical studies of AgNPs show that they possess cytotoxic activity toward a variety of cancer cell lines including breast [2–5], glioblastoma [6–8], cervical [9], liver [10], lung [11], and leukemia [12, 13].

AgNPs possess a strong affinity for sulfhydryl (thiol) groups [14, 15], and their physicochemical attributes can be easily tailored to produce different surface characteristics that are important for stability in physiological conditions and to aid in targeting [16, 17]. This unique property can be exploited to functionalize AgNPs with various targeting and tracking moieties that contain a

Purnima Dubey (ed.), *Reporter Gene Imaging: Methods and Protocols*, Methods in Molecular Biology, vol. 1790, https://doi.org/10.1007/978-1-4939-7860-1_16,

thiol group. It is well documented that the cytotoxic properties of nanomaterials are dependent upon characteristics including size, charge, and coatings, all of which affect the uptake [18]. Therefore after functionalization, it is imperative to characterize particles based on hydrodynamic dimeter and ζ-potential because these properties may affect stability and biodistribution of nanoparticles in addition to cytotoxicity [18].

Here, we describe how to functionalize AgNPs with the fluorescent tracking moiety Cyanine3, which is stabilized by a polyethylene glycol (PEG) group. PEG has been added to nanomaterials and small-molecule drugs to increase stability and bioavailability in physiological conditions [19, 20]. This fluorescent tracking moeity also contains a terminal thiol group that can readily interact with the AgNP. We demonstrate how ultraviolet/visible (UV/Vis) spectrophotometry can be used to monitor the reaction of the thiol group binding with the AgNP. Additionally, we describe how to purify the Cy3-PEG_{5000}-SH functionalized AgNPs (Cy3-AgNPs) from the starting materials (25 nm AgNPs and Cy3-PEG_{5000}-SH), and how to identify each using UV/Vis spectrophotometry. We demonstrate how dynamic light scattering (DLS) can further validate that the particles are functionalized based upon changes in hydrodynamic diameter and ζ-potential. Lastly, we describe how to visualize the Cy3-AgNPs in 2D cell monolayers and 3D tumor spheroids using confocal microscopy and the EVOS FL Auto Cell Imaging System, respectively.

2 Materials

Prepare all AgNPs and Cy3-PEG_{5000}-SH dispersions in deionized water at room temperature and store at 4 °C light protected.

2.1 Cy3-AgNP Synthesis and Purification Components

1. 25 nm PVP Redispersable Silver Nanoparticles (nanoComposix Inc.): dissolve 25 mg of AgNPs in 2.5 mL deionized water.
2. Cy3-PEG_{5000}-SH (Nanocs, Inc): dissolve in warm deionized water to make a 200 mM solution.
3. TCEP Bond Breaker solution (Thermo Scientific).
4. 100,000 MWCO column.
5. PD-10 Desalting Column 1.7 mL microcentrifuge tubes.

2.2 Characterization Components

1. UV/Vis Spectrophotometer.
2. Quartz cuvette.
3. Malvern Zetasizer Nano ZS90 (Malvern Panalytical).
4. Folded capillary Zeta cells.
5. Disposable, clear plastic cuvette.

2.3 2D and 3D cell culture imaging components

1. MDA-MB-231: were purchased from ATCC (American Type Culture Collection) (Manassas, VA, USA): Cells were grown in DMEM supplemented with 10% FBS (vol:vol), 2 mM l-glutamine, penicillin (250 U/mL), and streptomycin (250 μg/mL).
2. 1× Dulbecco's Phosphate-Buffered Saline (DPBS) without calcium or magnesium.
3. 16% Formaldehyde solution (w/v), Methanol-free: dilute 16% formaldehyde 1:4 (vol:vol) with 1× DPBS to make 4% formaldehyde solution.
4. Four well glass slide chamber slides.
5. Vectashield Hard Set Mounting Medium with DAPI.
6. Microscope Cover Glass.
7. Clear fingernail polish.
8. Confocal Microscope.
9. Round bottom 96-well plates.
10. Six-well tissue culture-treated plates.
11. Matrigel Matrix (Corning): dilute to 2% in growth medium for MDA-MB-231 cells outlined above.
12. EVOS FL Auto Cell Imaging System (Invitrogen) or similar equipment.

3 Methods

Perform all the steps at room temperature and protect from light unless otherwise specified.

3.1 Synthesis of Cy3-AgNPs

1. Disperse 25 nm AgNPs in deionized water via bath sonication for 5 min at 4 °C resulting in a brownish-gray opaque solution.
2. Dissolve Cy3-PEG_{5000}-SH in 1 mL warm deionized water at a 200 mM concentration via vortexing resulting in a pink solution.
3. Add TCEP bond breaker solution to the Cy3-PEG_{5000}-SH at a ratio of 50:1 (molarity) for 20 min (*see* **Note 1**).
4. Combine 2 mL of AgNPs with the Cy3-PEG_{5000}-SH + TCEP solution and additional deionized water to bring the final volume to 4 mL with a final concentration of 5 mg/mL AgNPs.
5. Monitor the reaction every 15 min by UV/Vis spectrophotometry (*see* **Note 2**) (Fig. 1).
6. After 45 min, concentrate the Cy3-PEG_{5000}-SH AgNPs dispersion using a 100,000 MWCO vivaspin column to approximately 1 mL volume via centrifugation at 3000.0 rcf for 10 min (*see* **Note 3**).

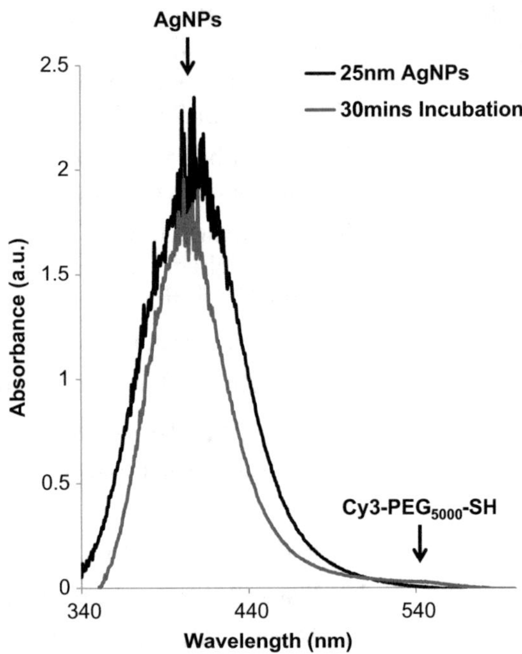

Fig. 1 UV/Vis spectrophotometry absorbance readings for monitoring the reaction of Cy3-PEG$_{5000}$-SH binding to AgNPs. Unfunctionalized AgNPs have a strong absorbance peak at 405 nm. When thiol binding occurs, a damping of the peak at 405 nm occurs along with the development of a peak at 550 nm where Cy3-PEG$_{5000}$-SH absorbs

3.2 Purification of Cy3-AgNPs

1. Remove the cap of the PD-10 desalting column and remove the column storage solution.
2. Cut the tip of the column at the indicated notch.
3. Fill the column with deionized water and allow it to enter the column completely. Repeat this **step 4** times, discarding the flow-through (*see* **Note 4**).
4. Filter the concentrated volume from **step 6** of the synthesis of Cy3-AgNPs through the equilibrated PD-10 desalting column with deionized water to separate free Cy3-PEG$_{5000}$-SH, unfunctionalized AgNPs, and Cy3-AgNPs (*see* **Note 5**).
5. Collect fractions in 1.7 mL microcentrifuge tubes in approximately 500–800 μL volumes (approximately 10 drops).
6. Analyze the fractions collected from the PD-10 column by UV/Vis spectrophotometry to identify fractions containing Cy3-AgNPs (*see* **Note 6**) (Fig. 2).
7. Combine fractions containing Cy3-AgNPs, and store light-protected at 4 °C.

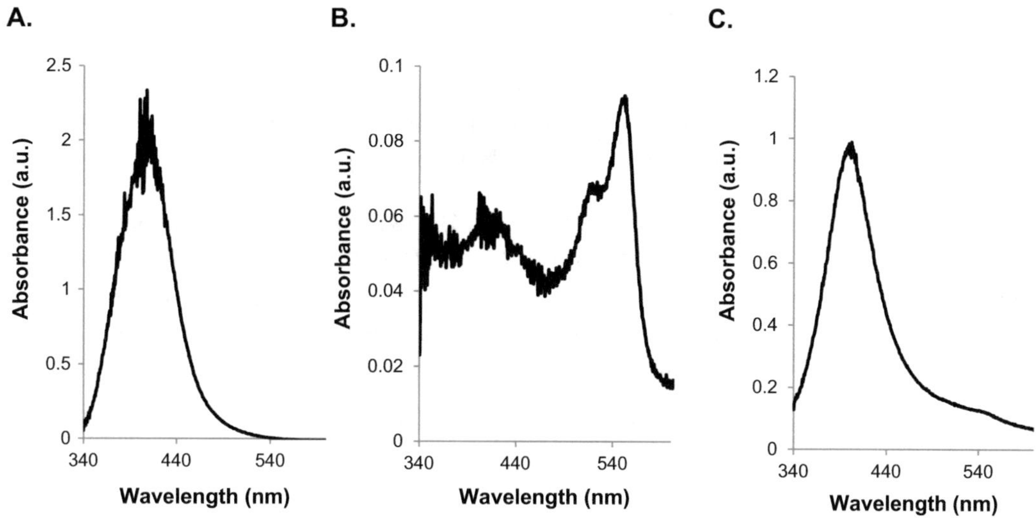

Fig. 2 UV/Vis spectrophotometry absorbance readings of various fractions obtained during the purification process utilizing the PD-10 desalting column. (**a**) Example of unfunctionalized particles: displays one absorbance peak at 405 nm. (**b**) Example of free (unbound) Cy3-PEG_{5000}-SH: displays one absorbance peak at 550 nm. (**c**) Example of Cy3-AgNPs: displays a large peak at 405 nm indicating the presence of AgNPs and a smaller peak at 550 nm indicating successful binding of the Cy3-PEG_{5000}-SH fluorescent moiety

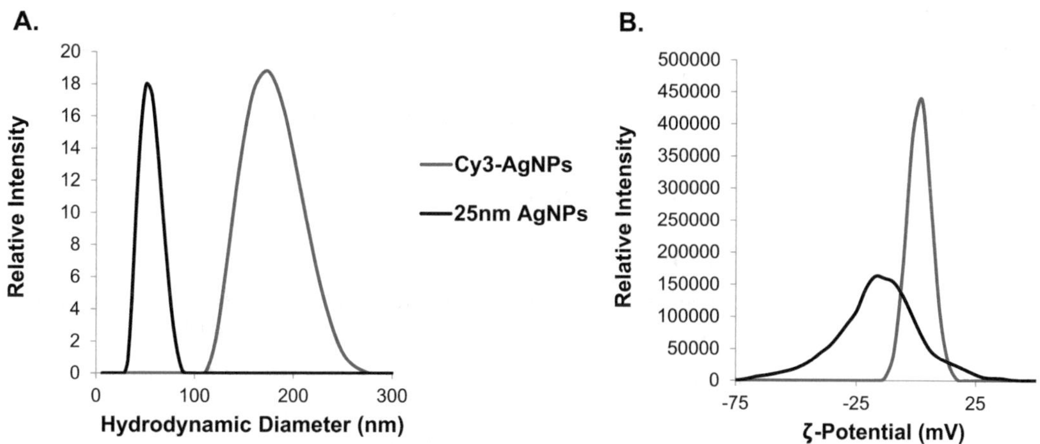

Fig. 3 Dynamic light scattering (DLS) data comparing unfunctionalized 25 nm AgNPs (black) and Cy3-AgNPs (red). (**a**) An increase in hydrodynamic diameter indicates the formation of Cy3-AgNPs. (**b**) Positive zeta potential shift indicates functionalization of AgNPs to form Cy3-AgNPs

3.3 Characterization of Cy3-AgNPs

3.3.1 Hydrodynamic Diameter of Cy3-AgNPs

1. Dilute 10 μl of Cy3-AgNPs in 1 mL of deionized water or 1× DPBS in a plastic cuvette.
2. Read the sample in triplicate on the Zetasizer Nano ZS90 with the following settings: 25 °C, automatic settings, adjust for refractive index of the dispersant (*see* **Note 7**) (Fig. 3a).

3.3.2 Zeta Potential of Cy3-AgNPs

1. Transfer the sample diluted in deionized water from the plastic cuvette to a folded capillary cell.
2. Read the sample in triplicate on the Zetasizer Nano ZS90 with the settings outlined above for the hydrodynamic diameter measurements (*see* **Note 8**) (Fig. 3b).

3.4 Imaging of Cy3-AgNPs in 2D Culture

1. Plate 5×10^5 MDA-MB-231 cells per well in a four-well glass slide chamber slide, and let it adhere for 48 h at 37 °C.
2. Treat cells with Cy3-AgNPs or unfunctionalized 25 nm AgNPs diluted in MDA-MB-231 growth medium for 1 h at 37 °C.
3. Wash cells twice with 1× DPBS.
4. Fix cells with 4% formaldehyde for 15 min at room temperature.
5. Remove chambers on the slide.
6. Add 2–3 drops of Vectashield Hard Set Mounting Medium with DAPI, and place a glass microscope cover on the slide.
7. Seal the edges with clear fingernail polish, and allow the mounting media to harden overnight, light-protected at 4 °C.
8. Image using a confocal microscope (*see* **Note 9**) (Fig. 4).

3.5 Imaging of Cy3-AgNPs in 3D Multicellular Spheroids (3D Culture)

1. Prepare MDA-MB-231 spheroids by plating 5000 MDA-MB-231 cells in a 96-well round bottom plate in 200 μL of 2% Matrigel matrix.
2. Allow spheroids to grow at 37 °C for 4 days.
3. Treat spheroids with 1× DPBS, Cy3-AgNPs, or Cy3-AgNP filtrate (obtained from the concentration of the particles (*see* Subheading 3.1, **step 6**) diluted in growth medium for 6 or 24 h.
4. Using a P1,000 pipette, transfer spheroids to a six-well plate containing fresh growth medium (*see* **Note 10**).
5. Image using the transmitted light and red fluorescent protein (RFP) lenses on the EVOS FL Auto Cell Imaging System or similar machine. Merge transmitted light and RFP images (*see* Fig. 5).

4 Notes

1. TCEP bond breaker solution is necessary to prevent disulfide bond formation among the Cy3-PEG_{5000}-SH fluorescent moieties. Disulfide bond formation between the moieties would prevent thiol binding of the AgNPs, and thus prevent functionalization of the particles.

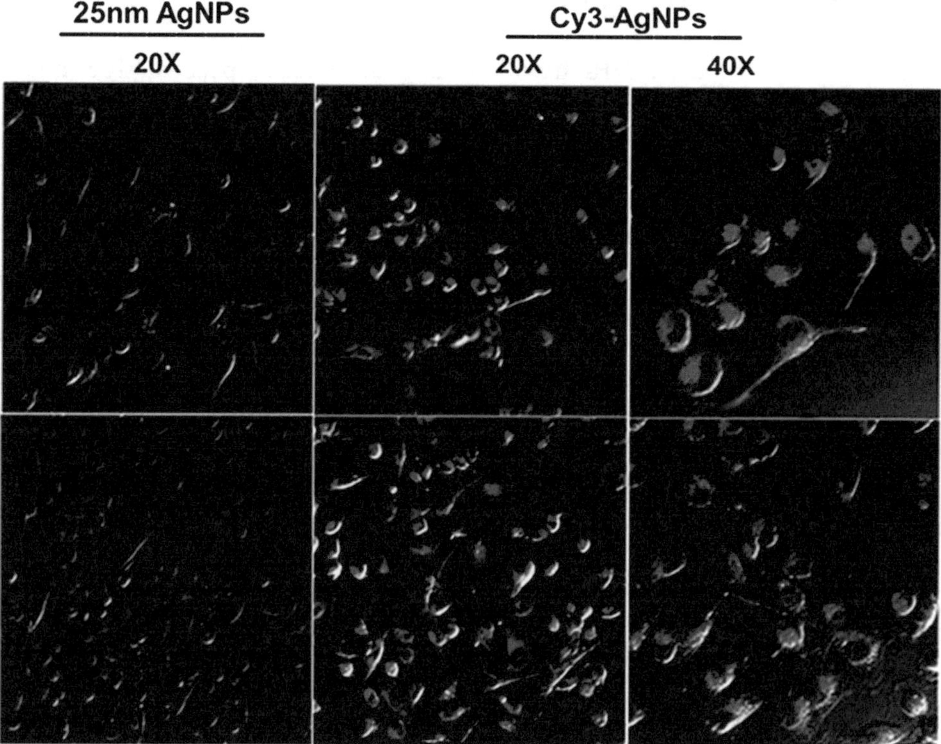

Fig. 4 Confocal images of MDA-MB-231 breast cancer cells after 1 h treatment with 25 nm AgNPs or Cy3-AgNPs. The first panel shows cells after 1 h treatment with 25 nm AgNPs at 20× magnification. The second and third panels show cells after a 1 h treatment with Cy3-AgNPs at 20× and 40× magnification, respectively

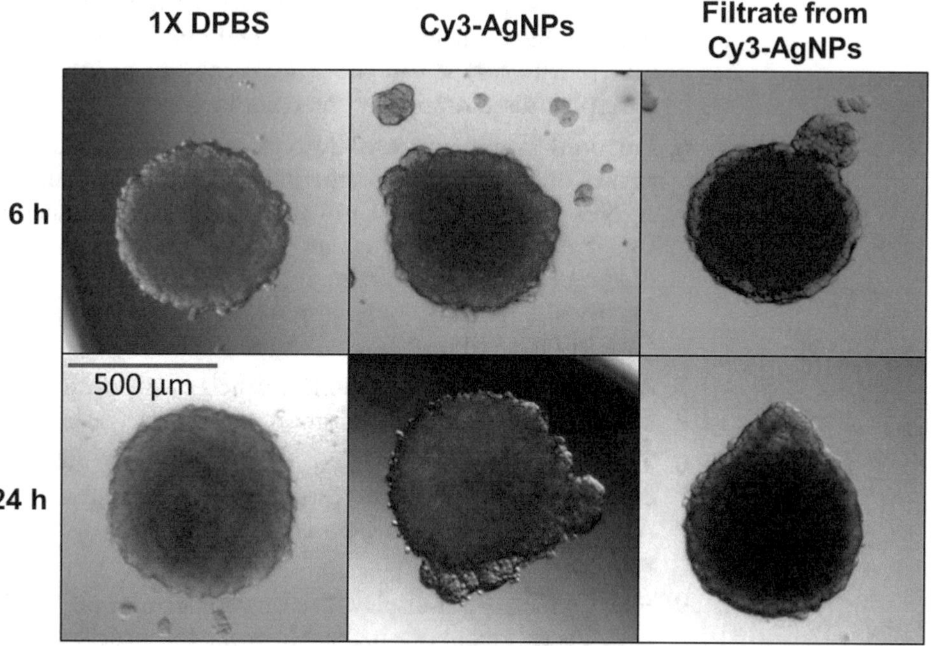

Fig. 5 EVOS images of MDA-MB-231 3D tumor spheroids treated for 6 or 24 h with 1× DPBS, Cy3-AgNPs, or filtrate collected from Cy3-AgNPs

2. AgNPs have a strong absorbance peak at 405 nm, while Cy3-PEG_{5000}-SH has a strong absorbance peak at 550 nm. Upon functionalization via thiol binding, a dampening of the AgNP peak at 405 will occur along with a red shift. Additionally, a small peak around 550 should be observed to indicate the presence of the Cy3-PEG_{5000}-SH.
3. Additional centrifugation may be required if the volume is still above 1 mL. Although the PD-10 desalting column specifies that larger volumes (up to 2.5 mL) may be used, smaller volumes provide better separation of unfunctionalized AgNPs, Cy3-AgNPs, and free Cy3-PEG_{5000}-SH. If the particles become entrapped in the membrane, a P200 gel loading tip can be used to loosen particles from the membrane.
4. Equilibration of the PD-10 desalting column may be performed while the reaction is occurring or while the reaction mixture is being concentrated. Ensure that the column does not dry out after equilibration by filling the column with deionized water and recapping the bottom of the column with the caps provided. When ready to filter the AgNPs, remove the cap and allow the deionized water to move into the packed bed of the column before adding the AgNPs.
5. Because the Cy3-AgNPs increase in size following functionalization, they will elute in the early fractions. The unfunctionalized AgNPs will elute in the middle fractions. The free Cy3-PEG_{5000}-SH will elute last because the small size will cause entrapment in the fenestrations of the column leading to a slow release from the column. Unbound Cy3-PEG_{5000}-SH may remain trapped in the PD-10 column as indicated by a light pink discoloration of the column.
6. Fractions containing Cy3-AgNPs will have two absorbance peaks: one peak at 405 nm indicating the presence of the AgNPs and one at 550 nm to indicate the presence of the Cy3-PEG_{5000}-SH fluorescent moiety. Fractions displaying only a peak at 405 nm contain unfunctionalized AgNPs, and fractions displaying only a peak at 550 nm contain free Cy3-PEG_{5000}-SH.
7. An increase in hydrodynamic diameter will occur, which is indicative of functionalization of the particle.
8. The ζ-potential of the Cy3-AgNPs becomes more neutral compared to negative ζ-potential for unfunctionalized AgNPs. This change in ζ-potential is indicative of functionalization via thiol binding.
9. Free Cy3-PEG-SH displays a strong absorbance peak at 550 via UV/Vis spectrophotometry. However for visualization of the Cy3-AgNPs in vitro, the optimal wavelength is between 565 and 665 nm.

10. When removing spheroids from the 96-well plates to the six-well plates, place all spheroids receiving the same treatment in one well of the six-well plate for imaging.

Acknowledgments

This work was supported in part by grant R00CA154006 (RS) from the National Institutes of Health, pilot funds from the Comprehensive Cancer Center of Wake Forest University supported by NCI CCSG P30CA012197, and by start-up funds from the Wake Forest School of Medicine Department of Cancer Biology. JS was supported in part by training grant T32CA079448 from the National Institutes of Health.

References

1. Chaloupka K, Malam Y, Seifalian AM (2010) Nanosilver as a new generation of nanoproduct in biomedical applications. Trends Biotechnol 28(11):580–588
2. Gurunathan S et al (2013) Cytotoxicity of biologically synthesized silver nanoparticles in MDA-MB-231 human breast cancer cells. Biomed Res Int 2013:535796
3. Jeyaraj M et al (2013) Biogenic silver nanoparticles for cancer treatment: an experimental report. Colloids Surf B Biointerfaces 106:86–92
4. Liu JH et al (2012) TAT-modified nanosilver for combating multidrug-resistant cancer. Biomaterials 33(26):6155–6161
5. Swanner J et al (2015) Differential cytotoxic and radiosensitizing effects of silver nanoparticles on triple-negative breast cancer and non-triple-negative breast cells. Int J Nanomedicine 10:3937–3953
6. Liu PD et al (2013) Silver nanoparticles: a novel radiation sensitizer for glioma? Nanoscale 5(23):11829–11836
7. Locatelli E et al (2014) Targeted delivery of silver nanoparticles and alisertib: in vitro and in vivo synergistic effect against glioblastoma. Nanomedicine 9(6):839–849
8. Sharma S et al (2014) Silver nanoparticles impregnated alginate-chitosan-blended Nanocarrier induces apoptosis in human Glioblastoma cells. Adv Healthc Mater 3(1):106–114
9. Miura N, Shinohara Y (2009) Cytotoxic effect and apoptosis induction by silver nanoparticles in HeLa cells. Biochem Biophys Res Commun 390(3):733–737
10. Kawata K, Osawa M, Okabe S (2009) In vitro toxicity of silver nanoparticles at noncytotoxic doses to HepG2 human Hepatoma cells. Environ Sci Technol 43(15):6046–6051
11. Beer C et al (2012) Toxicity of silver nanoparticles-nanoparticle or silver ion? Toxicol Lett 208(3):286–292
12. Guo DW et al (2014) The cellular uptake and cytotoxic effect of silver nanoparticles on chronic myeloid Leukemia cells. J Biomed Nanotechnol 10(4):669–678
13. Guo D et al (2013) Anti-leukemia activity of PVP-coated silver nanoparticles via generation of reactive oxygen species and release of silver ions. Biomaterials 34(32):7884–7894
14. Shrivas K, Wu HF (2008) Applications of silver nanoparticles capped with different functional groups as the matrix and affinity probes in surface-assisted laser desorption/ionization time-of-flight and atmospheric pressure matrix-assisted laser desorption/ionization ion trap mass spectrometry for rapid analysis of sulfur drugs and biothiols in human urine. Rapid Commun Mass Spectrom 22 (18):2863–2872
15. Liau SY et al (1997) Interaction of silver nitrate with readily identifiable groups: relationship to the antibacterial action of silver ions. Lett Appl Microbiol 25(4):279–283
16. Lynch I et al (2007) The nanoparticle - protein complex as a biological entity; a complex fluids and surface science challenge for the 21st century. Adv Colloid Interf Sci 134-35:167–174
17. Roa W et al (2012) Pharmacokinetic and toxicological evaluation of multi-functional thiol-

6-fluoro-6-deoxy-D-glucose gold nanoparticles in vivo. Nanotechnology 23(37):10

18. Oberdorster G (2010) Safety assessment for nanotechnology and nanomedicine: concepts of nanotoxicology. J Intern Med 267(1):89–105
19. Berti L et al (2010) Maximization of loading and stability of ssDNA:iron oxide nanoparticle complexes formed through electrostatic interaction. Langmuir 26(23):18293–18299
20. Mattheolabakis G et al (2014) Pegylation improves the pharmacokinetics and bioavailability of small-molecule drugs hydrolyzable by esterases: a study of phospho-ibuprofen. J Pharmacol Exp Ther 351(1):61–66

Index

Purnima Dubey (ed.), *Reporter Gene Imaging: Methods and Protocols*, Methods in Molecular Biology, vol. 1790, https://doi.org/10.1007/978-1-4939-7860-1, © Springer Science+Business Media, LLC, part of Springer Nature 2018

T

W

Printed in the United States
By Bookmasters